International Ophthalmology

Section 13
2004–2005

(First edition 2002–2003)

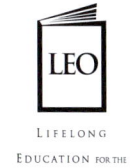

BASIC AND CLINICAL SCIENCE COURSE

AMERICAN ACADEMY OF Ophthalmology
The Eye M.D. Association

LEO

LIFELONG
EDUCATION FOR THE
OPHTHALMOLOGIST

LEO The Basic and Clinical Science Course is one component of the Lifelong Education for the Ophthalmologist (LEO) framework, which assists members in planning their continuing medical education. LEO includes an array of clinical education products that members may select to form individualized, self-directed learning plans for updating their clinical knowledge. Active members or fellows who use LEO components may accumulate sufficient CME credits to earn the LEO Award. Contact the Academy's Clinical Education Division for further information on LEO.

> The American Academy of Ophthalmology is accredited by the Accreditation Council for Continuing Medical Education to provide continuing medical education for physicians.
>
> The American Academy of Ophthalmology designates this educational activity for a maximum of 30 category 1 credits toward the AMA Physician's Recognition Award. Each physician should claim only those hours of credit that he/she actually spent in the activity.
>
> The American Medical Association has determined that non-US licensed physicians who participate in this CME activity are eligible for AMA PRA category 1 credit.

The Academy provides this material for educational purposes only. It is not intended to represent the only or best method or procedure in every case, nor to replace a physician's own judgment or give specific advice for case management. Including all indications, contraindications, side effects, and alternative agents for each drug or treatment is beyond the scope of this material. All information and recommendations should be verified, prior to use, with current information included in the manufacturers' package inserts or other independent sources, and considered in light of the patient's condition and history. Reference to certain drugs, instruments, and other products in this course is made for illustrative purposes only and is not intended to constitute an endorsement of such. Some material may include information on applications that are not considered community standard, that reflect indications not included in approved FDA labeling, or that are approved for use only in restricted research settings. The FDA has stated that it is the responsibility of the physician to determine the FDA status of each drug or device he or she wishes to use, and to use them with appropriate patient consent in compliance with applicable law. The Academy specifically disclaims any and all liability for injury or other damages of any kind, from negligence or otherwise, for any and all claims that may arise from the use of any recommendations or other information contained herein.

Copyright © 2004
American Academy of Ophthalmology
All rights reserved
Printed in the United States of America

Basic and Clinical Science Course

Thomas A. Weingeist, PhD, MD, Iowa City, Iowa, *Past President, American Academy of Ophthalmology*
Thomas J. Liesegang, MD, Jacksonville, Florida, *Senior Secretary for Clinical Education*
Gregory L. Skuta, MD, Oklahoma City, Oklahoma, *Secretary for Ophthalmic Knowledge*
Louis B. Cantor, MD, Indianapolis, Indiana, *BCSC Course Chair*

Section 13

Faculty Responsible for This Edition

Mylan VanNewkirk, MD, MPH, FRANZCO, *Chair*, Queenstown, New Zealand
Eduardo C. Alfonso, MD, Miami, Florida
Elaine L. Chuang, MD, Seattle, Washington
Mary Louise Collins, MD, Baltimore, Maryland
Sherwin J. Isenberg, MD, Los Angeles, California
Ronald Klein, MD, Madison, Wisconsin
Thomas M. Lietman, MD, San Francisco, California

Advisors

Alan C. Bird, MD, FRCS, FRCOphth, London, England
J. Donald M. Gass, MD, Nashville, Tennessee
Gullapalli N. Rao, MD, Hyderabad, India
Alfred Sommer, MD, MHSc, Baltimore, Maryland
Bruce E. Spivey, MD, New York, New York
Hugh R. Taylor, VC, Melbourne, Australia

Consultants

Richard L. Abbott, MD, San Francisco, California
Douglas R. Anderson, MD, Miami, Florida
Melissa Brown, MD, MBA, Flourtown, Pennsylvania
Janet L. Davis, MD, Miami, Florida
Harry W. Flynn, Jr, MD, Miami, Florida
Paul P. Lee, Jr, MD, Durham, North Carolina
Ivan R. Schwab, MD, Sacramento, California

Authors

Eduardo C. Alfonso, MD, Miami, Florida
Carlos e. L. Arieta, MD, São Paulo, Brazil
Alan C. Bird, MD, FRCS, FRCOphth, London, England
George W. Blankenship, MD, Hummelstown, Pennsylvania
Garry Brian, FRANZCO, Cairns, Australia
David G. Callanan, MD, Arlington, Texas
Elaine L. Chuang, MD, Seattle, Washington
August Colenbrander, MD, San Francisco, California
Mary Louise Z. Collins, MD, Baltimore, Maryland
Francisco Contreras, MD, Lima, Peru
Jamie Craig, MD, Adelaide, Australia
Emmett T. Cunningham, Jr, MD, PhD, West Brook, Connecticut
Yankum Dadzie, MD, Accra, Ghana
Lalit Dandona, MD, Hyderabad, India
Rakhi Dandona, PhD, Hyderabad, India
Paul J. Dubord, MD, Vancouver, British Columbia
John T. Flynn, MD, New York, New York
Paul J. Foster, FRCS(Ed), London, England
J. Donald M. Gass, MD, Nashville, Tennessee
Rubina Gillani, MBBS, MPH, Peshawar, Pakistan
Sherwin J. Isenberg, MD, Los Angeles, California
Newton Kara José, MD, São Paulo, Brazil
Ronald Klein, MD, Madison, Wisconsin
M. Cristina Leske, MD, MPH, Stony Brook, New York
Thomas M. Lietman, MD, San Francisco, California
David A. Mackey, MBBS, East Melbourne, Australia
C.A. McCarty, MPH, PhD, Marshfield, Wisconsin
Barbara Nemesure, PhD, Stony Brook, New York
Gullapalli N. Rao, MD, Hyderabad, India
Alan L. Robin, MD, Towson, Maryland
Todd A. Robin, MHS, Melbourne, Australia
Sanduk Ruit, FRANZCO, Kathmandu, Nepal
Alfredo A. Sadun, MD, PhD, Los Angeles, California
Alfred Sommer, MD, MHSc, Baltimore, Maryland
Einar Stefánsson, MD, PhD, Reykjavik, Iceland
Hugh R. Taylor, VC, Melbourne, Australia
James M. Tielsch, PhD, Baltimore, Maryland
Mylan VanNewkirk, MD, MPH, FRANZCO, Queenstown, New Zealand
Paul Vinger, MD, Concord, Massachusetts
Sheila West, PhD, Baltimore, Maryland
John P. Whitcher, Jr, MD, San Francisco, California
Mark Wood, MD, Moshi, Tanzania
Richard Wormald, FRCS, FRACOphth, London, England
Suh-Yuh Wu, MA, Stony Brook, New York
Xiao Bao Xiang, ProPH, Nanchang City, China

The authors state the following financial relationships:
Dr Cunningham is an employee of Eyetech Pharmaceuticals, Inc.
Dr Isenberg does not wish to disclose.

The other authors state that they have no significant financial interest or other relationship with the manufacturer of any commercial product discussed in the chapters that they contributed to this publication or with the manufacturer of any competing commercial product.

American Academy of Ophthalmology Staff

Richard A. Zorab, *Vice President, Ophthalmic Knowledge*
Hal Straus, *Director, Publications Department*
Carol L. Dondrea, *Publications Editor*
Christine Arturo, *Acquisitions Editor*
Maxine Garrett, *Administrative Coordinator*

Cover design: Paula Shuhert Design
Cover photograph: Choroidal folds, by Patrick J. Saine, MEd, CRA, Dartmouth-Hitchcock Medical Center

AMERICAN ACADEMY
OF OPHTHALMOLOGY
The Eye M.D. Association

655 Beach Street
Box 7424
San Francisco, CA 94120-7424

Contents

General Introduction xix
Foreword xxi

Objectives 1

1 Epidemiologic and International Aspects of Ophthalmology 3
Introduction 3
Epidemiology 5
Prevention of Blindness 5
    International Efforts 5
Health, Manpower, and Resources 7
    Socioeconomics of Vision Impairment 8
    Utilization of the Volunteer Ophthalmologist 8
    Resource Sustainability 8
Individual Contributions 9
Organizations With Prevention of Blindness Programs 9

PART I Ophthalmic Epidemiology Principles 15
Introduction 17

2 Evidence-based Ophthalmology 19
Background 19
Grading Scales of Evidence 20
Randomized Controlled Trials 21
    Efficacy versus Effectiveness: Trial Outcomes 22
    Adverse Event Reporting 23
    Measures of Risk and Benefit 23
    Stopping an RCT: Role of a Data-Monitoring and Ethics
        Committee 24
    CONSORT Statement 25
    RCT Registries 25
Systematic Reviews and Meta-Analysis 25
    Meta-analysis 27
Observational Studies 30
    Outcome Studies 30
    Cohort Studies 30
    Case-Control Studies 31
    Case Series 32
Measuring the Burden of Disease 33
    Cost–Benefit Analysis 34

Cost-Effectiveness Analysis 34
Cost–Utility Analysis 34
Audit 36
Conclusion 36

3 Aspects and Ranges of Vision Loss 37
Aspects of Vision Loss 37
Causes and Consequences, Choice of Tests 38
Ranges of Vision Loss 40
Ranges of Visual Acuity Loss. 40
Ranges of Visual Field Loss 41
Discussion of Individual Ranges 44
Visual Acuity Measurement 46
Chart Layout 47
Choice of Optotypes. 47
Presentation 49
Scoring 50
Choice of Test Distance 50
Tests for Near Vision 51
Visual Acuity Calculations. 52

4 Ophthalmic Survey Methodology. 55
Overview 55
Design Issues 55
Interpretation 56
Methodology 57
Ethical Standards and Informed Consent 57
Sampling Issues 57
Data Collection 58
Standardized Ophthalmologic Examination Using International
Diagnostic Classification and Grading Systems 60
Document Summarizing Results of Examination 62
Data Management and Analysis 62
Conclusion 62

5 Case Series Epidemiology 65
Overview 65
Applying the Approach: Diffuse Unilateral Subacute Neuroretinitis. . . .66
First Step: Defining the Disease. 66
Second Step: Determining the Etiology 67
Third Step: Identifying the Organism 68
Fourth Step: Treating the Disease 69
Acute Retinal Necrosis 71
Summary 71

PART II Prevalence and Prevention of Pediatric Vision Impairment ... 73
Introduction ... 75

6 Pediatric Blindness ... 77
Background ... 77
Methods for Assessing Childhood Blindness in a Population ... 79
Causes of Blindness ... 79
    Factors Affecting Blindness in Particular Regions ... 79
Suggestions for Reducing Childhood Blindness ... 82

7 Ophthalmia Neonatorum ... 85
Background ... 85
    History ... 85
    Context ... 85
    Economic Impact ... 85
Pathogenesis ... 86
Epidemiology ... 86
    Risk Factors ... 86
    Geographic, Environmental, Social Factors ... 86
    Ethnic Differences ... 86
    Surveys to Determine Prevalence/Incidence ... 86
Clinical Presentation and Findings ... 86
Prevention ... 88
Workup ... 88
Current Treatment Programs ... 89
    Screening ... 89
    Specific Recommendations in the Presence of Infection ... 89
    Success of Povidone-Iodine Prophylaxis ... 89

8 Retinopathy of Prematurity ... 91
Background ... 91
Economic Impact ... 92
Pathogenesis ... 92
Epidemiology ... 93
Clinical Presentation ... 95
Prevention ... 95
Current Treatment ... 96
Clinical Research ... 96

9 Vitamin A Deficiency Disorders ... 99
Background ... 99
    History ... 99
    Context ... 100
    Economic Impact ... 100
Pathogenesis ... 101

Epidemiology 101
   Surveys to Determine Prevalence/Incidence 101
   Risk Factors. 102
Clinical Presentation and Findings 103
   Measles Comorbidity 106
Prevention 107
Current Treatment Recommendations 108
Clinical Research Currently Under Way 108

10 Amblyopia 111
Background 111
   History 111
   Context 111
Epidemiology 112
   Economic Impact. 114
Pathogenesis 114
Clinical Presentation and Findings 115
Prevention 116
Current Treatment Programs 116
   Screening 116
   Treatment 117
   Recidivism 118
Conclusion 118

11 Ocular Trauma Epidemiology and Prevention 121
Background 121
   Context 121
   Economic Impact. 122
Ocular Trauma Terminology 122
Classification System for Mechanical Injuries of the Eye 122
Ocular Trauma Epidemiology 126
   Prevalence and Incidence 126
Risk Factors 128
   Bilateral Ocular Injuries 128
   Occupation 129
   Cultural 129
   Sport 130
Data Collection 130
Pathogenesis 131
Prevention Standards 131
   Prevention of Eye Injuries in Auto Accidents 133
   Prevention Educators 134
Conclusion 134

Contents • xi

PART III The Prevalence, Causes, and Prevention of Adult Vision Impairment 135

Introduction 137

12 Prevalence and Common Causes of Vision Impairment in Adults 139

Background 139
   History 139
   Context 140
      Importance of Complete Eye Examinations in Eye Disease Surveys 140
      Factors Influencing the Causes of Vision Impairment 140
      Comparison of Eye Disease Studies 141
      Economic Impact. 142
      Definitions of Blindness 143
Comparable Studies 143
Prevalence of Profound and Severe Vision Impairment 143
   Age as a Major Risk Factor 145
Causes of Vision Impairment 146
Causes of Severe and Profound Vision Impairment 147
Other Studies 148
   Asia 148
   Central and South America 148
   Africa 148
   Middle East 150
   South Pacific 150
Prevention 150
Conclusion 151

13 Uncorrected Refractive Error 153

Background 153
   History 153
   Context 153
   Economic Impact. 154
Epidemiology 155
   Risk Factors 155
   Surveys to Determine Prevalence/Incidence 156
Clinical Presentation and Findings 157
Prevention 157
Current Treatment Programs 158
   Screening 158
   Strengths, Weaknesses, and Results of Treatment Programs . . 158
Clinical Research Currently Under Way 160

14 Cataract 161

Background 161
Impact of Cataract 162

Magnitude of the Problem 162
　　　Economic Impact. 162
　　　Quality of Cataract Surgery 165
　　　Quality of Life 165
　　Epidemiology 166
　　　Prevalence 166
　　　Risk Factors 166
　　　Cataract and Mortality 169
　　Clinical Research Currently Under Way 170

15　Ethnic Differences in Primary Open-Angle Glaucoma 171
　　Background 171
　　Prevalence and Incidence 171
　　　Comparisons Among Studies 174
　　The Barbados Eye Study 174
　　Risk Factors 176
　　Conclusions 176

16　Primary Angle-Closure Glaucoma 177
　　Background 177
　　　History 177
　　　Context 177
　　Pathogenesis 179
　　　Pupillary Block 179
　　　Non–Pupillary Block 179
　　Epidemiology 179
　　　Incidence 179
　　　Prevalence 181
　　Risk Factors 181
　　Clinical Presentation and Findings 182
　　Prevention 183
　　　Screening 183
　　　Treatment 185
　　The Asymptomatic Narrow Angle and the "Fellow Eye" 186
　　Research Currently Under Way 187

17　Application of Findings in Diabetic Retinopathy Studies: The Iceland Experience 189
　　Background 189
　　Pathogenesis 190
　　Epidemiology 191
　　　Prevalence of Diabetic Retinopathy 191
　　　Incidence of Diabetic Retinopathy 192
　　Screening for Diabetes Mellitus 193
　　　Risk Factors 194
　　Treatment 194

The Iceland Experience 195
    Screening for Diabetic Retinopathy 195
    Outcomes 197
    Utilization of Eye-Care Services 198
    Study Strengths and Weaknesses 198
Conclusion 199

PART IV Preventable Infectious Causes of Vision Impairment 201

Introduction 203

18 Trachoma 205

Background 205
    History 205
    Context 205
    Economic Impact 205
Pathogenesis 206
Epidemiology 206
    Surveys to Determine Prevalence/Incidence 206
    Risk Factors 207
Clinical Presentation and Findings 209
Prevention 210
Current Treatment Programs 211
    Screening 211
    Strengths, Weaknesses, and Results of Treatment Programs . . . 212
Clinical Research Currently Under Way 213

19 Microbial Keratitis 215

Background 215
    History 215
    Context 215
    Economic Impact 215
Pathogenesis 216
Epidemiology 216
    Surveys to Determine Prevalence/Incidence 216
    Risk Factors 217
Clinical Presentation and Findings 218
Prevention 219
Current Treatment Programs 219
    Screening 219
    Strengths, Weaknesses, and Results of Treatment Programs . . . 220
Clinical Research Currently Under Way 220

20 HIV/AIDS and Global Blindness 223

Background 223
    History 223
    Context 223

xiv • Contents

        Economic Impact. 223
    Pathogenesis 226
    Epidemiology 228
        Surveys to Determine Prevalence 228
        Risk Factors. 229
        Contribution of HIV/AIDS to Global Blindness 232
    Clinical Presentation and Findings 232
    Prevention 233
    Current Treatment Programs 233
        Screening 233
        Therapy 233

21 Onchocerciasis 235
    Background 235
        Life Cycle of *O volvulus* 235
        History 236
        Context 238
        Economic Impact. 238
    Pathogenesis and Immune Response 239
    Epidemiology 240
        Surveys to Determine Prevalence/Incidence 240
        Risk Factors. 242
        Diagnosis 244
    Clinical Presentation and Findings 244
        Onchocercal Nodules 244
        Lymphatic System 244
        Skin Signs and Symptoms of Onchocerciasis 244
        Ocular Signs of Onchocerciasis 245
    Prevention 247
    Current Treatment Programs 247
        Screening 247
        Vector Control. 248
        Chemotherapy. 248
    Clinical Research Currently Under Way 250

PART V Collaborative Research 253
    Introduction 255

22 Ophthalmia Neonatorum Research as a Paradigm for Conducting Studies in Developing Countries . . . 257
    Background 257
    Pilot Data 257
    Mechanisms for Preparing a Foreign Study 258
    Findings 259

23 Epidemic Optic Neuropathy in Cuba 261
    Background 261
        History 261

Context 262
    Human Impact 262
Clinical Presentation and Findings 263
Epidemiology 263
    Surveys of Prevalence/Incidence. 263
    Risk Factors. 263
Pathogenesis 266
Prevention 268
Current Treatment Programs 268
Research Currently Under Way 269
Lessons Learned From This Epidemic 269

24 Glaucoma Inheritance Study in Tasmania: An International Collaboration 271
Background 271
Glaucoma Inheritance Study in Tasmania (GIST) 271
Study Methodology 273
Findings 274
Social Concerns 275
Future Treatment 275

25 Natural History of Sickle Cell Retinopathy in Jamaica 277
Background 277
Epidemiology 278
Natural History of Sickle Retinopathy 278
Findings From Jamaica 279
Treatment and Prevention of Visual Loss 281

26 Hong Kong Myopia 283
Background 283
Pathogenesis 284
Clinical Presentation and Findings 284
Findings From the Hong Kong Vision Study 284
Prevention 286
Conclusion 286

PART VI   Effective Health Care Delivery Systems . . 287
Introduction 289

27 The Aravind Eye Care System 291
Background 291
The Equitable Development Model 292
    Understanding the Model 292
    Number of Surgeries 293
Clinical Services 294

Demand Generation. 294
Understanding Sustainability and Cost Recovery in Eye Care 295
    Local Ownership and Financial Self-Sufficiency 295
    Social Marketing 296
    Economies of Scale 298
    Systems for Highly Efficient Service Delivery 298
Lions Aravind Institute of Community Ophthalmology (LAICO):
    Expanding Infrastructure 300
In-House Technology 301
Challenges in the Scaling-up Process 302

28 L.V. Prasad Eye Institute 303
Background 303
The L.V. Prasad Eye Institute 303
Overview of Challenges 304
    Finances 304
    Programmatic Focus 307
    Maintaining Quality 309
Conclusion 310

29 Kikuyu Eye Unit 311
Background 311
Epidemiology 311
Ophthalmic Infrastructure 312
Structure of the Kikuyu Eye Unit 312
    Personnel 313
    Services by Department 314
    Teaching 315
    Research 316
    Outreach 316
    Finance 317
Christoffel-Blindenmission 318
Conclusion 318

30 Cataract Care in Brazil and Peru 321
Background 321
Brazil 321
    Magnitude of the Problem 321
    Backlog of Unoperated Cataract 322
    Public Health System and Available Eye Care 322
    Personnel Training 323
Cataract-Free Zone Projects: Peru and Brazil 323
    Peru 324
    Brazil 325
    Surgical Techniques 326
    National Campaigns 327
    Supporting Organizations and Agencies 327

Contents • xvii

    Future Programs 327
    Conclusion 328

31 Cataract Management in Developing Countries 329
    Background 329
    Surgical Management of Cataract 330
    The Fred Hollows Foundation System of Cataract Management 331
        Does This Deliver? 333
    Conclusion 334

32 Global Eye Banking and Corneal Transplantation . . . 335
    Background 335
    Corneal Transplantation in the Developing World 336
    National Eye Banking Programs 337
    Eye Banking 338
        The "Best" Eye Bank Model 339
        Tissue Retrieval and Distribution Models 340
        Government Participation. 341
        Strategy 341
    Conclusion 342

    Credit Reporting Form 343
    Study Questions 347
    Answers 353
    Index 361

General Introduction

The Basic and Clinical Science Course (BCSC) is designed to meet the needs of residents and practitioners for a comprehensive yet concise curriculum of the field of ophthalmology. The BCSC has developed from its original brief outline format, which relied heavily on outside readings, to a more convenient and educationally useful self-contained text. The Academy updates and revises the course annually, with the goals of integrating the basic science and clinical practice of ophthalmology and of keeping ophthalmologists current with new developments in the various subspecialties.

The BCSC incorporates the effort and expertise of more than 80 ophthalmologists, organized into 14 section faculties, working with Academy editorial staff. In addition, the course continues to benefit from many lasting contributions made by the faculties of previous editions. Members of the Academy's Practicing Ophthalmologists Advisory Committee for Education serve on each faculty and, as a group, review every volume before and after major revisions.

Organization of the Course

The Basic and Clinical Science Course comprises 14 volumes, incorporating fundamental ophthalmic knowledge, subspecialty areas, and special topics:

1. Update on General Medicine
2. Fundamentals and Principles of Ophthalmology
3. Optics, Refraction, and Contact Lenses
4. Ophthalmic Pathology and Intraocular Tumors
5. Neuro-Ophthalmology
6. Pediatric Ophthalmology and Strabismus
7. Orbit, Eyelids, and Lacrimal System
8. External Disease and Cornea
9. Intraocular Inflammation and Uveitis
10. Glaucoma
11. Lens and Cataract
12. Retina and Vitreous
13. International Ophthalmology
14. Refractive Surgery

In addition, a comprehensive Master Index allows the reader to easily locate subjects throughout the entire series.

References

Readers who wish to explore specific topics in greater detail may consult the journal references cited within each chapter and the Basic Texts listed at the back of the book.

These references are intended to be selective rather than exhaustive, chosen by the BCSC faculty as being important, current, and readily available to residents and practitioners.

Related Academy educational materials are also listed in the appropriate sections. They include books, audiovisual materials, self-assessment programs, clinical modules, and interactive programs.

Study Questions and CME Credit

Each volume of the BCSC is designed as an independent study activity for ophthalmology residents and practitioners. The learning objectives for this volume are given on page 1. The text, illustrations, and references provide the information necessary to achieve the objectives; the study questions allow readers to test their understanding of the material and their mastery of the objectives. Physicians who wish to claim CME credit for this educational activity may do so by mail, fax, or online. The necessary forms and instructions are given at the end of the book.

Conclusion

The Basic and Clinical Science Course has expanded greatly over the years, with the addition of much new text and numerous illustrations. Recent editions have sought to place a greater emphasis on clinical applicability, while maintaining a solid foundation in basic science. As with any educational program, it reflects the experience of its authors. As its faculties change and as medicine progresses, new viewpoints are always emerging on controversial subjects and techniques. Not all alternate approaches can be included in this series; as with any educational endeavor, the learner should seek additional sources, including such carefully balanced opinions as the Academy's Preferred Practice Patterns.

The BCSC faculty and staff are continuously striving to improve the educational usefulness of the course; you, the reader, can contribute to this ongoing process. If you have any suggestions or questions about the series, please do not hesitate to contact the faculty or the editors.

The authors, editors, and reviewers hope that your study of the BCSC will be of lasting value and that each section will serve as a practical resource for quality patient care.

Foreword

"One World, One Vision"

Blindness knows no borders. Among the nearly 45 million people in the world with profound vision impairment, the prevalence is highest among those in developing nations. A high proportion of blindness is preventable through public health measures. Many other cases are treatable.

Malnutrition and retinopathy, as well as infectious diseases, including trachoma, onchocerciasis, and keratitis, continue to be major causes of blindness. Increases in life expectancy have resulted in more blindness from cataract, diabetic retinopathy, macular degeneration, and glaucoma in all nations.

The primary objectives of this first edition of Section 13 of the Basic and Clinical Science Course, *International Ophthalmology*, are to review the prevalence and causes of vision impairment around the world today and to introduce readers to the basic principles of evidence-based medicine by providing examples of clinically relevant efforts to combat blindness. In future editions, the American Academy of Ophthalmology will seek and welcome examples from other contributors.

Special thanks are due to the many volunteers who have contributed to the first edition. Many are acknowledged for their individual contributions. Others have worked tirelessly behind the scenes to make this volume possible.

The American Academy of Ophthalmology aspires to be a recognized leader in education for ophthalmologists and other health care professionals and a highly respected provider of educational resources dealing with the prevention of blindness. The Academy's Board of Trustees hopes the publication of *International Ophthalmology* will foster greater interest in combating blindness and enhance collaboration to this end among people thoughout the world.

Thomas A. Weingeist, PhD, MD
Past President
American Academy of Ophthalmology

Objectives

The overall objective of BCSC Section 13, *International Ophthalmology*, is to provide clinical knowledge to ophthalmologists in training and in practice about current research projects and local or regional practice issues specific to international ophthalmology in order to promote the prevention of visual loss worldwide.

Upon completion of BCSC Section 13, the reader should be able to:

- Outline the key concepts in statistics and epidemiology and their application to international ophthalmology.

- List the leading causes of visual loss in adult and pediatric populations around the world.

- Explain prevention and treatment strategies for ophthalmic conditions that contribute significantly to world blindness.

- Describe the social, geographic, and environmental factors and differences in ophthalmic disease worldwide.

- Present examples of outstanding clinical research in international settings.

- Obtain useful information about and through resource organizations that promote vision care on an international scale.

- Use the examples presented in this book to outline various local and regional factors that affect the success of current eye-care programs operating in different countries.

CHAPTER 1

Epidemiologic and International Aspects of Ophthalmology

Introduction

The Basic and Clinical Science Course (BCSC) is designed to provide ophthalmologists and ophthalmologists-in-training with a comprehensive yet concise curriculum of the field of ophthalmology. The current form is a widely used, self-contained text focused on basic science, diagnosis, and treatment. Section 13, which will expand the epidemiologic, international, and preventive aspects of ophthalmology in the BCSC, is organized into six parts.

Part I describes basic epidemiologic methods using published studies as examples to assist clinicians in gathering and analyzing medical evidence whose application improves patient outcomes. It includes brief discussions of the basic principles of evidence-based medicine, cost-effectiveness, quality of life, and the economic impact of blindness in various settings.

Part II discusses the prevalence and avoidable causes of childhood and young adult vision loss, such as ophthalmia neonatorum, retinopathy of prematurity, vitamin A deficiency, amblyopia, and trauma. It is estimated by the World Health Organization (WHO) that 1.5 million children around the world are blind, and another half million become blind each year. Childhood blindness accounts for major socioeconomic losses and is the second leading cause of blind-person-years.

Part III features the prevalence and causes of adult vision loss, ethnic differences in the epidemiology of open-angle glaucoma, and major avoidable causes of adult vision impairment: uncorrected refractive error, cataract, angle-closure glaucoma, and diabetic retinopathy. Major eye disease surveys using similar methodology in the developing and developed world have shown that uncorrected refractive errors are the leading cause of vision impairment. Unlike cataract, angle-closure glaucoma, and diabetic retinopathy, where 90% of blindness from these diseases often occurs due to health care delivery problems in the developing world, the rates of avoidable vision impairment due to uncorrected refractive errors are similar worldwide. Cataract is a major health challenge and second only to uncorrected refractive error as a cause of vision impairment. Well-designed epidemiologic studies have shown that angle-closure glaucoma in Asia is distinctly more complex than the occasional classic acute angle-closure glaucoma patient observed in emergency clinics in the predominantly white populations of the world. Well-designed epidemiologic studies have dramatically increased knowledge about and potential for preventing vision loss due to diabetes mellitus. Unfortunately, application of this knowledge and attainment of vision outcomes has been slow and disappointing in all parts of the world. Iceland provides an excellent example of how to apply epidemiologic findings effectively to a population to prevent vision impairment caused by diabetes.

Part IV is devoted to the diagnosis, treatment, and prevention of major infectious causes of vision loss in the developing world: trachoma, microbial keratitis, HIV/AIDS, and onchocerciasis. Trachoma causes vision impairment in approximately 6 million people, and the resulting trichiasis puts nearly twice that number at risk of vision loss. In the 20 years since AIDS was first recognized, the epidemic has been proceeding at an alarming rate, with nearly 95% of new cases occurring in developing countries. The number of HIV infections rose from 6 million in 1990 to more than 20 million in 1995 and approaches 60 million today. This disease poses a significant risk to vision as well as life, and although no cure has been discovered, prevention is possible.

> Cohen J. *Shots in the Dark: The Wayward Search for an AIDS Vaccine.* New York: Norton; 2001.

Part V provides snapshots of collaborative research projects around the world, including projects on ophthalmia neonatorum in Kenya and optic neuropathy in Cuba, the search for a glaucoma gene in Tasmania, and projects on sickle cell retinopathy in Jamaica and myopia in Hong Kong. These examples of successful clinical research projects may be a stimulus for others in the future. Collaborative research is possible in almost all clinical settings.

Part VI focuses on examples of effective health care delivery models in the developing world and addresses education in health, quality outcomes, manpower, and resources. These models, which could be applied to the developed world as well as developing nations, include Aravind Eye Hospital and the L.V. Prasad Eye Institute in India. Kikuyu Eye Unit in Kenya is a good example of a religious model, and the Fred Hollows Foundation approach to the treatment of cataract is a good example of a nongovernmental (NGO) organization model. The cataract-free zone projects in Brazil and Peru show how these South American countries respond to a major vision problem. The Eye Bank Association of India (EBAI) is a successful model of a comprehensive eye banking and corneal transplantation system in the developing world.

Cataract is estimated to cause impaired vision in approximately 20 million people around the world. The estimated worldwide annual cataract surgical rate is 9–10 million surgeries; unfortunately, there is increasing evidence that for many patients visual outcomes are unsatisfactory. It is important, therefore, not only to increase the rate of surgeries but to increase the quality of the surgical outcomes by incorporating thorough preoperative examinations and case selection, quality surgical technique, postoperative follow-up, and refraction. Quality, accessible care based on ability to pay is an important key to sustainability. In most parts of the world, the public places high value on quality eye-care services. Knowledge may lead to quality. A quality product increases demand. Demand promotes sustainability. Sustainability should lead to increased accessibility. This chain of events can reduce the avoidable blindness in all parts of the world.

Epidemiology

The epidemiologic principles discussed here are applicable to the developed as well as the developing nations. Many advances in ophthalmology, for example in the diagnosis and treatment of diabetic retinopathy, are based on the clinical application of epidemiologic findings. The best scientific evidence that can be used to evaluate the effects of preventive services comes from well-designed clinical trials and observational studies that link risk modification with improved outcomes. Recently, outcome measures have been developed incorporating quality-of-life measures that attempt to capture functional status and preference. Renewed focus on prevention of eye disease will improve the cost-effectiveness of eye care and reduce disability and suffering. Savings occur through reducing the costs of services, lost productivity, and morbidity and suffering.

Prevention of Blindness

Nearly 90% of the world's blind reside in sub-Saharan Africa and the Asian subcontinent, including China and India. The prevalence of avoidable vision loss is increasing in most of these regions because the incidence of avoidable vision loss exceeds the capability and resources of the communities to treat the conditions that cause it. The WHO estimates that 180 million people worldwide are vision impaired, including approximately 45 million persons who have profound vision loss (<20/400). The number is increasing and is expected to double by 2020, as world population and life expectancy increase. The WHO estimates that 80% of global vision loss is avoidable. Vision loss not only impacts the affected individuals and their families but also presents public health, social, and economic problems.

> VISION 2020: Global initiative for the elimination of avoidable blindness. WHO Fact Sheet 213. Revised February 2000.

Cataract causes nearly half of the world's vision loss. It was estimated in 1995 that more than 80% of people with cataract may die before they have a chance for surgery. Unfortunately, even the good intentions related to cataract surgery have created significant problems, such as blindness from complications of cataract surgery. In one study, almost half the patients operated on were dissatisfied with the outcome and more than one third were blind in the operated eye.

> Singh AJ, Garner P, Floyd K. Cost-effectiveness of public-funded options for cataract surgery in Mysore, India. *Lancet.* 2000;355:180–184.

International Efforts

The world has the resources to solve the problem of avoidable vision loss, and the progress that has been made through cooperative international effort is promising. Much of this promise can be credited to the efforts of international agencies, including the WHO and the International Agency for the Prevention of Blindness (IAPB). The IAPB was founded in 1975 by the International Federation of Ophthalmological Societies (IFOS) and the

World Blind Union (WBU) to lead a cooperative effort to reduce avoidable blindness throughout the world. The IAPB encouraged the establishment of national prevention of blindness committees, which now function as members of the IAPB in more than 80 countries. In addition to these country members, other members include the IFOS, the WBU, and international NGOs that actively support global programs for community eye care. The IAPB works with a consortium of NGOs and national committees to direct efforts and resources toward increasing public awareness and supporting sight conservation programs that largely implement WHO health care strategies against blinding diseases. The IAPB promoted the establishment of the WHO Program for the Prevention of Blindness, with which it has remained strongly linked.

In February 1999, the IAPB launched VISION 2020—The Right to Sight, a global initiative to eliminate avoidable blindness by the year 2020. This project and Section 13 of the BCSC share a focus: applying today's knowledge to prevent blindness around the globe. VISION 2020 has targeted five disorders in its avoidable blindness campaign: cataract, refractive error and low vision services, geographic focal blinding diseases such as trachoma and onchocerciasis, glaucoma, and diabetic retinopathy. Prevention of blindness from these conditions was deemed feasible and affordable. The goals of VISION 2020 may be achieved by using proven cost-effective strategies, maintaining close collaboration among all partners, and increasing global awareness, particularly at the community level (Table 1-1). VISION 2020 emphasizes disease prevention and control, training of personnel, strengthening existing eye-care infrastructure, use of appropriate and affordable technology, and mobilization of resources.

The initial phase of VISION 2020 is a global campaign to raise awareness among peoples and governments about the societal implications of vision loss, as well as to mobilize a strong, long-term political and professional commitment to eliminating avoid-

Table 1-1 VISION 2020 Partners

Task Force Members	The Carter Center
	Christoffel-Blindenmission (Christian Blind Mission International)
	The Fred Hollows Foundation
	Helen Keller Worldwide
	International Agency for the Prevention of Blindness
	International Federation of Ophthalmological Societies
	Lions Clubs International Foundation
	The Noor Al Hussein Foundation
	Operation Eyesight Universal
	ORBIS International
	Organisation pour la Prévention de la Cécité
	Sight Savers International
Supporting Members	The American Academy of Ophthalmology
	The Asian Foundation for the Prevention of Blindness
	The Canadian National Institute for the Blind
	Dark & Light
	International Centre for Eyecare Education
	Lighthouse International
	Perkins School for the Blind
	Seva Foundation

able blindness. National decision makers and donor agencies need to be convinced that financial and human resources provided for the elimination of avoidable blindness are a worthwhile investment. In recent years, these groups have spent about US$80 million per year on the prevention of blindness.

> Foster A. VISION 2020—The Right to Sight. International Agency for the Prevention of Blindness Newsletter. January 2001.

Health, Manpower, and Resources

Health is more attributable to prevention of disease and promotion of health than to treatment of a disease after it has occurred.

Health depends on consumer education, utilization and compliance, access to well-trained providers, and the resources necessary to fund the industry. A maldistribution of health care providers is typical in the developed world, whereas the number of providers and the distribution of health care are problems in most of the developing world. The Republic of South Africa demonstrates a serious problem in the distribution of ophthalmologists within the private and public sectors. Of its 275 ophthalmologists, 250 work in the private sector, caring for the needs of 8 million people; the remaining 25 work in a government practice that serves 32 million people. In most parts of Africa, the ratio of eye surgeon to population is less than 1 per 1,000,000.

Some countries have adequate numbers of eye-care providers who produce little because of inadequate education, equipment, and/or incentives. In 1994, for example, Bulgaria had 600 ophthalmologists for its 8.9 million inhabitants. This ratio is similar to that in the United States. However, only 120 of them (less than 20%) performed surgery.

In India, a country that has an estimated backlog of 4 million patients with cataract, there is approximately one ophthalmologist for every 100,000 people. Great Britain has a similar ratio of ophthalmologists per 100,000 people but essentially no cataract backlog. The National Program for Control of Blindness in India believes that the output of ophthalmologists in India is low because of underutilization and the low number of surgeons in rural regions, where the prevalence of blindness is high.

Thailand has been successful in reducing avoidable blindness from 1.1% in 1980 to 0.3% in 1997 by implementing a primary eye-care approach that improved access and quality of eye-care services within the eye-care networks of the national health scheme.

> Foster A, Johnson GJ. Treatable blindness: cataract. *Trop Doct.* 1988;18:112–115.
> Gieser SC, Vassileva P, West SK. Ophthalmology in Bulgaria. *Arch Ophthalmol.* 1994;112: 687–690.
> Jenchitr WT, Tansirikongkol V. Ophthalmology in Thailand 1997. *J Med Assoc Thai.* 2000; 83:107–116.
> Kumar R. Ophthalmic manpower in India—need for a serious review. *Int Ophthalmol.* 1993;17:269–275.
> Sommer A. Disease prevention and health promotion: a clinical primer. *Arch Ophthalmol.* 1995;113:419–420.

Socioeconomics of Vision Impairment

International evidence consistently demonstrates that groups with low socioeconomic status have significantly higher mortality and morbidity rates. The contributing factors include a higher rate of health-damaging behaviors, lower utilization of the health care system for preventive purposes, and a higher adverse risk factor profile. In a well-designed, population-based study of eye diseases in the state of Andhra Pradesh in India, vision loss was found to be more common in participants from the extreme lower socioeconomic strata than in others.

> Dandona L, Dandona R, Naduvilath TJ, et al. Is current eye-care policy focus almost exclusively on cataract adequate to deal with blindness in India? *Lancet.* 1998;351:1312–1316.

Utilization of the Volunteer Ophthalmologist

The International Council of Ophthalmology (ICO) is the governing body for the IFOS, which is composed of representatives from the primary ophthalmologic organizations in each country. The ICO was founded in 1927 in Scheveningen, The Netherlands, and the IFOS in 1933 in Madrid, Spain. The Academia Ophthalmologica Internationalis and the ICO hosted planning sessions in 1999 and 2000 to inform and involve ophthalmic organizations, government agencies, NGOs, and representatives of vision care companies in solving this global problem of vision impairment. These efforts produced the International Ophthalmology Strategic Plan to Preserve and Restore Vision: Vision for the Future, a program to assist and coordinate activities of the approximately 150,000 ophthalmologists and thousands of nonophthalmic physicians, health specialists, and community leaders in efforts to prevent avoidable vision loss throughout the world. The plan has great potential to enable all ophthalmologists to channel their energy and resources toward this global vision problem. The program will work with the WHO and IAPB in implementing the VISION 2020 program by facilitating education and clinical research, improving access to well-trained providers, and providing a liaison with governments and NGOs in allocating necessary resources.

Refer to the last section of this chapter for the addresses and web sites of agencies involved in the prevention of vision loss. These experienced organizations may provide the best opportunity for a volunteer ophthalmologist to contribute resources or personnel toward reducing avoidable vision loss around the world. Contact them. There are many valid approaches.

Resource Sustainability

India has two outstanding models of blindness prevention and treatment. Both have a significant, positive impact on preventable blindness, providing it at low cost in their regions, and both also function as outstanding teaching facilities. One of these is the Aravind Eye Hospital in Madurai, India, which has a long track record of providing sustainable high-quality eye care and education to the region. Aravind honors local customs and uses available resources efficiently to provide a system of high-quality, high-volume, cost-effective cataract surgery using screening eye camps and hospitals. Successful outcomes have created a demand for services that results in proper utilization of the facilities. Free eye care is provided to the needy; however, the high quality of service also generates a demand among people who are capable of paying for the services. Like L.V. Prasad, Aravind stresses community involvement, targeted screening, efficient utilization of both medical and paramedical personnel, and a streamlined diagnostic method approach. (See Part VI of this volume.) This system may be modified for use in other areas of the world.

Natchiar G, Robin AL, Thulasiraj RD, et al. Attacking the backlog of India's curable blind. The Aravind Eye Hospital model. *Arch Ophthalmol.* 1994;112:987–993.

Individual Contributions

The work of individuals and organizations who have made important contributions in preventing vision loss are featured in this Section 13 of the BCSC to show readers that it is possible to make a difference in our communities—that it is possible to improve the community by preventing vision loss. Every reader has the potential to make important contributions to his or her community or beyond.

Organizations With Prevention of Blindness Programs

The Asian Foundation for the Prevention of Blindness
248 Nam Cheong Street Shamshuipo
Kowloon, Hong Kong
Tel: 852 2778 8332, ext. 301
Fax: 852 2788 1336
Email: director@hksb.org.hk
www.hksb.org.hk

The Canadian National Institute for the Blind
1929 Bayview Avenue
Toronto, Ontario
Canada M4G 3E8
Tel: (416) 486-2500
Fax: (416) 480-7503
www.cnib.ca

The Carter Center
Office of Public Information
453 Freedom Parkway
Atlanta, GA 30307
Tel: (404) 331-3900
Fax: (404) 331-3900
Email: carterweb@emory.edu
www.cartercenter.org

Christoffel-Blindenmission (Christian Blind Mission International)
CBM/HQ
Nibelungenstrasse 124
D-64625 Bensheim
Germany
Tel: + 49 6251 131 0
Fax: + 49 6251 131 249
Telex: 468334 CBMB D
Email: overseas@cbm-i.org
who.int/ina-ngo/

Dark & Light
Stichting Dark & Light Blind Care
Postbus 672
3900 AR Veenendaal
The Netherlands
Tel: (0318) 561501
Fax: (0318) 561577
Email: info@darkandlight.org
www.darkandlight.org

The Fred Hollows Foundation
www.hollows.com.au

Australia
The Fred Hollows Foundation
Level 3, 414 Gardeners Road
Rosebery, NSW 2018
Tel: 61-2-8338 2111
Fax: 61-2-8338 2100
www.hollows.com.au

China
Jiangzi Material Supply Station
268 Fu Zhou Road
Nanchang City
Jiangxi Province
PR China 330006
Tel/Fax: 86-791-6257-569
Email: fhfchin@public.nc.jx.cn

Eritrea
The Fred Hollows IOL Factory
13 Fred Hollows Street
Asmara
Tel: 291-1-120293
Fax: 291-1-122532
Email: fhlab@eol.com.er

Nepal
The Fred Hollows IOL Laboratory
Tilganga Eye Centre
PO Box 561, Kathmandu
Tel: 977-1-493-775
Fax: 977-1-474-937
Email: tilganga@mos.com.np

New Zealand
The Fred Hollows Foundation
Private Bag, 56 908 Dominion Road
Auckland 1030
Tel: 64-9-630-7825
Fax: 64-9-630-2410
Email: f.hollows@xtra.co.nz

Pakistan
Fred Hollows House
H. No. 179, Street 8, Sector K-3, Phase 3
Hayatabad, Peshawar
North-West Frontier Province
Tel: 92-91-817-327
Fax: 92-92-818-862
Email: fhfpak@brain.net.pk

Vietnam
The Fred Hollows Foundation
No. 6F16 Thai Ha Alley
Thai Ha Road
Doug Ba District, Hanoi
Tel: 84-4-856-1416
Fax: 84-4-856-1545
Email: fredhn@netnam.org.vn

Helen Keller Worldwide
352 Park Avenue South
Suite 1200
New York, NY 10010
Toll-free tel: (United States) 1-877/KELLER-4 (1-877-535-5374)
Tel: (212) 532-0544
Fax: (212) 532-6014
Email: info@hkworld.org
www.hkworld.org

International Agency for the Prevention of Blindness (IAPB)
Dr. Gullapalli N. Rao
IAPB Secretariat
LV Prasad Eye Institute
LV Prasad Marg, Banjara Hills
Hyderabad - 500 034
India
Tel: + 91 40 354 5389
Fax: + 91 40 354 8271
Email: iapb@lvpeye.stph.net
www.iapb.org

International Centre for Eyecare Education
PO Box 328
RANDWICK NSW 2031
Australia
Tel: (612) 9385 7435
Fax: (612) 9385 7436
Email: icee@icee.org
www.icee.org

International Federation of Ophthalmological Societies (IFOS)
International Council of Ophthalmology (ICO)
Bruce E. Spivey, MD
Secretary-General
International Council of Ophthalmology
Spivey International
One Beekman Place
New York, NY 10022
Fax: (212) 326-8773
Email: bruce@spivey.org
www.icoph.org

Lighthouse International
111 East 59th Street
New York, NY 10022-1202
Toll-free tel: (800) 829-0500
Tel: (212) 821-9200
TTY: (212) 821-9712
Email: info@lighthouse.org
www.lighthouse.org

Lions Clubs International Foundation
Grant Programs Department
Tel: (630) 571-5466, ext. 292
Email: lehp@lionsclubs.org
www.lionsclubs.org

The Noor Al Hussein Foundation
P.O. Box 926687
Amman 11110 - Jordan
Tel: (962-6) 560-6992 or 560-6993
Fax: (962-6) 560-6994
Email: nhf@nic.net.jo
www.nhf.org.jo

Operation Eyesight Universal
National Office
4 Parkdale Crescent NW
Calgary, Alberta T2N 3T8
Canada
Toll-free tel: (800) 585-8265
Fax: (403) 270-1899
Email: oeuca@giftofsight.com
www.giftofsight.com

ORBIS International (Headquarters)
580 Eighth Ave., 11th floor
New York, NY 10018
Tel: (646) 674-5500
Fax: (646) 674-5599
Email: executive@ny.orbis.org
www.orbis.org

Organisation pour la Prévention de la Cécité
Email: opc@opc.assoc.fr
www.who.int/ina-ngo/ngo/ngo199.htm

Perkins School for the Blind
175 North Beacon Street
Watertown, MA 02472-2790
Tel: (617) 924-3434
Fax: (617) 926-2027
www.perkins.pvt.k12.ma.us/

Seva Foundation
1786 Fifth Street
Berkeley, CA 94710
Tel: (510) 845-7381
Fax: (510) 845-7410
Email: admin@seva.org
www.seva.org/

Sight Savers International
Grosvenor Hall
Bolnore Road
Haywards Health
West Sussex, RH16 4BX, UK
Tel: 07000 14 2020
Email: generalinformation@sightsavers.org
www.sightsavers.org/

World Blind Union
Email: umc@once.es
umc.once.es

World Health Organization
Avenue Appia 20
1211 Geneva 27
Switzerland
Tel: (+00 41 22) 791 21 11
Fax: (+00 41 22) 791 3111
Telex: 415 416
Telegraph: UNISANTE GENEVA
www.who.int

PART I

Ophthalmic Epidemiology Principles

Introduction

One of the basic purposes of ophthalmic epidemiology is to develop methods of clinical medicine that will help physicians make valid clinical decisions. Clinical observations are made by clinicians with variable skills and prejudices on patients with a wide spectrum of physical, cultural, and social variables. The use of epidemiologic principles helps clinicians deal with these variables, reduces bias, and allows estimates of the effect of chance on outcomes.

In Part I, we present a number of epidemiologic methods by using examples of ophthalmologic studies. In Chapter 2, Drs Wormald and Klein join me in presenting a review of the principles of evidence-based medicine (EBM) and the epidemiologic methods that assist in gathering and analyzing quality medical evidence. These tools include methods that help distinguish quality contributions required to maintain medical competency taken from the vast quantity of medical literature. In Chapter 3, Dr Colenbrander describes aspects of vision loss, as used in international classification systems, and ranges of vision loss, as defined by various scales. In Chapter 4, Drs Klein and Leske join me in presenting a review of survey methodologies for effectively collecting data on the frequency and distribution of eye diseases and for improving the comparability of studies from different populations of people. Dr Klein succinctly points out the pitfalls of global comparisons of diseases such as diabetic retinopathy (DR) and age-related macular degeneration (AMD) and shows how the reader may avoid these pitfalls. In Chapter 5, Drs Callanan and Gass describe case series methodology, which suits the study of rare diseases and is practical for the individual clinician. Clinical ophthalmology has been advanced by Gass's skillful use of this epidemiologic method.

These examples highlight the wide application of epidemiology in clinical and research ophthalmology. The principles are applicable in all parts of the world, and their use will help the clinician evaluate research methodology and the constant flow of medical information.

Mylan VanNewkirk, MD

CHAPTER 2

Evidence-based Ophthalmology

Background

Sight is such a critical human faculty that for centuries it has attracted the most astute inquiry and endeavor to correct defects such as cataract and refractive error. This may explain, in part, why ophthalmology is one of the oldest medical specialties. For many centuries, medical practice made slow progress, perhaps because rigorous scientific method was not applied to the relationship of cause and effect. Faith, chance, and the placebo effect are important confounders of the healing process, as even ineffective therapies can seem effective when the body heals itself. The doctor–patient relationship relies on an important tenet of the Hippocratic Oath: First, do no harm. For years it seemed possible to justify ineffective therapies as long as they were harmless, perhaps because the patient felt that something was being done.

Although an interest in medical evidence may have existed in Paris in the mid-19th century, the demand by physicians and patients for medical evidence has developed slowly. Today, pressure from payers, providers, and consumers challenges physicians to make informed clinical decisions that take into account both effectiveness and efficiency. In 1972, the British epidemiologist Archie Cochrane authored a book on this subject and in so doing became the namesake for the evidence-based Cochrane Library. Concerns about quality of care, effectiveness of health policy, the vast quantity of medical literature, and the use of scarce health care resources has prompted what is now regarded as a new movement: *evidence-based medicine (EBM).*

> Cochrane AL. *Effectiveness and Efficiency: Random Reflections on Health Services.* London: Nuffield Provincial Hospitals Trust; 1972.
> The Cochrane Library. Published quarterly and made available on both CD-ROM and the Internet at www.cochrane.org. Online access is provided by subscription through Update Software.

Evidence-based medicine is the application of clinical expertise and the best available clinical evidence to provide sound advice for health decisions. The foundation of clinical problem solving relies on clinical skills, including knowledge of anatomy and pathophysiology. In addition, compassion, sensitive listening, and social and cultural awareness are required for a clinician to relate appropriately to each individual patient. Evidence-based medicine does not provide a blueprint for decision making for all patients because each patient's point of view and best interest must be considered in the clinical decision the patient ultimately reaches. However, applying its principles should give both patient and physician a firmer foundation from which to choose a particular treatment. Although EBM is not new, many of the standards for gathering evidence and the tools for analyzing the evidence are new.

Grading Scales of Evidence

To apply a systematic approach to including or excluding evidence, a number of quality scales for evaluating evidence have been proposed. Three such scales follow. The quality of scientific evidence rating system was created by the US Preventive Services Task Force. The system is shown in Table 2-1, where quality of evidence is rated from top to bottom, with group I being the highest quality.

> US Preventive Services Task Force. *Guide to Clinical Preventive Services.* Washington, DC: US Department of Health and Human Services; 1996:862.

The *Users' Guides to the Medical Literature* has developed a hierarchy of preprocessed evidence. Table 2-2 shows this system, with evidence ranked from top to bottom, primary studies being the highest level of evidence.

Table 2-1 US Preventive Services Task Force Rating System of Quality of Scientific Evidence

I: Evidence obtained from at least one properly designed, randomized controlled trial

II-1: Evidence obtained from well-designed controlled trails without randomization

II-2: Evidence obtained from well-designed cohort or case-control analytic studies, preferably from more than one center or research group

II-3: Evidence obtained from multiple time series with or without the intervention, or dramatic results in uncontrolled experiments (such as results of the introduction of penicillin treatment in the 1940s)

III: Opinions of respected authorities, based on clinical experience, descriptive studies, or reports of expert committees

Table 2-2 A Hierarchy of Preprocessed Evidence

Primary Studies
Preprocessing involves selecting only studies that are both highly relevant and with study designs that minimize bias and thus permit a high strength of inference.

Summaries
Systematic reviews provide clinicians with an overview of all the evidence addressing a focused clinical question.

Synopses
Synopses of individual studies or of systematic reviews encapsulate the key methodologic details and results required to apply the evidence to individual patient care.

Systems
Practice guidelines, clinical pathways, or evidence-based textbook summaries of a clinical area provide the clinician with much of the information needed to guide the care of individual patients.

Guyatt G, Rennie D, eds. *Users' Guides to the Medical Literature: A Manual for Evidence-Based Clinical Practice*. Chicago: AMA Press; 2002.

In the *Evidence-Based Eye Care* journal, five levels of evidence are used to classify clinical studies, as suggested by David L Sackett in his text, *Evidence-based Medicine*. In Table 2-3, the evidence is again laid out from top to bottom, with Level 1 more likely to inform and less likely to mislead the reader.

Evidence relevant to the delivery of eye care exists in three domains. Understanding the magnitude and distribution of disease in populations, who is at risk, and what risk factors predispose to disease is the domain of descriptive and analytic epidemiology. Such evidence is relevant to public health programs and preventive interventions, including screening strategies. These issues are not of direct concern to the individual practitioner in dealing with a particular patient. Having access to up-to-date information on the effectiveness of treatments is, however, and that is the main focus of this chapter. Other concerns are implementing cost-efficient health care policy and monitoring outcomes according to established standards; these concern adherence to modern requirements of clinical governance in health care delivery.

Randomized Controlled Trials

Logically, the strongest evidence is an effect so obvious there is no doubt that it occurred—for example, the early results of penicillin use in bacterial infections. Ethics restrict further study of such evidence, but when there is doubt about effectiveness, the ethical concerns of withholding a possibly effective intervention from control trial participants must be carefully weighed against the ethics of failing to gather quality evidence of the effectiveness of this new intervention.

Though not the only source of evidence, *randomized controlled trials (RCTs)* are often said to be the gold standard for gathering evidence in clinical medicine. However, the evidence resulting from a systematic review of multiple RCTs with meta-analysis, when appropriate, may be superior to that resulting from one RCT. Other sources of evidence discussed in this chapter are meta-analysis, outcome studies, nonrandomized studies, and observational studies that include cohort and case-control designs.

The first RCT was published in 1948. Important aspects of RCT methodology are briefly discussed. The precise clinical objective of the RCT must be explicitly defined,

Table 2-3 Levels of Evidence Used in Evidence-based Eye Care

Level 1	Randomized clinical trial with an alpha of ≤.05 and a beta of ≤.20 (or power of ≥80%)
Level 2	Randomized clinical trial with a higher alpha and/or beta
Level 3	Nonrandomized clinical trial
Level 4	Case series
Level 5	Case report

(Adapted from Sackett DL, Richardson WS, Rosenberg W, et al. *Evidence-based Medicine: How to Practice and Teach EBM.* 2nd ed. New York: Churchill Livingstone; 2000.)

from the outset, in a scientific protocol. Random assignment of participants to experimental or control groups eliminates patient selection bias when properly administered. Random allocation is essential. To avoid selection bias, it is essential that no one know the next allocation. An external quality-control group for the trial, such as a datamonitoring and ethics committee, can monitor the actual and the intended allocation. Modern trials often use online or telephone allocation organized by a central trial administration center. An alternative is sealed, numbered envelopes, which must be opaque so that treatment allocation cannot be detected.

In addition, an estimate of the number of participants required to achieve statistically significant or nonsignificant results must be made before the clinical trial begins. The sample size calculation determines the power of the study to detect a given (clinically significant) effect of the intervention. Evaluation of an RCT with a negative outcome requires consideration of the role of chance and the probability of a false negative, also called *type II,* or β, *error.* The risk of a false negative study is particularly large in small RCTs. The probability that an RCT will find a statistically significant difference when a difference exists is its *statistical power.*

$$\text{Statistical power} = 1 - p_\beta$$

Power is analogous to the sensitivity of a diagnostic test. In other words, a study with high power has a high probability of detecting a difference of effect if a difference exists. To detect small differences in treatment outcome, it is necessary to have a large sample size; p_β of .20 is often chosen. This means that a study has a 20% chance of missing a true difference in an RCT.

A well-designed RCT collects data prospectively, masks participants and observers with regard to the intervention tested, and ensures no differential losses to follow-up in the treatment or control phases. A clinical trial with a dropout rate of less than 5% is excellent; if the rate is 20% or greater, any conclusion is suspect.

Randomized controlled treatment trials in individual patients provide the highest level of evidence for the individual patient. Results from RCTs must be judged carefully on generalizability from the study population to each individual patient. Excessively strict inclusion or exclusion criteria limit the external validity (applicability to the general population) of RCT results. Differences in diagnostic and/or surgical expertise, patient noncompliance, age, comorbidity, and concomitant therapy may make generalization of results outside the study unreliable. (See BCSC Section 1, *Update on General Medicine.*)

Aiello LM, Berrocal J, Davis MD, et al. The Diabetic Retinopathy Study. *Arch Ophthalmol.* 1973;90:347–348.

Medical Research Council. Streptomycin treatment of pulmonary tuberculosis. *BMJ.* 1948; 2:769–782.

Efficacy versus Effectiveness: Trial Outcomes

An explanatory trial measures the *efficacy* of an intervention in modifying the pathogenesis of a condition; outcomes are based on measures of the disease process. An example might be a trial to examine the effect of treatment of cystoid macula edema; the primary outcome would be based on fluorescein angiographic findings or measures of retinal thickness. A pragmatic trial measures the *effectiveness* of treatment, usually in terms of a patient-oriented outcome. What effect does the intervention have on the day-to-day functioning of the patient, and does the patient actually see better as a result of the intervention? Health services research requires pragmatic trials, whereas understanding the means of manipulating objective disease processes requires explanatory studies. The nature of the primary outcomes (upon which the power of the study is based) determines the predominant nature of the study. Often trials may attempt to include efficacy and effectiveness outcomes, but it is always essential to determine the priority outcomes of a study.

Adverse Event Reporting

A trial involving a new drug must demonstrate not only the effectiveness of the agent but also its safety. A standard adverse event reporting form is used to report adverse effects or toxicity. These reports are very important in drug trials where treatment is ongoing. Although less urgent, preoperative and postoperative complications encountered in trials should be reported in a similar way. The risks and benefits of all treatments should be reported in a balanced and complete fashion in order to allow clinicians and patients to choose the appropriate treatment. A recognized weakness of RCTs, however, is that serious but rare adverse events may not be detected with sufficient frequency in trials to inform this important issue. Other methods, such as surveillance systems, outcome studies, and case-control studies, may be necessary to provide the necessary evidence (see the following section).

Measures of Risk and Benefit

A useful concept in measuring risk and benefit is the *number needed to treat (NNT)* and the number needed to harm. The NNT is the number of patients a clinician needs to treat in order for one patient to benefit from the intervention. It is the reciprocal of the absolute risk difference between those treated and controls in a trial (1/ARR) and is therefore a measure of the change in risk status or benefit provided by the treatment. In the ocular hypertension treatment trial, 9% of the control group progressed to glaucoma, whereas only 4% of the treatment group progressed—a 5% ARR. The reciprocal of this difference is 20. Twenty patients with ocular hypertension need treatment for one patient to benefit. In the Diabetes Control and Complications Trial (DCCT) example in Table 2-4, for instance, we can say that for every two patients who are intensively treated with insulin for 9 years, one will be prevented from developing diabetic retinopathy (DR). Although NNT seems popular with clinicians, some statisticians question its use as a summary statistic to report the effectiveness of treatment because of the difficulty in representing the variance of the estimate.

Several measures of association between exposure and disease and the size and potential effects of treatment called *measures of effect* are used to compare risks. Some of these clinically useful measures include *absolute risk reduction (ARR)*; *relative risk reduction (RRR)*; and *relative risk,* or *risk ratio (RR)*. *Odds ratio (OR)* is sometimes used as an estimate of the risk ratio and is the measure of effect produced by case-control studies. A modification of the OR called the *Peto odds ratio* is also a common summary measure

Table 2-4 Clinically Useful Measures of the Effects of Treatment

Worsening of DR Type 1 DM, NO DR at Baseline	Event Rates (DR Progression After 9 Years Follow-Up)		Relative Risk Reduction (RRR)	Absolute Risk Reduction (ARR)	Number Needed to Be Treated (NNT)
	Usual Insulin Controls (CER*)	Intensive Insulin Treatment (EER†)	RRR = (CER − ERR)/CER	ARR = CER − EER	NNT = 1/ARR
DCCT	56%	11%	(56% − 11%)/56% = 80%	56% − 11% = 45%	1/45% = 2
LOW HYPO-THETICAL	0.0056%	0.0011%	(0.0056% − 0.0011%)/0.0056% = 80%	0.0056% − 0.0011% = 0.0045%	1/0.0045% = 20,000

* CER = control event rate
† EER = experimental event rate

(Adapted from Sackett DL, Richardson WS, Rosenberg W, et al. *Evidence-based Medicine: How to Practice and Teach EBM.* Melbourne: Churchill Livingstone; 1997.)

of effect in meta-analysis. When the event rate in a trial is low, OR and RR are similar; with more frequent outcomes, however, the RR is more appropriate.

The DCCT showed a highly statistically significant ($P \leq .001$) worsening of DR in type 1 diabetes mellitus (DM) without DR at baseline in patients with conventional insulin treatment compared with patients receiving intensive insulin treatment. How might this treatment effect be expressed in clinical terms? A traditional measure of effect has been RRR. Table 2-4 shows that in the DCCT cohort without DR at baseline, the RRR is 80%; intensive insulin treatment reduced the risk of worsening of DR by 80%. Unfortunately, RRR fails to distinguish between large treatment effects and much smaller ones, as illustrated in Table 2-4 when the actual DCCT data are compared with low hypothetical data. The ARR illustrates the absolute difference in effects.

Stopping an RCT: Role of a Data-Monitoring and Ethics Committee

The independent data-monitoring and ethics committee (DMEC) comprising clinicians and statisticians experienced in RCT design and conduct, and completely independent of the principal investigators, evaluates the interim data for effectiveness and side effects; such evaluation is often required by an Institutional Review Board or Research Ethics Committee. These committees have a responsibility to ensure that research on human subjects is conducted to the highest ethical standards according to the tenets of the Declaration of Helsinki, which has recently been updated and which can be viewed at www.wma.net.

Interim analysis is always planned prior to the start of recruitment. This plan should be based on a reasonable minimum sample size and include a defined power requirement and stringent stopping criteria. An important function of the data-monitoring and ethics committee is to stop an RCT when the study's interim data indicate a treatment benefit beyond a reasonable doubt ($P < .001$) in order to avoid recruiting patients who will receive an inferior standard of treatment. The committee may also occasionally stop the trial when the new treatment is actually ineffective or insufficiently convincing to change clinical practice or resolve important therapeutic issues. The committee must also carefully investigate the data for side effects of treatment in order to avoid putting patients at risk.

Pocock SJ. When to stop a clinical trial. *BMJ.* 1992;305:235–240.

Whitehead J. *The Design and Analysis of Sequential Clinical Trials.* 2nd ed. Chichester: Wiley; 1997.

CONSORT Statement

Although a trial may be well conducted, its findings, when reported in a peer-reviewed journal, may lack sufficient information for readers to be able to judge the quality of the study. To achieve a high standard of reporting on RCTs in the medical literature, a group of journal editors and clinicians have assembled guidelines for reporting about them. The guidelines are called the *CONSORT* (Consolidated Standards of Reporting Trials) *statement.* Details of this can be found at the website www.consort_statement.org. Leading journals such as *Ophthalmology, Archives of Ophthalmology,* and the *British Journal of Ophthalmology* are signatories to the CONSORT statement, and those conducting trials who wish to submit their papers to these journals will be expected to adhere to CONSORT guidelines.

RCT Registries

In recent years, the RCT has been used to evaluate a large number of interventions. The International Cochrane Collaboration maintains an electronic database of controlled trials and other health care interventions that serves as the best available resource for those preparing systematic reviews or searching for trials. The database, called CENTRAL, contains more than 300,000 records, including more than 5000 reports of controlled trials of interventions relevant to eyes and vision. CENTRAL includes citations that may not be indexed in MEDLINE or other bibliographic databases, citations published in languages other than English, and citations that are available only in conference proceedings or other hard-to-access sources. The database is continually updated and is published quarterly on the Cochrane Library.

Another RCT database index, published by the National Eye Institute, is accessible at www.nei.nih.gov.

The Ovid Evidence-based Medicine Reviews database is growing and offers a link to the Cochrane Library, the American College of Physicians Best Evidence 3, and to MEDLINE (www.ovid.com).

Systematic Reviews and Meta-Analysis

Although the cost of a properly powered RCT is often high, the cost-saving outcome measures—that is, the application of effective and the rejection of ineffective interventions—often help to recover the expense. Cost may be the reason many clinical trials are small. Sometimes, small trials may provide adequate evidence to challenge conventional therapy or authority when the observed effect size is large. Small, well-designed trials can be combined when the studies are sufficiently homogeneous and selection bias has been controlled by systematic retrieval, inclusion, and exclusion criteria. This systematic review method may include an "analysis of analyses" or "meta-analysis."

> Sackett DL, Cook DJ. Can we learn anything from small trials? *Ann N Y Acad Sci.* 1993;703: 25–31.

A systematic review is the entire process of developing a protocol that searches, sorts, and summarizes evidence and that goes on to apply that protocol to the conduct of the review. To maintain validity, a reviewer must use a systematic, scientific method to conduct the review.

Implicit in the theory of meta-analysis is the idea that a series of trials examining the effect of an intervention are samples from a "population" of trials on that intervention. All of them, no matter how large or small, are subject to the effects of random variation or chance. When they are put together, however, the effects of that variation are reduced and the overall estimate of effect is closer to the truth. The assumption that the trials all come from the same "population" is an important one and must be tested by closely examining both the intervention itself and the patient groups subjected to that intervention. This is a qualitative exercise that can be reinforced by a statistical test for heterogeneity using chi square.

The International Cochrane Collaboration has established centers for systematic review in nine countries, usually in association with an established medical center, such as the Australasian Cochrane Centre at the Flinders Medical Centre in South Australia. The common goal is to create, maintain, and disseminate systematic reviews of RCTs worldwide to provide clinicians with current and accurate medical evidence. The sustainability of the collaboration will depend largely on whether the Cochrane Database of Systematic Review methodology is timely, valid, and relevant.

Assessing the validity of a study is a critical task for the reviewer in deciding whether to include or exclude studies from the meta-analysis. Like any scientific clinical experiment, a meta-analysis should be conducted with an open mind regarding the outcome. The objective and scientific method of the review must be clearly stated in the context of the review so the validity of the findings is obvious. The search strategy is designed to be more sensitive than specific, so the result of the search is often a very long list of article citations that must be carefully sorted. The inclusion/exclusion criteria for sources of evidence should be clearly stated. Reviews should incorporate strategies that minimize bias and maximize precision, and they should be reported so explicitly that any interested reader would be able to replicate them. Here, a hierarchy of evidence will be applied and different reviews may have differing strategies. However, when a numerical synthesis of evidence is to be attempted, great caution must be applied in the meta-analysis of anything but the best-quality experimental evidence.

> Huston P. Cochrane Collaboration helping unravel tangled web woven by international research. *CMAJ.* 1996;154:1389–1392.

A recent systematic review of 44 studies identified 5 RCTs and 10 observational studies that met the inclusion criterion of providing the necessary information to assess the efficacy and costs of ambulatory cataract surgery. Outcomes of ambulatory surgery in Spain were compared with those of inpatient surgery, specifically postoperative visual acuity, surgical complications, and costs of the surgery. No difference was observed in vision, but a higher rate of elevated intraocular pressure (OR = 2.3; 95% CI: 1.3–3.9) was observed in outpatients. The ambulatory surgery costs ranged from 15% to 30% lower than inpatient costs. See BCSC Section 1, *Update on General Medicine,* and Chapter 4 of this volume.

> Castells X, Alonso J, Castilla M, et al. Efficacy and cost of ambulatory cataract surgery: a systemic review. *Med Clin (Barc).* 2000;114 (suppl 2):40–47.

Meta-analysis

A *meta-analysis* is a method whereby two or more comparable RCTs are combined to enhance the estimate of the direction and the strength of an intervention effect. The gold standard for meta-analysis is based on collecting individual outcomes from all the relevant trials and conducting a new analysis with all the combined data; this is called an *individual patient data (IPD)* meta-analysis. The method is a major endeavour, and because of the difficulties of retrieving and reanalyzing complete data sets, it is rare. Assuming all the relevant data are retrieved, this method avoids the effects of selection and publication bias that can affect meta-analysis that pools the results from separate study reports.

Meta-analysis is the method available in software produced by the Cochrane Collaboration (Revman–Update Software Inc) and other statistical packages. Results from individual studies are combined, and the summary effect size is estimated using fixed or random effects modeling, weighting the contribution of individual studies according to their study power. This method depends on collecting the numbers of people successfully (or unsuccessfully) treated and the denominators for each arm of the trials. The software calculates an overall effect size, which can be reported in terms of Peto OR, RR, or AR. It also tests the individual outcomes with a chi-square test for heterogeneity, which will warn the reviewer of the possibility that the trials are actually from different populations and that use of a summary effect is inadvisable. Examples of such reviews can be seen on the Cochrane Database of Systematic Reviews.

The Stockholm Diabetes Intervention Study, an RCT, demonstrated the beneficial effect of intensive glycemic control on diabetic retinopathy in 102 participants with type 1 diabetes. The data were combined with data from five other trials (271 participants) by meta-analysis. The increased number of participants improved the power of the study to show that the risk of progression of diabetic retinopathy was lower in the intensive insulin therapy group than in the conventional insulin treatment group after 2 years (OR = 0.49; 95% CI: 0.28–0.85). Early data from RCT studies on tight control of blood glucose in type 1 diabetes were inconsistent. A meta-analysis of data from these studies demonstrated the association between tight control and a reduced risk of diabetes complications.

> Reichard P, Nilsson BY, Rosenqvist U. The effect of long-term intensified insulin treatment on the development of microvascular complications of diabetes mellitus. *N Engl J Med.* 1993;329:304–309.

Wang PH, Lau J, Chalmers TC. Meta-analysis of effects of intensive blood-glucose control on late complications of type I diabetes. *Lancet.* 1993;341:1306–1309.

A reviewer must determine how well each RCT meets established methodologic criteria before including it in a meta-analysis. A meta-analysis will not improve a poorly designed and executed RCT. Like all RCTs, the meta-analysis depends on the quality of evidence collected. It does not eliminate the role that chance plays even in the largest and most well-designed trial. A critical strength of meta-analysis is that it reduces the possibility that several well-conducted trials will, by the same twist of fate, reach the wrong conclusion. The greater the number of good trials combined, the greater the chance that the meta-analysis will get closer to the truth. For example, 16 RCTs involving 2898 eyes examining the effectiveness of medical prophylaxis of cystoid macular edema (CME) and 4 RCTs involving 187 eyes testing the effectiveness of medical treatment of chronic CME were studied by meta-analysis. Results indicated that prophylactic intervention was effective in reducing the incidence of both angiographic CME (OR = 0.36; 95% CI: 0.28–0.45) and clinically relevant CME (OR = 0.49; 95% CI: 0.33–0.73). The intervention also revealed a statistically significant positive effect on improving vision (OR = 1.97; 95% CI: 1.14–3.41). However, the reviewers concluded that the overall quality of the trials was so poor that it was not possible to conclude on the basis of the meta-analysis that the evidence was of sufficient strength to implement the therapy and that further properly powered high-quality trials were required.

Rossetti L, Chaudhuri J, Dickersin K. Medical prophylaxis and treatment of cystoid macular edema after cataract surgery. The results of a meta-analysis. *Ophthalmology.* 1998;105: 397–405.

If there is any doubt of the homogeneity of trials, a meta-analysis should not be attempted; however, the systematic review is still of value, as are the findings of individual studies presented without pooling. Even a complete absence of trials of adequate quality is an important finding because this serves as a powerful stimulus for the initiation of future trials, which are needed to answer a reviewer's question.

Bias in meta-analysis

Selection bias in various forms is the main problem with meta-analysis. Systematic searching of the world literature is an attempt to prevent bias by language or time. Use of an a priori protocol with explicit inclusion and exclusion criteria, as well as standardized methods for assessing trial quality for the selection of trials for the review by two or more independent reviewers, should prevent selection bias. When reviewers differ in their selection, resolution by consensus or arbitration is recommended. Duplicate data extraction from included studies reduces the risk of transcription error. Cochrane reviews are subject to peer review at the protocol and review stages.

Publication bias may occur when editors and authors give preference in publication and submission to trials with a positive outcome. Failure to publish trials with negative results may lead to incorrect conclusions—usually overestimation of the size of effect—from meta-analysis and systematic reviews.

The effect of bias of any kind can be managed if, first, it is known to exist and, second, it is quantifiable. One such method allows for the qualitative assessment of publication bias in a meta-analysis by representation in a funnel plot, which is a graphic display of the trial's effect estimates against sample size. The funnel plot assumes that the precision in estimating the underlying treatment effect will increase as the sample size of the studies in the meta-analysis increases. Thus, in the absence of bias, small studies will be scattered at lower precision levels and larger studies will show less scatter and higher precision, thus resembling a symmetrical inverted funnel. Figure 2-1 shows a symmetrical funnel plot comparing the precision against the odds ratio observed in the DCCT with smaller studies by Wang and colleagues.

> Wang PH, Lau J, Chalmers TC. Meta-analysis of effects of intensive blood-glucose control on late complications of type I diabetes. *Lancet.* 1993;341:1306–1309.

A problem facing all modern clinicians is that the medical literature is enormous and is continually expanding so that keeping up to date is impossible. Systematic reviews take a long time to complete, and hard copy publication can often mean that the review is out of date by the time it is published. This is why the Cochrane Library is electronically published quarterly and why all Cochrane reviewers have made a commitment to continuously update reviews, including new evidence as and when it emerges. Most review groups have a policy of running new searches at least every 2 years. Reviews that have not been updated for more than 2 years are flagged with a warning on the library and ultimately removed.

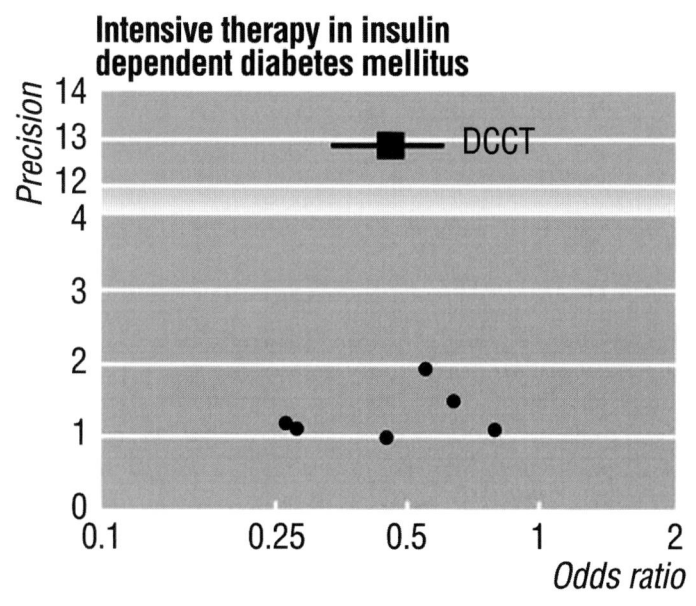

Figure 2-1 Funnel plot comparing precision against odds ratio in the Diabetes Control and Complications Trial (DCCT). *(Modified from Egger M, Davey Smith G, Schneider M, et al. Bias in meta-analysis detected by a simple, graphical test.* BMJ. *1997;315:629–634. Reproduced with permission from the BMJ Publishing Group.)*

Observational Studies

Observational studies are by definition not experimental and there is, therefore, no prospective random allocation to intervention or control groups. These studies are prone to many sources of bias and confounding and, as a result, contribute less to the evidence base. Meta-analysis of observational studies, except perhaps well-conducted outcome studies and sample surveys, should be interpreted with care. Observational studies that may be called upon to inform the evidence base are outcome studies, cohort studies, case-control studies, and case series.

Outcome Studies

Because RCTs are conducted under restricted conditions, the observed effects of a new treatment may sometimes be greater than those observed in the real world. Trials therefore do not provide a complete picture of the effectiveness of interventions. Studies describing the outcome of treatment as actually delivered are of value in establishing standards for clinical practice. In order to be valid, outcome studies must include all relevant cases and be representative both temporally and geographically of actual clinical practice. Outcome studies may be designed to measure the impact of disease, treatment cost-effectiveness, and the patient's functional status and quality of life.

Cataract surgical outcomes have been most frequently studied in many health care systems, such as those in the United States, United Kingdom, Sweden, and Denmark. These outcome studies have provided the basis for the establishment of standards against which individual clinicians can measure their own outcomes in day-to-day practice in audit.

> Desai P, Minassian DC, Reidy A. National cataract surgery survey 1997–8: a report of the results of the clinical outcomes. *Br J Ophthalmol.* 1999;83:1336–1340.
> Lundstrom M, Stenevi U, Thorburn W. Outcome of cataract surgery considering the preoperative situation: a study of possible predictors of the functional outcome. *Br J Ophthalmol.* 1999;83:1272–1276.
> Steinberg EP, Tielsch JM, Schein OD, et al. National study of cataract surgery outcomes. Variation in 4-month postoperative outcomes as reflected in multiple outcome measures. *Ophthalmology.* 1994;101:1131–1141.
> Wegener M, Alsbirk PH, Hojgaard-Olsen K. Outcome of 1000 consecutive clinic- and hospital-based cataract surgeries in a Danish county. *J Cataract Refract Surg.* 1998;24: 1152–1160.

Cohort Studies

Prospective cohort study

Cohort studies are usually used to investigate risk factors and thus to shed light on the etiology of disease in populations. Some of the most important cohorts have studied occupational exposures to disease in industry, comparing the incidence of disease in industrially exposed and unexposed cohorts. In terms of measuring the effectiveness of an intervention, the exposure may be an intervention but the allocation to that intervention is not random. This type of study is the same as a nonrandomized parallel group prospective trial, where a treated group is compared with an untreated group without randomization. In a sequential prospective design, one series of patients might receive treatment A and a subsequent group, treatment B, in a nonparallel comparison.

Retrospective cohort study

In a retrospective study, the investigator goes back in history to define a risk group and follows the cohort up to the present to see what outcomes have occurred. An intervention group may be compared to a historical control cohort unexposed to the intervention. This type of historical cohort study is less costly than prospective cohort studies, and results are available more quickly. However, the investigator loses the ability to control the criteria used in determining the outcome.

An example of a retrospective study is a review of the national Danish hospital registry for endophthalmitis following cataract surgery, 1985 to 1987. Of 19,426 patients who were 50 years of age or older undergoing surgery, 61 were rehospitalized with endophthalmitis, a 12-month estimated cumulative risk of 0.18% (95% CI: 0.09–0.26). When the sample was restricted to patients 65 years of age or older in order to compare it with the US National Study of Cataract Outcomes, the Danish study's estimated 12-month risk of endophthalmitis following cataract surgery was 0.17% (95% CI: 0.08–0.251), which was not a statistically significant difference from the US estimate of 0.12%.

> Norregaard JC, Thoning H, Bernth-Petersen P, et al. Risk of endophthalmitis after cataract extraction: results from the International Cataract Surgery Outcomes study. *Br J Ophthalmol.* 1997;81:102–106.

Case-Control Studies

The efficiency of a population-based study or observational study may be improved by designing a case-control study "nested" within the framework of the overall study. This technique allows the relationship between risk factors and disease to be evaluated statistically by comparing the prevalence of exposure in the control group with that in the cases. Case-control studies can provide information on a range of potential risk factors that might relate to a specific disease. The population must have a case group with a clearly defined case definition and a control group that is disease-free but otherwise similar (drawn from the same population) as the case group. The sample size must be sufficiently large to reduce the effect that chance may play in the observed results.

Risk factors are the attributes associated with target conditions. They can help predict outcomes but may not cause the target condition. Risk factors include demographic variables such as gender, ethnicity, or age; behavioral risk factors such as smoking or driving without seatbelts; and environmental factors such as the area of residence. When there are exposures that might act as powerful confounding factors between cases and controls, such as age or gender, these can be controlled by matching cases and controls for those factors. Matching for any risk factor, however, prevents an evaluation of its effect on risk for disease, and when matching has been used, a matched analysis is usually required. Ascertaining the presence or absence of risk factors (risk assessment) is accomplished through thorough patient histories, targeted examinations, and laboratory tests. Risk of disease is not measured directly; the relative risk of exposure is estimated by the OR. (See BCSC Section 1, *Update on General Medicine.*)

Case-control studies are at serious risk of bias by the selection of cases and, especially, controls. They are not generally used for the estimation of effectiveness of interventions; rather they are used to explore risk factors and etiology; they can be of value in exploring the relationship of exposure and outcome when the exposure might be a preventive effect, such as health-seeking behavior or immunization. An example is a case-control study for risk factors for late presentation of glaucoma in the United Kingdom. Regular attendance for a sight test proved to be highly protective. In general, though, this method can generate hypotheses that then require more rigorous scientific evaluation.

> Fraser S, Bunce CV, Wormald R, et al. Deprivation and late presentation of glaucoma; case-control study. *BMJ*. 2001;322:639–643.
>
> Wallace DK, Kylstra JA, Chesnutt DA. Prognostic significance of vascular dilation and tortuosity insufficient for plus disease in retinopathy of prematurity. *J AAPOS*. 2000;4:224–229.

Case Series

One of the commonest types of study reported in the ophthalmic literature is the uncontrolled case series. Such series are commonly found throughout the surgically dominated specialties. In the past, presenting a successful series of a new surgical technique was thought sufficient evidence of both its safety and effectiveness. However, with nothing to compare it against, no estimate of effectiveness (in terms of effect size) can be determined, and no explicit mechanisms for controlling bias exist. Only when an effect is so dramatic and obvious can this sort of evidence be admissible for evidence-based practice.

Case series are of value in initial small-scale investigations of new treatments, where they act as a pilot study for a larger trial. A good example of this kind of study is one that tested the theory that ionizing radiation may destroy the endothelial cells of proliferating new blood vessels and thereby inhibit neovascularization. Although the toxic ocular effects of radiation are well known, the effect of ionizing radiation on the choroidal neovascular membranes (CNVM) of age-related macular degeneration (AMD) was unknown. The results of a prospective, nonrandomized study of 19 AMD patients in England with subfoveal CNVM treated with low-dose radiation to the macular region suggested that visual acuity was maintained or improved in almost two thirds of the patients. The seven patients who refused treatment and served as a comparison group showed steady deterioration of vision and enlargement of the neovascular membranes.

Similar small prospective, nonrandomized series from Turkey and California showed encouraging results, although some radiation retinopathy was observed in a group treated with 14 Gy. A similar study in Munich of 56 patients did not find a beneficial effect of radiation in AMD patients.

> Chakravarthy U, Houston RF, Archer DB. Treatment of age-related subfoveal neovascular membranes by teletherapy: a pilot study. *Br J Ophthalmol*. 1993;77:265–273.
>
> Roesen B, Scheider A, Kiraly A, et al. Choroid neovascularization in senile macular degeneration. 1 year follow-up after radiotherapy. [Article in German.] *Ophthalmologe*. 1998;95:461–465.

Although techniques and dosage differed in all these AMD studies, all authors encouraged a prospective, randomized study to test this hypothesis. A small RCT of 27 AMD patients with subfoveal choroidal neovascularization randomized to either observation or 1 fraction of 7.5 Gy found slightly less loss of vision in the radiation group, a finding of borderline statistical significance, but no difference in the fluorescein angiographic findings. The RAD clinical trial study of subfoveal choroidal neovascularization consisted of 205 AMD patients with 89% completing the 1-year follow-up. Both the patients and the ophthalmologists were masked to the applied treatment. Patients were randomized to 8 fractions of 2 Gy or to 8 fractions of 0 Gy (sham treatment). At 1 year, no difference was observed in the 16 Gy treatment group compared with the control sham treatment group. Observation versus radiation was also studied in an RCT of 101 elderly Japanese using 20 Gy in 10 fractions of 2 Gy. The 2-year follow-up data consisted of 84% of the original participants and showed less change in area of CNVM and best-corrected visual acuity in the treatment group than in the control group. The best outcome effects were in cases of occult CNVM, small CNVM, and better visual acuity.

> Char DH, Irvine AI, Posner MD, et al. Randomized trial of radiation for age-related macular degeneration. *Am J Ophthalmol.* 1999;127:574–578.
> Kobayashi H, Kobayashi K. Age-related macular degeneration: long-term results of radiotherapy for subfoveal neovascular membranes. *Am J Ophthalmol.* 2000;130:617–635.
> RAD Study Group. A prospective, randomized, double-masked trial on radiation therapy for neovascular age-related macular degeneration (RAD Study). Radiation Therapy for Age-related Macular Degeneration. *Ophthalmology.* 1999;106:2239–2247.

Although chance and bias may play a major role in the conclusions of nonrandomized studies, other risk factor variables, such as nature of the lesion (occult, mixed, classic), size of the CNVM, and visual acuity may also influence the outcome effects. Additional RCT studies with larger sample sizes and long-term follow-up, with systematic review to evaluate the fractional dosage effect and more fully define the outcome effect of radiation treatment for choroidal neovascular membrane in AMD, are now being conducted.

A retrospective case series report is improved in value by a consecutive series and little loss of cases to follow-up. An excellent example is a report on the results of 134 consecutive cases of vitrectomy for proliferative diabetic retinopathy.

> Michels RG. Vitrectomy for complications of diabetic retinopathy. *Arch Ophthalmol.* 1978; 96:237–246.

Measuring the Burden of Disease

The frequency of illness and health in defined populations is estimated by sample surveys of prevalence that describe the magnitude of the problem and who is at risk. Measuring the impact of illness or disability on populations in terms of function and economics is more complicated. A 1993 report proposed using disability-adjusted life-years (DALYs) for measuring the global burden of disease. This indicator, which measures the time lived with a disability and the time lost due to premature mortality, provides a useful measure of burden of disease, risk factors, and injuries. Disparities in health between the developed and the developing world become evident with this measure. Developed regions account for 12% of the worldwide burden from all causes of death and disability and account for 90% of health expenditure worldwide. Nearly 45% of the worldwide DALY total is a result of communicable, maternal, perinatal, and nutritional disorders; noncommunicable causes account for over 40%; and injuries, a significant 15%.

> Murray CJ, Lopez AD. Global mortality, disability, and the contribution of risk factors: Global Burden of Disease Study. *Lancet.* 1997;349:1436–1442.

A study conducted by the World Bank found that of the 1362 million DALYs lost to all illnesses in 1990, 7.97 million were lost to diabetes. Estimates of the global cost of diabetes based on these studies reveal that diabetes accounts for 2%–3% of the total health care budget in every country; therefore, an increase in diabetes incidence and prevalence translates into a significant economic impact.

> Jonsson B. The economic impact of diabetes. *Diabetes Care.* 1998;21(suppl 3):C7–C10.

Cost–Benefit Analysis

Of the methods used to evaluate the economics of health care interventions, cost–benefit analysis lists all the costs and benefits related to an intervention for a specified time, expressed in monetary terms. If the total benefits are greater than the total costs, the result is a positive net present value. This method is most useful in comparing two interventions, but it may be used to indicate the economic effect of a single intervention or to evaluate peripheral costs or benefits such as time expended by family members caring for an ill relative.

Cost-Effectiveness Analysis

A cost-effectiveness analysis of clinical preventive services is a potential means to aid public health resource allocation. This method expresses the net direct and indirect costs and cost savings in terms of a predefined health care outcome, such as lives saved or cases of illness avoided. This method is best used when comparing two or more health care interventions in the same population—for example, vaccination versus chemoprophylaxis. A serious limitation of this method is that no numerical value of the health care outcome results.

Cost–Utility Analysis

Cost–utility analysis is a specific form of cost-effectiveness analysis, where results are expressed in terms of cost per gains in quality-adjusted life-year ($/QALY). The health care outcomes in the denominator are valued in terms of utility or quality.

> Meltzer MI. Introduction to health economics for physicians. *Lancet.* 2001;358:993–998.

The economic burden of blindness in India for the year 1997 was calculated using a cost-of-illness approach. This approach was based on estimates of profound vision impairment in 1% of the population (9.61 million people) and the per capita annual gross national product (GNP) of Rs. 11,160 (US$310) growing at 5% per year. The lost production was calculated assuming the following:

- The average number of working years lost due to adult blindness is 10 years.
- The average working years lost of blind children is 33 years.
- 10% productivity is lost for one caring family member.
- 20% of all those who are blind are economically productive at 25% the productivity level of a sighted member of the labor force.
- 75% of adult blindness and 50% of childhood blindness are either curable or preventable.

This method estimates that the economic burden of blindness in India is Rs. 159 billion (US$4.4 billion), and the cumulative loss over the lifetime of the blind is Rs. 2787 billion (US$77.4 billion). Childhood blindness accounts for 28.7% of this lifetime loss. If we assume that almost half the blindness in India is due to cataract, and if we use Rs. 1750 (US$48.60) as the cost for one ECCE with IOL, then the cost of treating all cases of cataract blindness in India is Rs. 8.4 billion (US$0.23 billion). If we assume that surgery is available to half of the cataract blind at a cost of Rs. 5.3 billion (US$0.15 billion) and 80% of the cataract surgeries successfully restore working vision, then savings in the annual GNP due to cataract surgeries would be Rs. 40 billion (US$1.1 billion). This would make cataract surgery in India very cost effective.

Shamanna BR, Dandona L, Rao GN. Economic burden of blindness in India. *Indian J Ophthalmol.* 1998;46:169–172.

Utility theory is applied in medicine to study the changes in quality of life in relation to disease. A utility value scale ranges from 1.0, perfect health, to 0.0, death. The better the quality of life, the closer the utility value is to 1.0; the worse the quality of life, the closer the utility value is to 0.0. Utility values associated with vision loss are proportional to vision in the better-seeing eye. Therefore, visual acuities in the better-seeing eye of 20/40 and 20/400 are equal to utility values of 0.80 and 0.54, respectively.

Brown GC. Vision and quality-of-life. *Trans Am Ophthalmol Soc.* 1999;97:473–511.

When a health care intervention improves the utility value, and the new utility value is multiplied by the duration of the benefit, the result is the number of quality-adjusted life-years (QALYs) gained from the intervention. This methodology incorporates both the improvement in quality of life and/or length of life occurring as a result of the intervention. The improvement can then be assimilated with discounted cost to yield expenditures per QALY gained.

Brown GC, Brown MM, Sharma S. Cost–utility analysis. *Ann Intern Med.* 2001;134:625–626.

Expenditures per QALY gained is a measure that allows a comparison between patient-perceived value of virtually all health care interventions and dollars expended. In comparing cost-effectiveness values, it is important that all parameters entering into the calculations be standardized. Medical therapies having favorable cost-effectiveness ratios include immunizations and chemoprophylaxis. Preventive services are more cost-effective when they target a high-risk population. The cost-effectiveness of some medical therapies is shown in Table 2-5.

Table 2-5 Cost-Effectiveness of Medical Therapy

Therapies	US$/QALY
Laser therapy for threshold ROP	688
Screening and treatment of diabetic retinopathy	3130*
Laser grid therapy for diabetic macular edema	3655†
Coronary artery bypass, left main coronary artery	6985
Intensive therapy of type 1 diabetes mellitus	9626‡
Liver transplant	332,413

* From Javitt JC, Aiello LP. Cost-effectiveness of detecting and treating diabetic retinopathy. *Ann Intern Med.* 1996:124(1 Pt 2):164–169.
† From Sharma S, Brown GC, Brown MM, et al. The cost-effectiveness of grid laser photocoagulation for the treatment of diabetic macular edema: results of patient-based cost-utility analysis. *Curr Opin Ophthalmol.* 2000;11:175–179.
‡ From Meltzer D, Egleston B, Stoffel D. Effect of future costs on cost-effectiveness of medical interventions among young adults: the example of intensive therapy for type 1 diabetes mellitus. *Med Care.* 2000;38:679–685.

(Adapted from Brown GC. Vision and quality of life. *Trans Am Ophthalmol Soc.* 1999;97:473–511.)

Audit

The final step in establishing evidence-based practice is to audit outcomes from medical practice against an established standard of "best practice." Audit is the means by which local health services can be compared within the community or country. Audits must use epidemiologic tools and monitor large numbers of patient interventions. An efficient audit depends on efficient information retrieval and applies inclusiveness and representation as used for outcome studies. Audits compare a specific set of outcomes with an established standard. It is important to establish standards in ophthalmology, but few such standards exist in the developing countries. One example of an attempt to establish standard parameters in cataract outcomes was used in a training course conducted in Nigeria by members of the faculty of the Aravind Eye Hospital. Outcome data were collected on all 175 consecutive cataract patients who had ECCE/IOL during the transitional training of six ophthalmic surgeons experienced in ICCE. Postoperative results showed that uncorrected vision of 20/200 was observed in 87% (152 of 175 patients).

> Alhassan MB, Kyari F, Achi IB, et al. Audit of outcome of an extracapsular cataract extraction and posterior chamber intraocular lens training course. *Br J Ophthalmol.* 2000;84:848–851.

Conclusion

The tools and standards for gathering and analyzing medical evidence are evolving and providing assistance to clinicians and patients in choosing beneficial cost-effective treatments. Well-designed epidemiologic studies provide data that need to be clinically appraised by physicians for validity, applicability, and efficacy. The study of epidemiologic data, including systematic review and meta-analysis, is designed to assist the lifelong learning of the physician and ultimately result in improved patient care.

CHAPTER 3

Aspects and Ranges of Vision Loss

To compare the results from different surveys, it is essential that the data be categorized in a consistent manner. This chapter summarizes guidelines that have evolved over the last quarter century.

Aspects of Vision Loss

The causes and consequences of vision loss can be approached from different points of view and, depending on the point of view, different aspects will be seen. It is useful to distinguish four main aspects (Table 3-1). These aspects were used in the *International Classification of Impairments, Disabilities and Handicaps (ICIDH)* and are used in its successor, the *International Classification of Functioning (ICF)*, two WHO classifications that supplement the *International Classification of Diseases*.

International Classification of Diseases, 9th revision: ICD-9. Geneva: WHO; 1978. The international classification for statistical reporting.

International Classification of Diseases, 9th revision, Clinical Modification: ICD-9-CM. Washington, DC: Department of Health and Human Services; 1978. With regular updates. The US modification of ICD-9 for more detailed hospital indexing and diagnostic reporting.

International Classification of Diseases and Related Health Problems, 10th revision: ICD-10. Geneva: WHO; 1992. The successor of ICD-9 for international reporting.

International Classification of Functioning, Disability and Health. (ICF; was also known as ICIDH-2 during its development.) Geneva: WHO; 2001. The successor of the original ICIDH.

International Classification of Impairments, Disabilities and Handicaps. (ICIDH, also known as ICIDH-80.) Geneva: WHO; 1980. Developed for coding the consequences of disease.

Of the four main aspects, two refer to the organ system. The first aspect relates to physical and anatomical changes at the organ level. It describes diseases and disorders and is the aspect most familiar to physicians.

The next aspect describes the resulting functional changes, or impairments, at the organ level. With regard to vision, we measure these changes by measuring *visual functions*, such as visual acuity, visual field, color vision, dark adaptation, and so on.

The next two aspects refer to the whole person. The ability aspect refers to the ability of the person to perform activities of daily living (ADL). With regard to vision, we refer to *functional vision*, which can be described in terms of reading ability, orientation and mobility, self-care ability, and so on.

Table 3-1 Aspects of Vision Loss

	The Organ		The Person	
ASPECTS	Structural change at the organ level	Functional change at the organ level	Skills, abilities (ADL) of the individual	Social, economic consequences
Loss, limitation	Disorder, injury	Impairment	Ability loss (dis-ability)	Handicap
Neutral terms	Health condition	Organ function	Skills, abilities	Social participation
Application to VISION	Eye health	**"Visual Functions"** measured quantitatively	**"Functional Vision"** described qualitatively	Vision-related quality of life
		Categorized as ranges of **"Vision Loss"**		
Tests		Performance on eye tests (eg, visual acuity)	Performance on ADL skills (eg, reading ability)	Performance on job-related tasks and in social roles
Ambiguous terms (eg, "Disability")		Disability = impairment, as in "Americans with Disabilities Act" (ADA)	Dis-ability = ability loss, as in "disabled veterans"	Disability = economic status, as in "being on disability"

The fourth aspect is that of societal and economic consequences. ICIDH referred to this aspect as the handicap aspect; ICF refers to it as the participation aspect. Others may refer to it as vision-related quality of life.

For our discussion, the distinction between visual functions and functional vision is most important. The visual functions of each eye are measured with eye tests, such as visual acuity tests (a measure of visual angle). Functional vision of the person is measured with ADL tests, such as reading ability (including reading fluency, speed, and comprehension). Caution needs to be used when the same or similar terms can be used for different aspects. Table 3-1 shows that the term *disability* can have at least three different meanings; we will avoid using this term.

Causes and Consequences, Choice of Tests

Although the four aspects are clearly related, the links are not fixed but can be influenced by various interventions. Medical and surgical care can help minimize the functional effect of various disorders. For any given visual impairment, visual aids and devices can improve the ability to perform various activities. Education, training, and workplace adaptations can reduce the social and economic impact of the ability loss (Table 3-2).

The fact that the links can be modified makes rehabilitation possible. Because of the many external influences, individual performance across links cannot be predicted; only statistical averages can be considered. For instance, the mere presence of a cataract cannot predict the amount of visual acuity loss. Some people will have better skills than others

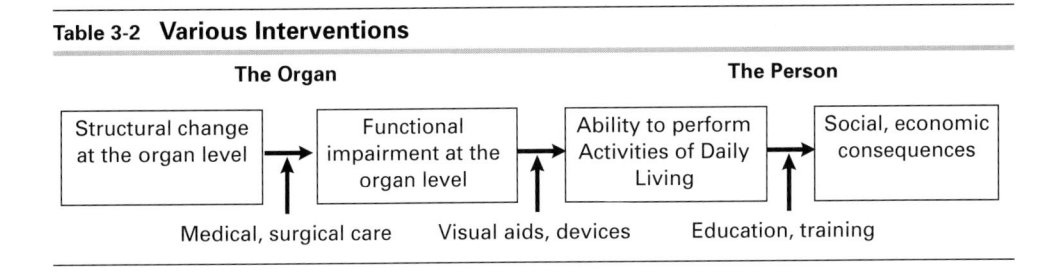

Table 3-2 Various Interventions

The Organ		The Person	
Structural change at the organ level →	Functional impairment at the organ level →	Ability to perform Activities of Daily Living →	Social, economic consequences
↑	↑	↑	
Medical, surgical care	Visual aids, devices	Education, training	

with the same acuity loss. Some people cope better with the social and economic consequences than others with the same disability. A general statement such as "As a group, people with vision loss are less employable than those with normal vision" may be possible, but an individual prediction such as "An individual with >20/200 (>0.1, >6/60) acuity is employable, whereas a person with <20/200 (<0.1, <6/60) is not" is not justifiable. Some totally blind individuals are gainfully employed, whereas some normally sighted ones are not.

The statistical correlation is less for aspects that are farther apart in the diagram. This must be kept in mind when designing a survey. When the goal is to detect *causes* of vision loss (as it is in many surveys), measuring visual acuity and other visual functions provides a useful marker. When the goal is expanded to studying the societal *consequences* of vision loss, measurement of functional vision and various visual abilities would be more appropriate. However, because visual functions are usually measured anyway, they are often used as a substitute for the measurement of skills and abilities, even though they are farther removed from the aspect of social and economic consequences.

The objective of the survey may also influence the choice of test. For instance, when the objective is to detect even slight genetic color vision deficiencies, the Ishihara test will be the test of choice. When the objective is to detect color vision deficiencies that may have vocational consequences, the Farnsworth D15 will be a better choice. When the objective is to detect disorders such as early glaucoma, a static field test of the central 30° will provide the most information. If the objective is to predict orientation and mobility problems, a field test that includes far peripheral vision will be more appropriate, and even a simple confrontation test may reveal significant problems.

The objective of the survey may also influence the choice of test. For instance, when the objective is to detect even slight genetic color vision deficiencies, the Ishihara test will be the test of choice. When the objective is to detect color vision deficiencies that may have vocational consequences, the Farnsworth D15 will be a better choice. When the objective is to detect disorders such as early glaucoma, a static field test of the central 30° will provide the most information. If the objective is to predict orientation and mobility problems, a field test that includes far peripheral vision will be more appropriate, and even a simple confrontation test may reveal significant problems.

Ranges of Vision Loss

Having defined the aspects of interest, we must classify our findings as to the severity of the deficits found. This can be done on scales of greater or lesser detail.

The simplest scale is a dichotomous one such as *legally sighted/legally blind*. Dichotomous scales are often used for benefit eligibility but are too coarse for clinical use.

A more detailed scale is a three-level classification such as *normal vision/low vision/blindness*. In the 1970s, this scale was introduced in ICD-9 to replace the hodgepodge of definitions used in various countries. A recent review of 50 surveys of vision loss showed that, a quarter of a century later, the WHO definitions have taken hold, with 95% of the surveys reporting on the WHO definitions of low vision (<20/60, <0.3, <6/18) and blindness (<20/400, <0.05, <3/60). A few reported on smaller subdivisions, but those subdivisions were not used consistently. The comprehensive chart in Table 3-3 provides a guideline for more detailed reporting.

For many purposes, a classification with three ranges is still too coarse. Because visual acuity is the visual function that is measured most often, we start with a discussion of visual acuity ranges. Note that we use the word *loss* as a generic term; for congenital conditions, the term *deficit* would be more appropriate.

Ranges of Visual Acuity Loss

Visual acuity is the reciprocal of the magnification needed to bring a subject to a standard performance. If an individual needs letters that are twice as large or twice as close, visual acuity is said to be one half (20/40, 0.5, 6/12). If the letters need to be five times closer or five times larger, visual acuity is said to be one fifth (20/100, 0.2, 6/30), and so on.

If decimal notation is used, the progression of letter sizes often is 0.1, 0.2, 0.3, ..., 0.8, 0.9, 1.0, 1.1. This progression suffers from steps that are too large at the lower end and too small at the upper end. A progression with equal increments of the Snellen denominator would suffer from the opposite effect: 20/10, 20/20, 20/30 would be too coarse, whereas 20/200, 20/210, 20/220 would be too fine. Only a geometric (logarithmic) progression can cover a wide range with equal steps.

The series ... 0.8, **1.0, 1.25, 1.6, 2.0, 2.5, 3.2, 4.0, 5.0, 6.3, 8.0, 10.0,** 12.5 ... is based on the tenth root of 10. It fits with the decimal system because ten steps equal a factor 10×; after ten steps, the same values repeat with only a shift in the decimal position. Three steps equal a factor 2×. This series, also known as the "preferred numbers series," is widely used in international standards. Its use for a letter chart was first proposed in 1868 by Green, an American ophthalmologist who had worked with Snellen in 1866 (Snellen had invented the letter chart in 1862). Subsequently, it was forgotten and reinvented several times. Presently, it is best known through the ETDRS charts, promoted by the National Eye Institute for its clinical studies.

Table 3-3 shows how groups of four lines on this mathematically derived series result in a useful classification of vision loss in six ranges. These six ranges fit well with the ranges proposed by the WHO in the 1960s, which were largely based on socioeconomic categories. They also fit with a generic classification of ranges of ability loss based on rehabilitative needs. That such different starting points can lead to the same ranges may be taken as mutual reinforcement for their validity.

Even when a geometric progression is used, visual acuity values cannot be simply averaged. Clinicians have long recognized this by speaking of "lines lost" or "lines gained"; in mathematical terms, this means converting the geometric progression to a linear one. The Visual Acuity section of Table 3-3 shows two linear scales. In 1976 Bailey and Lovie introduced the layout that is now used in the ETDRS charts. They also introduced the term *logMAR* (logarithm of the minimum angle of resolution). The logMAR scale is a scale of vision *loss* because higher logMAR indicates poorer vision; its decimal values do not make it very user friendly. Bailey later introduced the "letter count" score, which is more intuitive. This score assigns 5 points to each line and 1 point to each letter read on an ETDRS-type chart. Standard vision (20/20, 1.0, 6/6) is assigned the value 100, and 20/200 (0.1, 6/60) receives 50 points. Zero is reached only at 20/2000 (0.01, 6/600), so negative values are avoided. Because letter count scores use smaller increments than the line scores used in most clinical settings, they can detect smaller differences and are better suited for statistical manipulations.

Bailey IL, Bullimore MA, Raasch TW, et al. Clinical grading and the effects of scaling. *Invest Ophthalmol Vis Sci.* 1991;32:422–432.

Bailey IL, Lovie JE. New design principles for visual acuity letter charts. *Am J Optom Physiol Opt.* 1976;53:740–745.

The Ability section of Table 3-3 lists various ranges of reading ability. On one side, these ranges fit well with the reading distance for 1 M print (average newsprint), as calculated from the visual acuity values. On the other side, they also fit with a set of generic ability ranges. These ability ranges can be fitted with a scale from 0 to 100, which in turn fits the letter count score in the Visual Acuity section.

The Handicap/Participation section describes some of the consequences of vision loss. This section also follows the six ranges. Sometimes ranges are grouped to provide broader categories. The U.S. concept of "legal blindness" includes the lower three ranges. The WHO definition of blindness covers only two ranges. In ICD-9-CM, only the lowest range is designated as blindness.

Ranges of Visual Field Loss

The Visual Field section of Table 3-3 provides a similar classification for visual field loss. The lower three ranges are based on ICD-9 and ICD-9-CM; the upper three ranges (not covered in ICD-9-CM) are based on the new visual field grid in the AMA *Guides to the Evaluation of Permanent Impairment,* 5th edition. On this grid, 1 point is scored for every grid point seen, resulting in a score similar to the letter count score for visual acuity. Although most regulations consider only concentric losses, grid systems such as in the AMA *Guides* also allow consideration of irregular losses. On this grid, a concentric restriction to an average radius of 10° (20° diameter) is considered equally disabling (50 points) as an acuity restriction to 20/200. A homonymous hemianopia also scores 50 points.

Cocchiarella L, Anderson GBJ, eds. *Guides to the Evaluation of Permanent Impairment.* 5th ed. Chicago: AMA; 2001. Chapter 12.

Table 3-3A Aspects and Ranges of Vision and Vision Loss Visual Acuity and Reading Ability

Ranges of Vision	Impairment Aspect (how the eye functions)							Ability Aspect (how the person functions)		Generic Ability Ranges
	Visual Acuity				Linear scales				
	U.S. notation	Decimal notation	6 m notation	Letter score	Log MAR	Reads 1M at:	Reading Ability	
Range of Normal Vision	20/12.5 20/16 **20/20** 20/25	1.6 1.25 **1.0** 0.8	6/3.8 6/4.8 **6/6** 6/7.5	110 105 **100** 95	−0.1 −0.2 0 +0.1	160 cm 125 cm 100 cm 80 cm	Normal reading speed Normal reading distance Reserve capacity for small print	Normal performance with reserve 100 ± 10
Minimal Vision Loss Mild Vision Loss	20/32 20/40 20/50 20/63	0.63 0.5 0.4 0.32	6/9.5 6/12 6/15 6/18	90 85 80 75	0.2 0.3 0.4 0.5	60 cm 50 cm 40 cm 30 cm	Normal reading speed Reduced reading distance No reserve for small print	Normal performance losing reserve 80 ± 10
Moderate Vision Loss	20/80 20/100 20/125 20/160	0.25 0.2 0.16 0.125	6/24 6/30 6/36 6/48	70 65 60 55	0.6 0.7 0.8 0.9	25 cm 20 cm 15 cm 12.5cm	Near-normal with appropriate reading aids Low-power magnifiers or large-print books	Near-normal performance with aids 60 ± 10
Severe Vision Loss	**20/200** 20/250 20/320 20/400	**0.1** 0.08 0.063 0.05	**6/60** 3/60 	**50** 45 40 35	**1.0** 1.1 1.2 1.3	10 cm 8 cm 6 cm 5 cm	Slower than normal with reading aids High-power magnifiers (restricted field)	Restricted performance with aids 40 ± 10
Profound Vision Loss	20/500 20/630 20/800 20/1000	0.04 0.032 0.025 0.02	2/60	30 25 20 15	1.4 1.5 1.6 1.7	4 cm 3 cm 2.5 cm 2 cm	Marginal with aids Uses magnifiers for spot reading but may prefer talking books for leisure	Marginal performance with aids 20 ± 10
Near-Blindness	less	less	1/60 less	10 5 0	1.8 1.9 2.0	1 cm	No visual reading Must rely on talking books, Braille, or other nonvisual sources	Must rely on substitution skills 0 – 10
Blindness	0.0	NLP	NLP					

Table 3-3B Aspects and Ranges of Vision and Vision Loss Handicap/Participation and Visual Field

Ranges of Vision	Handicap / Participation Aspect (how the person participates in society)			Visual Field (score based on new AMA grid)				Generic Ability Ranges
	Use of Aids	Social Consequences	Broader Ranges	Grid score	Average rad.(diam.)	O & M Abilities (Orientation & Mobility)		
Range of Normal Vision	No aids	Note that normal adult vision is better than 20/20 (1.0). Average acuity does not drop to 20/20 (1.0) until age 60 or 70.	Legally Sighted – USA / (no code) / (Near-)normal	110 / 105 / 100 / 95	70° (140°) / 60° (120°)	Normal Orientation Normal Mobility		Normal performance with reserve 100 ± 10
Mild Vision Loss	↓ vision enhancement aids	Many functional criteria fall within this transitional range (whether for a driver's license or for cataract surgery).		90 / 85 / 80 / 75	50° (100°) / 40° (80°)	Normal O&M performance needs more scanning		Normal performance losing reserve 80 ± 10
Moderate Vision Loss		In the U.S. children in this range qualify for special-education assistance.	Low Vision – WHO / Low Vision – ICD-9-CM	70 / 65 / 60 / 55	30° (60°) / 20° (40°) hemianopia	Near-normal performance must scan for obstacles		Near-normal performance with aids 60 ± 10
Severe Vision Loss	↓	In the U.S. individuals in this range are considered "legally blind" and qualify for a tax break and for disability benefits.	"Legal Blindness" – USA	50 / 45 / 40 / 35	10° (20°) / 8° (16°)	Visual mobility is slower than normal may use cane as adjunct		Restricted performance with aids 40 ± 10
Profound Vision Loss	vision substitution aids	The WHO (ICD-9, -10) includes this range under "blindness." In ICD-9-CM it is considered profound Low Vision.	Blindness – WHO	30 / 25 / 20 / 15	6° (12°) / 4° (8°)	Must use cane for detection of obstacles may use vision as adjunct for identification		Marginal performance with aids 20 ± 10
Near-Blindness / Blindness		In this range residual vision becomes unreliable, but may still be used as an adjunct to vision substitution skills.		10 / 5 / 0	2° (4°) / NLP	Visual orientation not reliable – must use blind mobility skills, long cane, hearing, guide dog		Must rely on substitution skills 0 – 10

Discussion of Individual Ranges

The ranges, summarized in Table 3-3, can serve multiple purposes. They are recommended for use in population surveys. They can also be helpful for estimating the amount of functional loss resulting from vision loss, as in the new 5th edition of the AMA *Guides*. The ability ranges can be helpful in documenting progress in individual vision rehabilitation programs.

The following sections provide a brief description of each of the ranges. Although the ranges may be sharply divided on the visual acuity scale, the distinctions are much fuzzier on the ability scale. The cut-off points may be compared to mile markers along a road. The markers provide useful reference points, but the landscape does not change abruptly at each marker.

Range of normal vision

In the normal vision range, the visual system (like most body systems) has reserve capacity. The reference standard for visual acuity (20/20, 1.0, 6/6) is defined as the ability to recognize a standard letter (1 M-unit) at a standard distance (1 meter). In normal reading, newsprint (about 1 M) is read at about 40 cm, an ample reserve.

Average visual acuity decreases with age. Figure 3-1 shows that adult acuity does not drop to the 20/20 "standard" level until age 60 or 70. It is an error to describe 20/20 as "normal" or as "average" acuity, let alone as "perfect" vision. Visual acuity measurements should never be truncated at the 20/20 level.

Minimal and mild vision loss

The minimal and mild vision loss range is a transitional range between normal vision and more pronounced vision loss, classified as "Low Vision." In this range, the reserve capacity is gradually lost. Reading distances for newsprint drop from 60 to 32 cm; print may be held slightly closer, but general reading performance is still adequate. Normal reading adds of up to 3 D suffice. Many functional criteria fall within this range, with some tasks requiring stricter cut-offs than others. For example, a 20/20 cut-off may be used for pilots, whereas a 20/40 cut-off is commonly used for driver's license requirements. This cut-off divides the range into two subranges: minimal loss (20/30, 20/40) and mild loss (20/50, 20/60). Cataract surgeons may consider "less than 20/40" an indication for surgery. Refractive surgeons may consider "20/40 or better" a satisfactory outcome. U.S. students qualify for special education assistance when visual acuity drops to 20/80 (the top of the next range).

Some caution is warranted when setting priorities for health care delivery programs based on prevalence levels in population surveys. It has been shown that half of those who do not reach the 20/40 cut-off with presenting correction would do so when best-corrected. This means that differences found might reflect differences in eye health as well as differences in health care delivery. It also means that prevailing causes of vision loss will be different for different ranges. In the mild vision loss range, undercorrected refractive error will be dominant, even in developed countries; in the severe and profound range, more serious conditions will dominate, which may vary from country to country.

CHAPTER 3: Aspects and Ranges of Vision Loss • 45

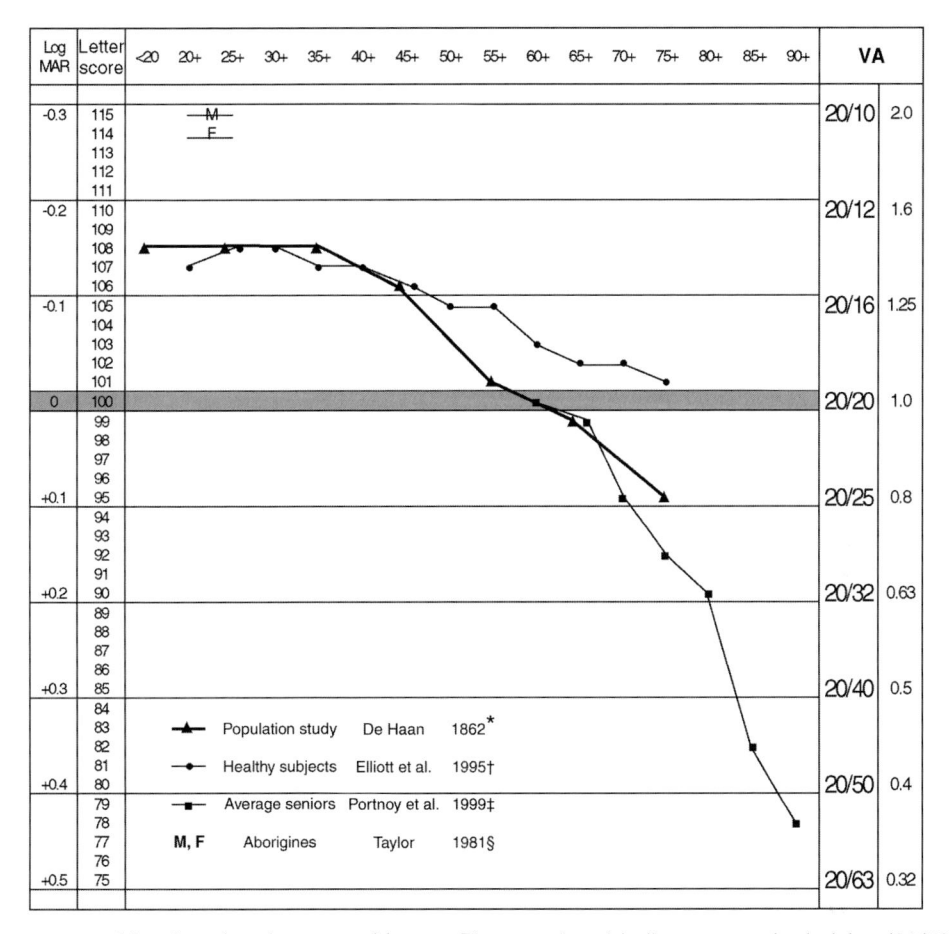

Figure 3-1 Visual acuity changes with age. The gray band indicates standard vision (20/20, 1.0, 6/6). The chart demonstrates that it is a mistake to consider 20/20 as "average," "normal," or "perfect" vision. Average adult visual acuity is significantly better than 20/20, not dropping to 20/20 until after age 60.

The ▲ markers represent a study using prototypes of Snellen's test letters, published in 1862. The ● markers represent a recent meta-analysis of healthy eyes from several research studies. The ■ markers represent recent findings from an elderly population (including eyes with age-related changes). The M and the F markers represent data from male and female Australian Aborigines, who were found to have statistically significant better acuity than comparable Caucasians.

The 1862 findings are remarkably similar to the recent data for healthy adults in the younger age groups and to those for unselected seniors in the older groups.

*de Haan V. Onderzoekingen naar de invloed van de leeftijd op de gezichtsscherpte [Research on the influence of age on visual acuity; doctoral dissertation]. Utrecht; 1862.

†Elliott DB, Yang KC, Whitaker D. Visual acuity changes throughout adulthood in normal, healthy eyes: seeing beyond 6/6. *Optom Vis Sci*. 1995;72:186–191.

‡Haegerstrom-Portnoy G, Schneck ME, Brabyn JA. Seeing into old age: vision function beyond acuity. *Optom Vis Sci*. 1999;76:141–158.

§Taylor HR. Racial variations in vision. *Am J Epidemiol*. 1981;113:62–80.

(Courtesy of August Colenbrander, MD.)

Moderate vision loss

In the moderate vision loss range, support from large-print materials or moderate power magnifiers is required to enhance the available vision. Binocular reading at 25 cm or less (the traditional reference distance for magnifiers) requires the use of prisms. Reading adds must be 4 D or more.

The lower end of this range is an important transition point in the United States. When visual acuity changes from just better than 20/200 to just worse, a person's abilities do not change dramatically but the person's benefits do. In the United States, individuals in this range qualify for tax and rehabilitation benefits. They are often labeled as legally "blind," a misnomer, because 90% of the "legally blind" have residual vision.

Severe vision loss

When visual acuity drops to 20/200 (0.1, 6/60) or below, reading performance is compromised. The reading distance for newsprint becomes 10 cm or less. At this distance, reading is definitely possible with appropriate magnifiers, but reading endurance is limited and reading speed is reduced because of the small field of strong magnifiers. The short reading distance makes binocularity impossible.

Profound vision loss

In the profound vision loss range (<20/400, <0.05, <3/60), visual reading becomes marginal; it may be used for spot reading but not for recreational reading. In Europe, many benefits do not start until this level is reached. The WHO (ICD-9 and ICD-10) includes this range in its "blindness" category; ICD-9-CM in the United States labels it as "profound low vision." In rehabilitation, the emphasis shifts from vision enhancement aids to aids that substitute the use of other senses.

Near-total vision loss, or near-blindness

In the near-blindness range (<1/50, CF [counting fingers] 1 m [3 ft] or less), vision becomes unreliable and use of vision substitution skills becomes dominant.

Total blindness

Use of vision substitution skills is the only option.

Similar ranges are shown for visual field loss. Note that the visual field score used here is aimed at estimating the effect on orientation and mobility (O & M) skills, not at facilitating the diagnosis of the underlying condition.

Visual Acuity Measurement

(See also BCSC Section 3, *Optics, Refraction, and Contact Lenses,* Chapters 3 and 8.)

When Snellen published his letter chart in 1862, he effectively made letter or symbol recognition the standard for clinical visual acuity measurement. In a century and a half, this measurement principle has not changed, but various refinements have been introduced to make the measurements more reliable and more reproducible. In 1982, the National Eye Institute introduced a new chart for its Early Treatment Diabetic Retinopathy Study. This chart combined the proportional layout promoted by Bailey and Lovie with the Sloan letter set. Since that time, ETDRS-type charts have become the acknowledged standard for visual acuity measurement.

>Bailey IL, Lovie JE. New design principles for visual acuity letter charts. *Am J Optom Physiol Opt.* 1976;53:740–745.
>Ferris FL 3rd, Kassoff A, Bresnick GH, et al. New visual acuity charts for clinical research. *Am J Ophthalmol.* 1982;94:91–96.
>Sloan LL. New test charts for the measurement of visual acuity at far and near distances. *Am J Ophthalmol.* 1959;48:807–813.

Chart Layout

Traditional charts, like Snellen's original one (Figure 3-2A), combined lines of a few large letters with smaller lines of many letters and did not standardize the letter spacing. On such charts, the recognition task is not the same at all levels because variable spacing affects the recognizability of the symbols through crowding or contour interaction. Bailey and Lovie eliminated these differences through standard spacing (horizontally equal to the letter width, vertically equal to the height of the row below), an equal number of letters on each line, and a geometric progression of letter sizes (Figure 3-2B). A very similar design had been proposed by Green in 1868 but was completely forgotten (see Figure 3-2C).

Choice of Optotypes

Snellen coined the term *optotypes* for symbols that are specifically designed for visual acuity measurement. Roman letters are the most widely used optotype. Snellen used letters with serifs on a 5-×-5 grid. Sloan designed letters without serifs on a 5-×-5 grid. The British standard chose nonserif (sans serif) letters on a 4-×-5 grid. In 1868, Green's sans serif letters were rejected "because they looked unfinished"; in 1968, the British standard rejected letters with serifs "because they look old fashioned."

>Colenbrander A. Measuring vision and vision loss. In: Tasman W, Jaeger EA, Parks MM, et al. *Duane's Clinical Ophthalmology.* Vol. 5: chap 51. Philadelphia: Lippincott Williams & Wilkins; 2002 ed.

Numbers

Using letters on the test has the advantages of offering obvious validity for the patient who wants to read and of allowing the examiner to memorize the sequence. However, they cannot be used for illiterate patients. For illiterate adults, charts with numbers are often used.

For children, various other symbols must be used.

Lea symbols

Lea symbols (house, square, apple, circle) have been specifically designed to blur equally and have been calibrated against Landolt Cs. They are available in different chart formats and as games for young children. Various studies indicate that they give the most reliable results, especially for young children.

48 • International Ophthalmology

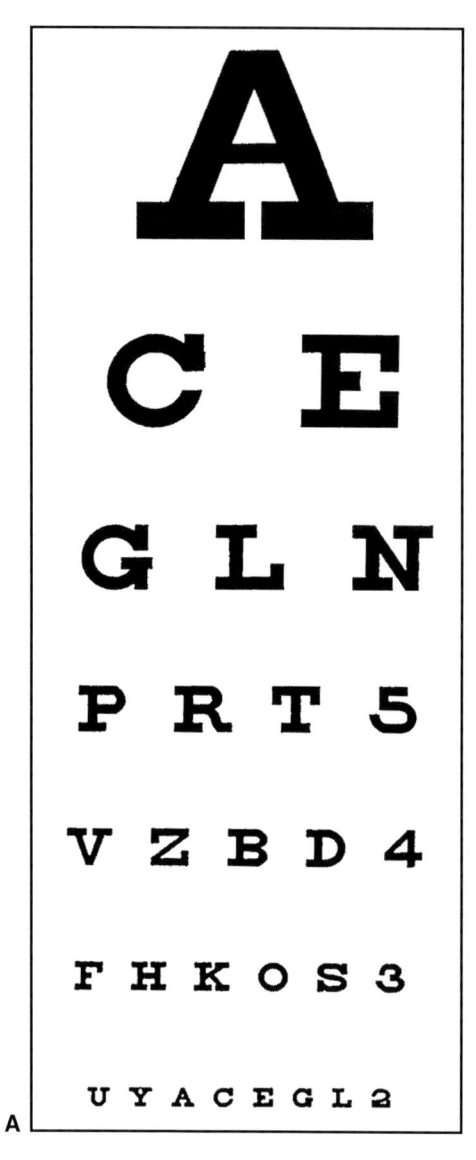

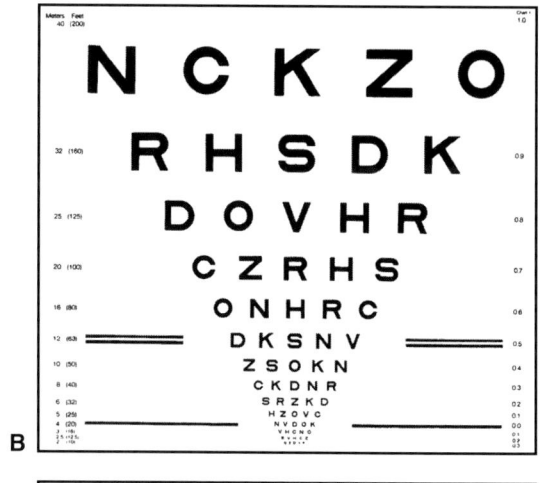

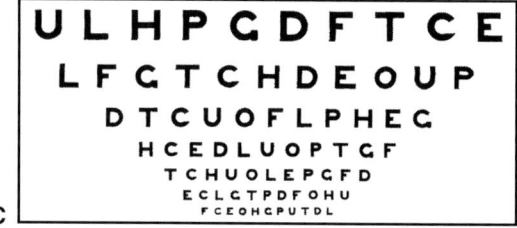

Figure 3-2 A, Snellen's original chart (1862), using specially designed letters rather than existing fonts. Note the irregular progression of sizes. **B,** ETDRS chart, combining the Bailey-Lovie layout with the Sloan letter set. Note the logarithmic progression, sans serif letters, proportional spacing of letters and lines, and five letters on every line (which makes the chart much wider than traditional charts). **C,** Segment of Green's chart (1868). Note the logarithmic progression, sans serif letters, proportional spacing of letters and lines, and the same number of letters on each line (not maintained for the larger sizes; see top line). Note too that the three charts are shown to demonstrate layout differences; they are not shown to scale in relation with each other. *(Charts courtesy of August Colenbrander, MD.)*

HOTV test

The HOTV test also uses four symbols, and, like the Lea symbols, they do not require a sense of laterality (see Figure 3-3A).

Tumbling Es

The tumbling E test is widely used but has the disadvantage of requiring a sense of laterality, which may not be fully developed in young children or in developmentally delayed individuals.

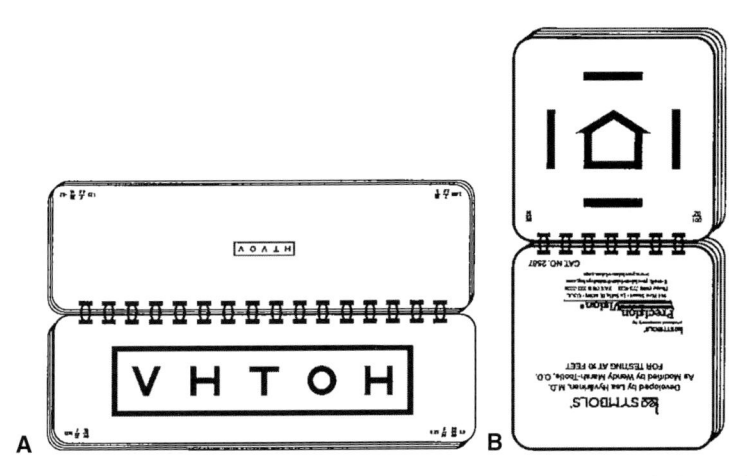

Figure 3-3 A, When presentation in a chart format is not feasible, symbols (such as these HOTV symbols) may be presented a line at a time. A frame may be added to simulate the crowding effect of surrounding letters in the chart format. **B,** When presentation in a line format is not feasible, symbols (such as this Lea symbol) may be presented one at a time. Crowding bars may be added to compensate for the lack of contour interaction from surrounding symbols. *(A and B courtesy of Precision Vision.)*

Landolt Cs

Developed in 1888, Landolt Cs (or Landolt broken rings) have the advantage that the symbol has only one element of detail. These symbols are widely used in laboratory settings and are recognized as the standard against which the recognizability of other optotypes should be calibrated.

> International Council of Ophthalmology. Visual acuity measurement standard, 1984. *Ital J Ophthalmol.* 1988;II/I:1–15.

Pictures

Pictures have often been used as optotypes. However, it is hard to standardize their recognizability, and children may vary in their picture-naming ability. Picture charts should be used only as a last resort if none of the other tests are available or workable.

Presentation

Recognizing isolated letters or symbols is a simpler task than recognizing them in a chart format. Thus, for standardized measurements, the chart format is preferred. A printed chart with the full ETDRS-type layout is preferred over the small screen with fewer letters of a projector chart.

Pointing to letters or isolating letters should be avoided if the objective is to assess the patient's fixation ability. If pointing or isolating improves the measured acuity, this suggests difficulties with fixation or attention. Guessing may be encouraged for subjects who tend to give up too early. Spontaneous corrections may be accepted, but the examiner should not ask for corrections after an error is made because this too would change the difficulty of the task.

With children, it is often difficult to keep their attention on a full chart. When a single line of characters is presented, the crowding effect of the chart may be simulated with a frame around the line (Figure 3-3A). For single characters, four crowding lines may be used (see Figure 3-3B).

In field surveys in developing countries, testing to the full ETDRS standard may not be feasible. A much abbreviated test might present tumbling Es at only two levels: 20/60 (0.3, 6/18) (Low Vision, WHO) and 20/400 (0.05, 3/60, 1/20) (Blindness, WHO).

Scoring

Traditionally, visual acuity is scored as the last line on which "more than half" of the characters are read correctly. On non-ETDRS charts, this requirement varies with the number of characters per line. For an occasional office visit, this may be accurate enough.

On non-ETDRS charts, the accuracy also varies with the line interval. For example, on an ETDRS-type chart with lines at 20/100, 20/125, 20/160, and 20/200, "20/200 or less" is correctly interpreted as "less than 20/160." On a traditional chart, with no lines between 20/100 and 20/200, "20/200 or less" erroneously becomes "less than 20/100." This can be avoided by bringing the traditional chart to 10 ft, where "less than 20/160" can be interpreted as "less than 10/80."

In addition to line-by-line scoring, ETDRS-type charts also offer a more accurate option: letter-by-letter scoring. Here, 1 point is given for every letter read, or 5 points per line. In this case, reading all letters on one line and none on the next receives the same score as reading three letters on one line and two on the next. In cases where the visual acuity of one patient must be followed accurately over time, or where the visual acuities of different patients must be averaged, this method provides greater accuracy.

Bailey and Lovie chose five letters for each line. For line-by-line scoring, the criterion to read "better than half" thus becomes 3 out of 5, or 60%. It has been shown that more than five symbols would not significantly increase the accuracy of letter-by-letter scoring.

Bailey IL, Bullimore MA, Raasch TW, et al. Clinical grading and the effects of scaling. *Invest Ophthalmol Vis Sci.* 1991;32:422–432.

Choice of Test Distance

Snellen's original chart (1862) was calibrated for 20 Parisian feet. After the adoption of the Treaty of the Meter (1875), he switched to charts for 6 m (close to 20 ft) and 5 m (easier in the decimal system). These distances were chosen because they relax the accommodation when used for refraction. For the ETDRS charts, a distance of 4 m was chosen to limit the width of the chart and because the distance can be halved and halved again to 2 m and 1 m. These shorter distances pose no problem in measuring visual acuity; however, for refractive use, the 0.25 D of accommodation at 4 m can no longer be ignored. A 3-m (10-ft) distance may be used for children, whose attention may not be held at 6 m (20 ft). This distance may also be used for patients with moderate vision loss, particularly to interpret "20/200 or less" appropriately as "less than 10/80 (20/160)" on a traditional chart.

At 4 m, the ETDRS charts can measure from 4/40 (20/200, 0.1, 6/60) to 4/2 (20/10, 2.0, 6/3). At 2 m, the lowest level is 2/40 (20/400, 0.05, 6/120); at 1 m, it is 1/40 (20/800,

0.025, 6/240). When measuring in the ranges of severe and profound vision loss, it is desirable that the cut-off values do not fall at the limit of the chart (in other words, the chart should always start with at least one line the patient can read and end with at least one line the patient cannot read). Thus, if the subject cannot read the largest line on the distance chart, it is advisable to skip a 2-m or 3-m distance and to go directly to testing at 1 m, where the largest possible range can be covered. At this distance, presbyopes need a 1 D reading add, and the proper distance should be monitored with a cord attached to the chart (see Figure 3-4).

Tests for Near Vision

Statements about reading vision come in two flavors. A statement such as "The patient can read newsprint (1 M)" is a statement about functional vision. It tells us that the patient can meet an important ADL requirement. For patients in the normal or near-normal range, this statement may be sufficient. However, stating only the letter size does not tell us how the patient does it, whether with the naked eye, with reading glasses, with a magnifier, or even with a videomagnifier. To make a statement about reading acuity as a visual function, we also need the reading distance. This allows us to calculate the reading performance for nonstandard distances (see the following section), to compare it to distance acuity, and to estimate the amount of magnification required for low vision patients.

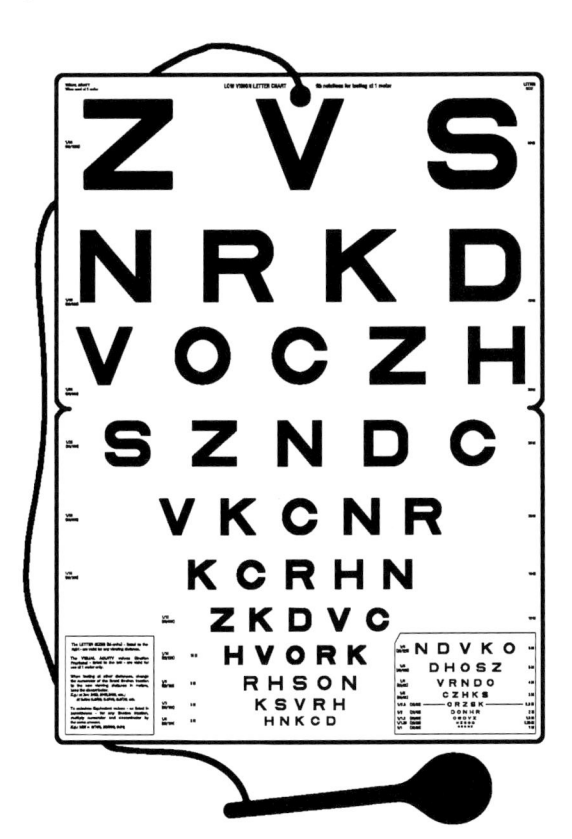

Figure 3-4 Letter chart for use at 1 m, with cord and occluder to maintain the 1-m distance. At 1 m, the visual acuity values range from 1/50 (20/1000) to 1/1 (20/20). *(Courtesy of Precision Vision.)*

Near vision is often tested with a miniature letter chart. This test does not provide much information that could not be obtained from the distance test except for a verification of the reading add. More functional information can be obtained from a test with continuous text. If the text is presented in paragraphs of a standard length (see Figure 3-5), it is possible to measure not only *reading acuity* but also *reading speed*. The critical print size is the print size below which reading slows down; this usually is somewhat larger than the threshold print size below which reading is impossible. The threshold print size should correspond to the threshold value for distance acuity. The extra magnification from the threshold to the critical print size is also known as the "magnification reserve for reading fluency."

Visual Acuity Calculations

Snellen marked each line on his chart with a number indicating the distance at which the letters subtend five minutes of arc. To make the definition less verbose, Louise Sloan coined the term *M-unit* for this value. The visual acuity is then expressed as the well-known Snellen fraction:

V = viewing distance *(in meters)*/letter size *(in M-units)*

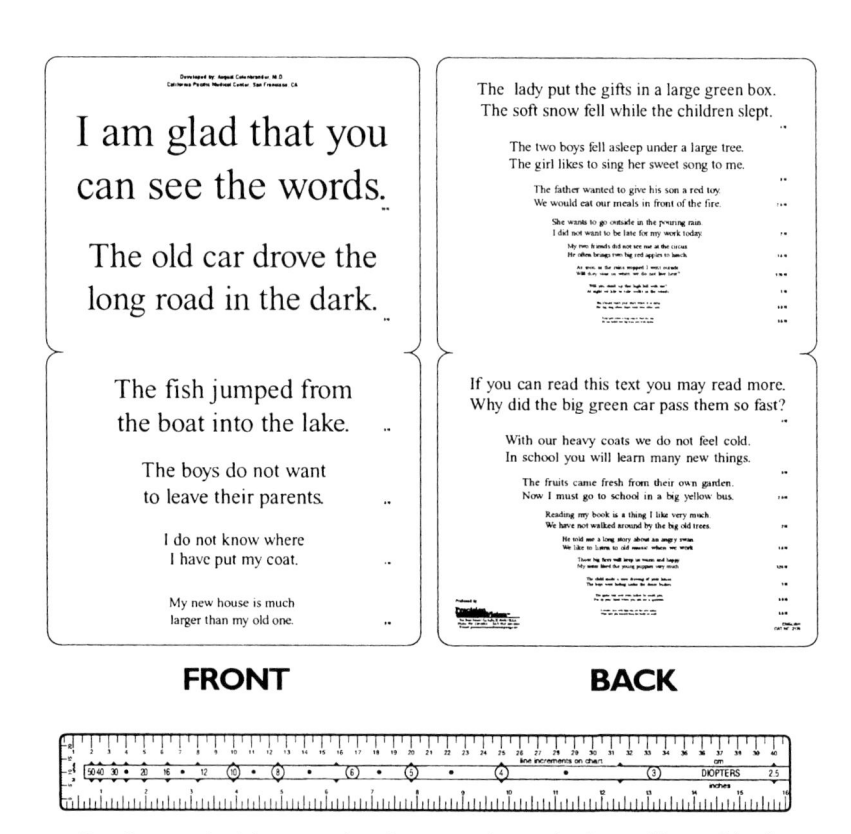

Figure 3-5 Reading card with proportional paragraphs and ruler, calibrated in diopters. Letter sizes range from 10 M to 0.6 M. Charts with the same design are available in a number of languages. *(Courtesy of Precision Vision.)*

This formula is useful for distance vision but becomes awkward for reading vision when the viewing distance becomes a fraction within a fraction. This can be overcome by a simple inversion:

$$1/V = \text{letter size/viewing distance} = \text{letter size} \times 1/\text{viewing distance}$$

Because the reciprocal of a metric distance is the diopter, we can write:

$$1/V = \text{letter size } (in\ M\text{-}units) \times \text{viewing distance } (in\ diopters) = M \times D$$

or

$$V = 1/(M \times D)$$

For near vision, this modified Snellen formula replaces the awkward fractional calculation with a multiplication, which is easier to calculate and has the advantage that the reading distance in diopters relates directly to the reading add. Recording the reading distance directly in diopters is simple with a special ruler, as provided with most phoropters or with the reading card shown in Figure 3-5.

This formula uses the M-unit to express print size. The M-unit, based on Snellen's formula, is the only letter size unit that is well defined and the only unit that allows a comparison of distance and near vision. The Jaeger numbers that are still used quite often have no numerical meaning because they refer to item numbers in a printing catalogue from Vienna in the 1850s. Because they have no other external definition, their implementation with fonts from other catalogues is extremely variable. Printers' points (N rating in Britain) refer to line height rather than to letter height. Because the ratio of line height to letter height may vary for different fonts, their point size designations may differ also (for example, 8 pt Arial = 9 pt Times Roman).

For patients in the normal and near-normal range, a standardized reading distance can be used (usually 40 cm, 2.5 D, 16 inches). This usage has led to the habit of expressing letter sizes as visual acuity values. However, this is incorrect because the same letter size that would represent one acuity level at 40 cm would represent double that acuity at 80 cm and only half that at 20 cm. For example, at 40 cm (2.5 D), 2 M represents 20/100 because $V = 1/(M \times D) = 1/(2 \times 2.5) = 1/5 = 20/100$, but at 80 cm (1.25 D), 2 M represents $V = 1/(2 \times 1.25) = 1/2.5 = 20/50$, and at 20 cm, 2 M represents $V = 1/(2 \times 5) = 1/10 = 20/200$.

For patients in the low vision range, who require nonstandard reading distances, such acuity calculations are essential. Only the use of M-units and the modified Snellen formula, given earlier, allow such calculations. Compare the statement, "The patient could read 2 M at 20 cm (5 D)," with the statement, "The patient could read at 20 cm a letter size that would have represented 20/100 if presented at 40 cm."

CHAPTER 4

Ophthalmic Survey Methodology

Overview

The goal of this chapter is to describe the various methods of collecting epidemiologic data on ophthalmic diseases using survey methods that will provide accurate estimates to be used to

- Define the prevalence, severity, incidence, and progression of eye diseases
- Investigate associated risk factors
- Plan appropriate eye health care services
- Develop prevention and rehabilitation programs
- Project costs of these programs

A *survey* is an observational epidemiologic study based on examination of all persons in a given population or a specifically defined subgroup of the population. It is most commonly used to estimate the prevalence and incidence (if there is follow-up) of a disease. *Prevalence* is estimated by cross-sectional studies that assess the presence of disease in a specific population at a point in time. As such, prevalence studies provide information on the magnitude or impact of the condition in the population but do not determine incidence or risk of developing the disease. *Incidence* is estimated by follow-up of the population cohort to assess the probability of developing the disease over a period of time. Population surveys often have an initial cross-sectional phase to measure prevalence, which is followed by a second, longitudinal phase to assess incidence (eg, Beaver Dam Eye Study, Barbados Eye Studies).

Design Issues

A critical step in conducting a survey is to obtain a representative sample of the population to be studied. Nearly complete participation of the cohort members is important to ensure the validity of the estimates obtained and governs the ability to generalize findings beyond the study population. The study design must attempt to minimize the influence of biases that may result from the methods used to measure endpoints and risk factors, as they will affect the interpretation of the data collected. (See BCSC Section 1, *Update on General Medicine.*) Several of the potential biases of surveys are nonresponse bias; recall bias; detection bias, or observation bias; and sampling bias.

Nonresponse bias occurs if participants are not representative of the proposed study population due to selective nonparticipation. For example, the presence of disease may be underestimated in a large population if persons with that disease or its complication (eg, persons with severe proliferative diabetic retinopathy) are less likely to participate than those without. To minimize this bias, attempts must be made to ensure the participation of all those eligible, as well as to make special efforts to include sicker individuals—for example, to perform home and institutional examination visits. Whenever possible, it is useful to collect information about the health of all persons eligible for the study.

Recall bias may occur when participants with a disease (eg, cataract or age-related macular degeneration) are questioned about historical information, such as ultraviolet light exposure or family history, as they may tend to remember and report such information more readily than persons without the condition.

Detection bias, or *observation bias,* may occur if the examiner is not masked as to a specific condition that may affect the measurement of an endpoint or a risk factor. For example, knowing a patient has poor visual acuity may influence the diagnosis of cataract on clinical examination. Similarly, knowing that a patient has cataract may influence the interviewer to ask more questions on the extent of light exposure or use of specific medications. To minimize variation in observations collected, it is essential to evaluate intra- and interobserver reproducibility and to conduct rigorous training, pretesting, and quality assurance of measurements (eg, intraocular pressure) throughout the study.

A clinical observation is *valid* if it reflects the true state of the parameter being measured. For the observation to be valid, it must be neither biased nor incorrect due to chance. *Internal validity* is a necessary feature of useful observational studies and is threatened by bias and chance. *External validity* is the degree to which the results of an observation apply to another setting—that is, comparing like with like.

Sampling bias occurs when observations and conclusions based on a sample of people are generalized to dissimilar groups. Worldwide comparisons within and among surveys provide important information, but they depend on using standardized protocols that are comparable and observations with internal and external validity.

Interpretation

Observational studies can provide unique information regarding prevalence, incidence, and the impact of eye diseases in the general population. Although hypotheses of cause and effect of relationships may be implied, they cannot be proven by this type of study design. For example, a relationship between glycemic control and retinopathy may be difficult to evaluate in an observational study due to the "parallel" effects of severe diabetes. A randomized, controlled clinical trial would best be suited to address this issue. However, participants in these trials are self-selected, may be more highly motivated, may have different illness patterns, and, in general, may be unrepresentative of all persons with the condition. Thus, interventions (eg, strict use of vitamin supplements) in a trial may have a different impact on the incidence or progression of eye diseases—for example, age-related macular degeneration—than they would in the general population of persons with this condition. Thus, clinical trials and observational incidence studies complement each other in providing information to assess the potential public health impact of a therapeutic intervention.

Methodology

Basic survey methodology, used in major surveys in the United States, Europe, the Caribbean, Australia, and India, is described, with brief comments, in the following sections.

Ethical Standards and Informed Consent

Guidelines on the general conduct of biomedical research are published in the World Medical Association Declaration of Helsinki and in *Ethics and Epidemiology: International Guidelines*. Informed consent must be voluntarily given and obtained prior to participating in a study, and participants must have the right to withdraw from the study at any time. Detailed features of the study should be printed in an operations manual and submitted to the appropriate institutional ethics committee for its approval.

> Bankowski Z, Bryant JH, Last JM, eds. *Ethics and Epidemiology: International Guidelines.* Geneva: Council for International Organizations of Medical Sciences (CIOMS); 1992.

Sampling Issues

Sample selection

Observational population-based studies are "representative" in that persons are selected from a sampling frame according to specific procedures because they reside in the population and meet the criteria for the study. The eligibility criteria for the study must be defined prior to recruitment and examination and must be adhered to strictly. The sampling can be simple, such as everyone 43–84 years of age and living in Beaver Dam during a citywide census (as in the Beaver Dam Eye Study) or drawing a simple random sample of all residents of Barbados, West Indies, ages 40–84 years (as in the Barbados Eye Study).

Alternatively, sampling may be very intricate, as in the Melbourne Visual Impairment Project, in which urban elderly institutionalized residents and rural residents are oversampled and complex statistical approaches are required when reconstituting the whole population.

In general, a large sample size is necessary if the observations in a survey are to provide meaningful conclusions. It is important for the sample size to be sufficient to make chance an unlikely explanation for the differences observed.

Use of a pilot study may be helpful in accurately projecting a reasonable sample size and assessing the feasibility of the survey. The data obtained by the pilot study are used to calculate the optimal sample size for obtaining accurate prevalence estimates, as well as to estimate the ability to detect risk factors. The smallest detectable odds ratios may be calculated, based on the prevalence of the risk factors observed in the pilot study.

> Leske MC, Connell AM, Kehoe R. A pilot project of glaucoma in Barbados. *Br J Ophthalmol.* 1989;73:365–369.
>
> VanNewkirk MR. The Hong Kong Vision Study: a pilot assessment of visual impairment in adults. *Trans Am Ophthalmol Soc.* 1997;95:715–749.

Identification of the population sample

A *sampling frame* is required to identify eligible persons in the population. Some studies—for example, the Baltimore Eye Survey, the Beaver Dam Eye Study, the Blue Mountains

Eye Study, and the Melbourne Visual Impairment Project—have used a household census conducted by trained interviewers to identify eligible residents.

Other studies, such as the Barbados Eye Study and the Salisbury Eye Evaluation Project, have successfully used large population databases to identify the population.

Participation

The estimated rates from observational studies may be adversely influenced by moderate nonparticipation. Participation rates of at least 80% should be achieved whenever possible. High participation rates, it should be noted, reduce selection bias but do not eliminate it. Achieving high participation is a major challenge for incidence studies, which require follow-up of a cohort and are susceptible to losses to follow-up due to deaths of cohort members, refusals, or other reasons for nonparticipation.

Demographic and historical data on all eligible persons may be available from the sampling frame itself or may be collected by self-report during the household census. Such data are valuable for assessing possible biases resulting from nonparticipation. Biases may result if responders differ from nonresponders in an observational study. The initial visit for a household census provides the opportunity to encourage participation, either by scheduling appointments for further examination at a convenient site or, when appropriate, scheduling home examination visits.

Data Collection

The study should establish a detailed protocol for examination, measurements, disease gradings, and disease classification. A complete but streamlined examination protocol should be used in the study to avoid delays and minimize inconvenience to the participants. All protocols should be detailed in a manual of procedures, and examiners should be standardized in all measurements prior to the beginning of the study.

Interview

Initial home visit If the study includes an initial home visit, interviewers can collect the following types of useful data:

- Demographic characteristics
- History of ocular conditions
- History of systemic conditions
- Family history
- Primary eye-care providers

Carefully prepared standardized questionnaires can be given to the participants at the doorstep, or home, interview to facilitate further data collection at the examination center.

Study visit When participants attend the study visit at the examination site, additional information can be collected on a number of variables and potential risk factors. Such detailed information is usually obtained through the use of standardized questionnaires that elicit personal and other data such as

- Use of medications
- Use of vitamins and nutritional supplements
- Diet
- Smoking (eg, packs/years of use)
- Alcohol consumption (eg, average annual volume and type)
- Sunlight exposure (eg, average annual ambient light exposure)
- Socioeconomic history, including occupation, employment status, education, income, and marital status

These data are most efficiently collected by having participants enter them during the examination visit directly into computers using well-designed software packages; computers should be located at conveniently accessible sites.

Ocular examination

Refraction A number of studies, including the Baltimore Eye Survey, Beaver Dam Eye Study, Blue Mountains Eye Study, Andhra Pradesh Eye Disease Study, and the Melbourne Visual Impairment Project, named uncorrected refractive error as the leading cause of visual impairment. Therefore, a survey methodology without refraction providing best-corrected visual acuity would grossly overestimate the rates of visual impairment.

The standard method of visual acuity measurement in ophthalmic research is based on the ETDRS chart, with the aim of obtaining best-corrected logMAR visual acuity (logarithmic minimum angle of resolution). These charts provide reproducible visual acuity data that are easily used in quantitative analysis.

> Ferris FL 3rd, Kassoff A, Bresnick GH, et al. New visual acuity charts for clinical research. *Am J Ophthalmol.* 1982;94:91–96.

For categories of vision impairment, see Chapter 3 of this volume.

Automated perimetry Many methods are available to screen for visual field defects using automated perimetry. Suprathreshold field testing has been successfully used for glaucoma screening. In the Barbados Eye Study, this method had a sensitivity of 91% and a specificity of 60% in detecting open-angle glaucoma. In the Baltimore Eye Survey, of all the screening parameters, a combination of age, race, IOP, family history of glaucoma, history of diabetes, cup–disc ratio, narrowest rim width, and field analyzer defect(s) resulted in the best specificity (90%) and the best sensitivity (75%).

Although the majority of survey participants provide reliable automated perimetry data, it is important to anticipate difficulties with participants, especially elderly participants with severe and profound vision loss and media opacities. Unreliable automated visual fields must be repeated.

Frequency-doubling technology perimetry shows promise as a faster, more user-friendly screening tool; it has been adopted for screening by Prevent Blindness America and the Glaucoma Foundation.

> Cioffi GA, Mansberger S, Spry P, et al. Frequency doubling perimetry and the detection of eye disease in the community. *Trans Am Ophthalmol Soc.* 2000;98:195–202.

Heijl A, Lindgren G, Olsson J. The effect of perimetric experience in normal subjects. *Arch Ophthalmol.* 1989;107:81–86.

Trible JR, Schultz RO, Robinson JC, et al. Accuracy of glaucoma detection with frequency-doubling perimetry. *Am J Ophthalmol.* 2000;129:740–745.

Standardized Ophthalmologic Examination Using International Diagnostic Classification and Grading Systems

Studies should strive to use standardized, generally accepted methods to achieve comparability of results. The World Health Organization (WHO) has been responsible for the organization, coordination, and execution of activities related to the International Statistical Classification of Diseases, Injuries, and Causes of Death (ICD) since 1948. The 43rd World Health Assembly approved the 10th Revision of the International Classification of Diseases (ICD-10) in May 1990 and recommended its implementation by January 1, 1993. At first intended primarily to classify causes of death, the ICD scope has been progressively widening to include coding and tabulating causes of morbidity, as well as medical record indexing and retrieval. The ability to exchange comparable data from region to region and from country to country, to allow comparison from one population to another, and to permit the study of diseases over long periods, is one of its strengths.

Accuracy in diagnosis requires a complete ophthalmologic examination. However, examination time, expense, and participant comfort must be considered in designing the standardized examination and special testing. An examination should include slit-lamp biomicroscopy of the lids, tear film, conjunctiva, cornea, and iris.

Lens

Several similar slit-lamp biomicroscopy methods of standardized classification of nuclear, cortical, and posterior subcapsular cataract are in use, each with good inter- and intraobserver reproducibility.

In addition, other, more complex classification methods, such as the Lens Opacities Classification System III, or LOCS III, can be applied to lens photographs.

Chylack LT Jr, Leske MC, McCarthy D, et al. Lens opacities classification system II (LOCS II). *Arch Ophthalmol.* 1989;107:991–997.

Chylack LT Jr, Wolfe JK, Singer DM, et al. The Lens Opacities Classification System III. The Longitudinal Study of Cataract Study Group. *Arch Ophthalmol.* 1993;111:831–836.

Sparrow JM, Bron AJ, Brown NA, et al. The Oxford Clinical Cataract Classification and Grading System. *Int Ophthalmol.* 1986;9:207–225.

West SK, Taylor HR. The detection and grading of cataract: an epidemiologic perspective. *Surv Ophthalmol.* 1986;31:175–184.

Optic nerve

Reliable stereoscopic assessment of the vertical cup–disc ratio (VCDR) is important for the diagnosis and monitoring of glaucoma. Visible structural alterations of the optic nerve or retinal nerve fiber layer frequently occur before visual field defects can be measured.

VCDR estimates using stereophotography of the optic disc have been reported to be larger than estimates from ophthalmoscopy in some studies. Stereophotography assessment of the optic disc cup has greater intraobserver and interobserver agreement.

Klein BE, Moss SE, Magli YL, et al. Optic disc cupping as clinically estimated from photographs. *Ophthalmology.* 1987;94:1481–1483.

Sommer A, Pollack I, Maumenee AE. Optic disc parameters and onset of glaucomatous field loss. I. Methods and progressive changes in disc morphology. *Arch Ophthalmol.* 1979;97: 1444–1448.

Macula

The preferred technique for evaluating the macula is magnified stereoscopic biomicroscopic visualization through a dilated pupil.

Gonioscopy

Of the major surveys, a study in the Hovsgol province of Mongolia performed gonioscopy on the entire sample of 942 participants. This examination is essential for accurately diagnosing angle-closure glaucoma. The Andhra Pradesh Eye Disease Study also included gonioscopy in its methodology.

Foster PJ, Baasanhu J, Alsbirk PH, et al. Glaucoma in Mongolia. A population-based survey in Hovsgol province of northern Mongolia. *Arch Ophthalmol.* 1996;114:1235–1241.

Indirect ophthalmoscopy

Indirect ophthalmoscopy is essential for retinal disease detection and is very helpful in assigning vision loss in eyes with media opacities, such as cataract, and retinal disease.

Stereophotography

The many advantages of fundus photography include the following:

- Slide film or digital imaging creates a permanent record that enables accurate follow-up comparisons.
- Photographs allow the addition of new items to the grading scheme.
- Graders are easily masked.
- It enables intra- and interobserver comparisons.
- Detection of diabetic retinopathy and age-related maculopathy are enhanced.

Masked photographic grading

Fundus photographs graded by experienced graders are reported to be a reliable measure of diabetic retinopathy and provide a more sensitive and objective method than direct ophthalmoscopy for detecting diabetic retinopathy.

Data from Klein et al suggest that the most sensitive and specific method for detecting and classifying age-related maculopathy is the grading of 30° stereoscopic fundus photographs.

Based on photographic data, diagnostic grading classifications have been established for diabetic retinopathy and age-related maculopathy.

Diabetic Retinopathy Study Research Group. Report 7. A modification of the Airlie House classification of diabetic retinopathy. *Invest Ophthalmol Vis Sci.* 1981;21 (pt 2):210–226.

The International ARM Epidemiological Study Group. An international classification and grading system for age-related maculopathy and age-related macular degeneration. *Surv Ophthalmol.* 1995;39:367–374.

Klein R, Meuer SM, Moss SE, et al. Detection of drusen and early signs of age-related maculopathy using a nonmydriatic camera and a standard fundus camera. *Ophthalmology.* 1992;99:1686–1692.

Schachat A, Hyman L, Leske MC, et al. Comparisons of diabetic retinopathy detection by clinical examinations and photograph gradings. Barbados (West Indies) Eye Study Group. *Arch Ophthalmol.* 1993;111:1064–1070.

Document Summarizing Results of Examination

A brief summary of the results of the ophthalmic examination, which is given to each participant at the conclusion of the testing, is appreciated by the participants and facilitates communication with the participants' own physicians.

Data Management and Analysis

Software packages for data entry and analysis are available and may be essential in this type of research. The computer has greatly facilitated collection and management of data. Regardless of how the data are managed, however, it is extremely important that they be as complete as possible.

Proper analysis of epidemiologic data must address the possibility of biases. For example, to address the question of a possible association of cataract with macular degeneration, age is an important confounder that must be dealt with, as it affects both variables of interest. The investigator must determine the putative risk that cataract is associated with age-related macular degeneration while controlling for the effects of age.

Restriction of participants to a narrow range of characteristics may reduce confounding by creating a homogeneous group, but this usually reduces external validity. Stratification in the analysis and presentation of data according to subgroups of participants is commonly used to reveal confounding. Multivariate adjustment is used to control for the effects of many variables in order to determine the independent effects of one variable.

Conclusion

Adopting and implementing well-designed survey methodology leads to invaluable evidence in the study of ophthalmic disease. Continued application of these methods around the world will bring improved understanding of eye diseases.

Andhra Pradesh Eye Disease Study

Dandona L, Dandona R, Naduvilath TJ, et al. Burden of moderate visual impairment in an urban population in southern India. *Ophthalmology.* 1999;106:497–504.

Dandona R, Dandona L, Naduvilath TJ, et al. Design of a population-based study of visual impairment in India: The Andhra Pradesh Eye Disease Study. *Indian J Ophthalmol.* 1997; 45:251–257.

Baltimore Eye Survey

Katz J, Tielsch JM, Quigley HA, et al. Automated suprathreshold screening for glaucoma: the Baltimore Eye Survey. *Invest Ophthalmol Vis Sci.* 1993;34:3271–3277.

Tielsch JM, Sommer A, Witt K, et al. Blindness and visual impairment in an American urban population. The Baltimore Eye Survey. *Arch Ophthalmol.* 1990;108:286–290.

Barbados Eye Study

Leske MC, Connell AM, Schachat AP, et al. The Barbados Eye Study: Prevalence of open angle glaucoma: the Barbados Eye Studies. *Arch Ophthalmol.* 1994;112:821–829.

Leske MC, Connell AM, Wu SY, et al. Incidence of open-angle glaucoma. *Arch Ophthalmol.* 2001;119:117–118.

Beaver Dam Eye Study

Klein R, Klein BE, Lee KE. Changes in visual acuity in a population. The Beaver Dam Eye Study. *Ophthalmology.* 1996;103:1169–1178.

Klein R, Klein BE, Linton KL, et al. The Beaver Dam Eye Study: visual acuity. *Ophthalmology.* 1991;98:1310–1315.

Blue Mountains Eye Study

Attebo K, Mitchell P, Smith W. Visual acuity and the causes of visual loss in Australia. The Blue Mountains Eye Study. *Ophthalmology.* 1996;103:357–364.

Melbourne Visual Impairment Study

Livingston PM, Guest CS, Bateman A, et al. Cost-effectiveness of recruitment methods in a population-based epidemiological study: the Melbourne Visual Impairment Project. *Aust J Publ Health.* 1994;18:314–318.

VanNewkirk MR, Weih L, McCarty CA, et al. Cause-specific prevalence of bilateral visual impairment in Victoria, Australia: The Visual Impairment Project. *Ophthalmology.* 2001; 108:960–967.

Weih LM, VanNewkirk MR, McCarty CA, et al. Age-specific causes of bilateral visual impairment. *Arch Ophthalmol.* 2000;118:264–269.

Salisbury Eye Evaluation Project

Munoz B, West S, Rubin GS, et al. Who participates in population based studies of visual impairment? The Salisbury Eye Evaluation Project experience. *Ann Epidemiol.* 1999;9: 53–59.

CHAPTER 5

Case Series Epidemiology

Overview

Prospective clinical trials using a large patient population are considered the gold standard for evaluating common diseases. A large number of patients increases the power and accuracy of statistical analyses. However, diseases that have a low frequency of occurrence in the population cannot be studied using large clinical trials. It is difficult to obtain epidemiologic information about etiology and prognosis when only a few cases are seen by any one clinician. It is also difficult to do randomized treatment trials when the prevalence of a disease is low. For rare diseases, case series epidemiology is useful in collecting data.

In case series methodology, small numbers of patients seen by only one or a few clinicians are carefully identified and followed in order to develop an information database about the disease. Compiling information on each unusual case can be done with something as simple as a 3-×-5 index card or as sophisticated as a computerized database. In most cases, the clinician must have the initiative to pursue these data without research funding. A different approach must be used for each disease, depending on the specific characteristics of that condition. The clinician must decide whether the disease is inflammatory, infectious, neoplastic, or genetic. This early hypothesis helps direct subsequent investigations. As data are collected, the presumed etiology can change or even become multifactorial. The effects of new treatments must be assessed on small numbers of patients, which is difficult.

Despite these drawbacks, case series epidemiology has made significant contributions to the discipline. Numerous diseases such as diffuse unilateral subacute neuroretinitis (DUSN), acute posterior multifocal placoid pigment epitheliopathy, multiple evanescent white dot syndrome, and acute retinal necrosis have been characterized using this approach.

Fisher JP, Lewis ML, Blumenkranz M, et al. The acute retinal necrosis syndrome. Part 1: Clinical manifestations. *Ophthalmology*. 1982;89:1309–1316.

Gass JD. Acute posterior multifocal placoid pigment epitheliopathy. *Arch Ophthalmol*. 1968; 80:177–185.

Gass JD, Gilbert WR Jr, Guerry RK, et al. Diffuse unilateral subacute neuroretinitis. *Ophthalmology*. 1978;85:521–545.

Jampol LM, Sieving PA, Pugh D, et al. Multiple evanescent white dot syndrome. I. Clinical findings. *Arch Ophthalmol*. 1984;102:671–674.

Applying the Approach: Diffuse Unilateral Subacute Neuroretinitis

First Step: Defining the Disease

The first step in identifying a new disease entity is recognizing its clinical features. This requires that one or several investigators accumulate a few cases that are distinctly different from known disease entities but similar to each other. Every disease has some variability, so the clinical parameters of the disease have to be carefully discerned over time and validated with each new case. The idea is to develop definite criteria for the clinical features of the disease that separate it from other entities and that allow for its recognition in both early and late stages. Diffuse unilateral subacute neuroretinitis, studied and identified at the Bascom Palmer Eye Institute, is a good example of how this can be done.

Before 1973, 13 cases of unusual, unilateral visual loss in children or young adults had been seen at the Bascom Palmer Eye Institute. Patients presented with severe visual loss associated with focal areas of pigment epithelial atrophy, mild vitritis, optic atrophy, and narrowing of the retinal vessels. Electroretinography showed moderate to marked reductions in the B wave and lesser effects on the A wave. No etiology was apparent in these patients despite thorough medical and ocular examinations. The condition was initially named the *unilateral wipe-out syndrome.*

By 1975, it had become clear that some patients who presented with mild papilledema, vitritis, and central visual loss developed, over time, the later characteristics just described. In 1976, the next step in characterizing the disease occurred. A few new patients presented with evanescent crops of small yellowish white infiltrates in the deep retina and retinal pigment epithelium (RPE), mild vitritis, and unilateral visual loss. These small infiltrates were generally confined to a zone of about 5 to 6 disc diameters. Typically, the lesions faded within 7 to 10 days, usually leaving no trace of their presence in the fundus. They were often replaced by a new crop of lesions in the nearby retina. On some occasions, initial follow-up examination showed no lesions, only to have them reappear at a later time. Occasionally, focal atrophic lesions similar to those in the presumed ocular histoplasmosis syndrome developed.

When followed over time, the patients developed the typical picture of unilateral wipe-out syndrome. It was through careful follow-up of each new patient and comparison with the previous cases that the link was made between the early- and late-phase presentations as one disease. Patients with these crops of inflammatory loci and mild vitritis represented the early stages of the disease; over time they developed optic atrophy, narrowed vessels, focal RPE atrophy, and the severe visual loss that represents the late stage of the disease. The follow-up and comparison allowed the various stages of DUSN to be recognized.

Some time later, an eye with DUSN was enucleated and examined at the Bascom Palmer Institute 15 months after the onset of the disease. The eye showed extensive degeneration of the retina, optic nerve atrophy, and mild degenerative changes of the RPE. Patchy areas of low-grade, nongranulomatous choroiditis and perivasculitis were also seen. The newer term of *diffuse unilateral subacute neuroretinitis* was proposed. The clinical spectrum of this disease was now understood. This advance in understanding the disease occurred because of the careful cataloguing of unusual cases with similar features.

Second Step: Determining the Etiology

The next step in understanding a disease is to elucidate the etiology. In an ideal situation, all of Koch's postulates regarding the etiology of a disease can be fulfilled (Table 5-1). Doing so generally takes many years and is not accomplished for even infectious disease. In some cases, only a category of etiology can be determined. If the disease can be identified as inflammatory, infectious, or neoplastic, then some general approaches to treatment can be attempted. Medications such as steroids can be tried if the disease appears inflammatory in nature, whereas these would not be used if the disease were felt to be an infection. Once the disease is described, all clinicians and investigators can contribute to the effort of finding the etiology.

In late 1977, Dr J. Donald M. Gass at the Bascom Palmer Eye Institute was preparing a lecture concerning toxocariasis. In a fundus photograph of a subretinal nematode presumed to be *Toxocara canis,* Gass noted the presence of multiple white subretinal lesions near the nematode. The patient had presented several weeks before the discovery of the nematode with acute visual loss and vitritis attributed to optic neuritis. This led to the hypothesis that perhaps a motile nematode in the subretinal space was responsible for the recurrent crops of white lesions and the later picture of unilateral wipe-out syndrome.

Soon after this, Gass received photographs of another patient with a subfoveal nematode. Some years earlier, this patient had presented with acute visual loss associated with a crop of multifocal yellowish white subretinal lesions and multiple chorioretinal scars in one eye. The patient had been hospitalized because of suspected active ocular histoplasmosis chorioretinitis. During the hospitalization, before the subfoveal nematode was discovered, it was noted that some lesions faded and new lesions appeared. Initially these two subfoveal nematodes were presumed to be *T canis*.

With this new information, Gass searched the Bascom Palmer Institute photography files for all patients presenting with multifocal chorioretinitis simulating that seen in the early stages of DUSN. Follow-up information was obtained on these patients, as well as on the two originally seen with subfoveal nematodes. In addition, he obtained follow-up information on all patients with subretinal nematodes previously reported in the literature. By 1983, this information provided further evidence that

- DUSN was caused by a nematode that probably was not *T canis*
- Nematodes of two different sizes were involved
- There were at least two endemic areas for DUSN
- These areas were related to the nematode size

Table 5-1 Koch's Postulates, 1882

1. The organism must be present in every case of the disease.
2. The organism must be isolated and grown in pure culture.
3. The organism must, when inoculated into a susceptible host, cause the specific disease.
4. The organism must then be recovered from the host animal and identified.

- The nematode could remain viable in the human eye for at least 3 years
- Thiabendazole and diethylcarbamazine citrate were ineffective therapeutically
- Laser photocoagulation of the nematode was effective in destroying the nematode and preventing further progression of the disease

Since that time, numerous cases have confirmed that a motile, subretinal nematode is in fact the etiologic agent of DUSN and what was formerly called the unilateral wipe-out syndrome. Over the last 2 decades, the clinical characteristics of DUSN and the role of the subretinal nematode have been confirmed by other investigators around the world.

> de Souza EC, da Cunha SL, Gass JD. Diffuse unilateral subacute neuroretinitis in South America. *Arch Ophthalmol.* 1992;110:1261–1263.
>
> Gass JDM. *Stereoscopic Atlas of Macular Diseases: Diagnosis and Treatment.* 4th ed. St. Louis: Mosby; 1997:622–628.
>
> Gass JD, Braunstein RA. Further observations concerning the diffuse unilateral subacute neuroretinitis syndrome. *Arch Ophthalmol.* 1983;101:1689–1697.
>
> Harto MA, Rodriguez-Salvador V, Avino JA, et al. Diffuse unilateral subacute neuroretinitis in Europe. *Eur J Ophthalmol.* 1999;9:58–62.

Third Step: Identifying the Organism

Once the association between DUSN and a subretinal nematode was made, the hunt to identify the specific nematode was on. It is difficult even for parasitologists to determine the type of nematode from fundus photographs alone. The geographic incidence and relative size of the worm can help guide these efforts. The progress made in this area centered around two approaches: one that used associated clues and findings and one that involved obtaining a specimen directly from the eye.

Serologic testing and size of the nematode were reviewed in 18 patients. Only 6 had serologic evidence of *T canis* infection. Stool examination for ova and parasites was negative in the 8 patients tested. Eosinophilia was present in only 1 patient. Serologic tests for filariasis were negative in 2 patients. *T canis* did not appear to be the etiologic agent.

Baylisascaris procyonis, the raccoon ascarid, was a likely candidate based on its appearance and its ability to produce similar findings in experimental animals. Monkeys, mice, hamsters, squirrels, and woodchucks were inoculated with *Baylisascaris* eggs and developed ocular findings. However, large doses of the eggs were used and several of the animals died. In mice and hamsters, the infection produced retinal and vitreal hemorrhages and hyphema. Two deaths in children were also reported about this same time from *Baylisascaris* infection, although there were no reported cases of typical DUSN leading to death in humans. There was still some question, therefore, whether *Baylisascaris* caused DUSN. In 1993, a case of DUSN was reported in which Western blot analysis suggested infection with *Baylisascaris,* and raccoons in the area were shown to be infected with the parasite.

> Fox AS, Kazacos KR, Gould NS, et al. Fatal eosinophilic meningoencephalitis and visceral larva migrans caused by the raccoon ascarid Baylisascaris procyonis. *N Engl J Med.* 1985; 312:1619–1623.

Goldberg MA, Kazacos KR, Boyce WM, et al. Diffuse unilateral subacute neuroretinitis. Morphometric, serologic, and epidemiologic support for Baylisascaris as a causative agent. *Ophthalmology*. 1993;100:1695–1701. [See comments in *Ophthalmology*. 1994;101:971–972.]

Gass suggested *Ancylostoma caninum*, the dog hookworm, as a possible candidate. A few patients with DUSN reported a syndrome compatible with cutaneous larva migrans prior to their eye symptoms and *Ancylostoma* is a known cause of this condition. The size of third-stage larvae of *Ancylostoma* matches that of the nematode seen in patients.

Gass JDM. *Stereoscopic Atlas of Macular Diseases: Diagnosis and Treatment*. 3rd ed. St. Louis: C. V. Mosby, 1987:474.

Each of the above investigations to determine the identity of the nematode was made without invading the eye. Unfortunately, none were conclusive. The most reliable way to identify the nematode would be to obtain a living specimen from a human eye. The first two specimens were obtained by eye wall resections. However, the specimens were preserved for electron microscopy; the best method to use for identifying these nematodes is light microscopy. A nematode was removed from a patient in Germany, but only half of the organism was obtained. Another was removed from a child in Brazil and identified as a third-stage larva of *T canis*, although some suggested that it was more likely to be *A caninum*. As a result, it is still not certain which parasite is predominantly responsible for DUSN. It appears that more than one nematode can produce the clinical picture. The current candidates remain *Ancylostoma*, *Baylisascaris*, and, in some cases, *Toxocara*. The chorioretinitis caused by the subretinal filarial nematode *Onchocerca volvulus* is also very similar in appearance. (See Chapter 21 of this volume.)

de Souza EC, Nakashima Y. Diffuse unilateral subacute neuroretinitis. Report of transvitreal surgical removal of a subretinal nematode. *Ophthalmology*. 1995;102:1183–1186.

Meyer-Riemann W, Petersen J, Vogel M. An attempt to extract an intraretinal nematode located in the papillomacular bundle. *Klin Monatsbl Augenheilkd*. 1999;214:116–119.

Fourth Step: Treating the Disease

The ultimate goal of case series epidemiology is to determine a treatment for the disease or develop a preventive strategy. Knowing the etiology obviously makes this much easier. However, in some cases, treatment can be tried without understanding the pathophysiology. Many inflammatory diseases respond to treatment with corticosteroids, for example, but it is very important not to exacerbate an infectious disease with steroids or immunosuppressants. Each proposed treatment regimen must be tried in a handful of cases and then judged as to whether it alters the known natural history of the disease.

The realization that a subretinal nematode was the culprit in DUSN immediately provided a possible treatment. If the single nematode could be killed, the disease might not progress further. Laser treatment was noninvasive and therefore an ideal choice. Over many years, this has proven to be the case. If the nematode can be found on careful examination, laser destruction of the worm halts the disease. Once the nematode is killed by laser, the inflammation gradually subsides and progression of the disease stops. If the macula has been directly affected, the central acuity does not always improve. If, however, the nematode has not damaged the macula directly, acuity can improve to 20/20 in some cases.

In a significant number of patients, the nematode cannot be visualized. This prompted the trial of oral antihelminthic drugs. The first ones tried were thiabendazole and diethylcarbamazine, as they were proven agents in other cases of parasitic infestation. Both were ineffective in immobilizing the subretinal nematodes under observation. Thiabendazole was effective in some patients with 3 to 4+ vitreous cells. Within 7 to 10 days after treatment, the yellowish white lesions disappeared and a new large focus of retinitis, believed to be caused by the dead nematode, developed. In these cases, the inflammation cleared and the disease progression was stopped. Thiabendazole can cause significant nausea accompanied by emesis. A few patients could not tolerate the medication. In other cases, the medication was ingested, but it had no observable effect on the nematode and the disease continued to progress. After reviewing the limited series, it appeared that thiabendazole was effective only in cases with significant vitreal inflammation. If the eye was relatively quiet, the medication had no effect.

In cases where repeated fundus contact lens examination and fundus photographic examination failed to find the nematode, Gass used scatter laser treatment in the region of the whitish outer retinal lesions to break down the blood–retina barrier, along with giving either thiabendazole or albendazole. This treatment was successful in three of four cases. The inflammation resolved and there was no further progression of visual loss. This type of treatment should be reserved for patients showing the typical clinical picture and course of DUSN and only after several examinations have failed to find the nematode.

Gass JD, Callanan DG, Bowman CB. Oral therapy in diffuse unilateral subacute neuroretinitis. *Arch Ophthalmol.* 1992;110:675–680.

Ivermectin is an antihelminthic drug that is quite successful in treating onchocerciasis, where significant side effects occur only in cases of massive infestation. Use of ivermectin in DUSN has been limited and it appears to be ineffective, particularly in cases of limited inflammation.

Casella AM, Farah ME, Belfort R Jr. Antihelminthic drugs in diffuse unilateral subacute neuroretinitis. *Am J Ophthalmol.* 1998;125:109–111.
Greene BM, Taylor HR, Cupp EW, et al. Comparison of ivermectin and diethylcarbamazine in the treatment of onchocerciasis. *N Engl J Med.* 1985;313:133–138.

Research into the structure of the blood–brain barrier provided more clues as to the restricted effectiveness of both thiabendazole and ivermectin. The P-glycoprotein molecule is now known to be part of the entity known as the blood–brain barrier. Neither thiabendazole nor ivermectin is capable of crossing this barrier, presumably because of their interaction with the P-glycoprotein molecule. This is the reason these agents were unsuccessful in patients with limited inflammation. Presumably patients with significant vitreal inflammation had a breakdown in the blood–brain barrier that allowed the agents to reach the nematode. Those with limited inflammation probably had an intact blood–brain barrier that limited the concentration of the drugs reaching the nematode.

Jolliet-Riant P, Tillement JP. Drug transfer across the blood–brain barrier and improvement of brain delivery. *Fundam Clin Pharmacol.* 1999;13:16–26.

This information, as well as the availability of a new pharmacologic agent, has led to the latest drug to be tried: albendazole. This drug is known to cross the blood–brain barrier and is an effective antihelminthic agent. It is currently being studied for its effectiveness in DUSN. Once again, a small number of cases will be treated to provide information regarding the effectiveness of a new treatment modality.

Because of the rarity of DUSN, it is difficult to do a randomized trial of new therapeutic approaches. However, each drug can be compared with laser treatment, which is known to successfully kill the nematode if it is directly visualized. The drawback of this approach is that the inadequacy of any drug tried is not known until the disease progresses.

Acute Retinal Necrosis

Another clinical disease that demonstrates the techniques of case series epidemiology is acute retinal necrosis. In the 1980s, ophthalmologists collected several unusual cases they had seen and reviewed similar cases reported in the literature. They proposed the term *acute retinal necrosis* for an entity that included necrotizing retinitis, vitritis, and retinal vasculitis. They continued to focus attention on this new disease and eventually obtained both vitreous samples and enucleated eyes to determine the possible etiology. They found evidence of both herpes simplex and herpes zoster in these eyes, which led to treatment with antiviral medicines. Persistent evaluation of clinical cases and pathologic material turned an unrecognized disease into a well-characterized, treatable condition.

> Culbertson WW, Blumenkranz MS, Haines H, et al. The acute retinal necrosis syndrome. Part 2: Histopathology and etiology. *Ophthalmology*. 1982;89:1317–1325.
> Culbertson WW, Blumenkranz MS, Pepose JS, et al. Varicella zoster virus is a cause of the acute retinal necrosis syndrome. *Ophthalmology*. 1986;93:559–569.
> Lewis ML, Culbertson WW, Post JD, et al. Herpes simplex virus type 1. A cause of the acute retinal necrosis syndrome. *Ophthalmology*. 1989;96:875–878.

Summary

Diseases with a low frequency of occurrence like DUSN cannot be studied using large randomized trials. Case series epidemiology is an extremely useful approach to these rare diseases. With careful documentation and follow-up, information can be collected that allows the disease to be characterized. Over a period of years, clues can be obtained and pursued that help elucidate the pathogenesis. The prognosis can be ascertained from prolonged follow-up of the patients. This type of research requires a concerted and sustained effort on the part of one or a few investigators and patients who return for follow-up examinations. As can be seen from the examples of DUSN and acute retinal necrosis, this process can take years to yield the needed information. The treatment of these conditions is also problematic. Each new treatment modality must be tried on a small number of patients and the outcome compared with the known prognosis. Despite all these drawbacks, case series epidemiology remains a useful tool for dedicated clinicians and investigators in the fight to combat disease and preserve sight.

PART II

Prevalence and Prevention of Pediatric Vision Impairment

Introduction

Pediatric vision impairment is a problem in both developing and developed countries. The consequences of blindness (<20/400) are especially tragic in the least developed countries, where the lifespan is already reduced. Not only do young people in these countries have a shorter lifespan, but many of them will spend it unable to see. In this section, we discuss the prevalence and prevention of childhood blindness. Dr Sherwin Isenberg begins with an overview of the available worldwide data regarding the causes of pediatric blindness, the methods used to assess childhood blindness in a population, and the factors contributing to pediatric blindness in particular regions. Once we understand this subject matter on a global scale, we can begin to develop an ordered approach to prevention and treatment.

Following the chapter on prevalence, we cover some of the specific major causes of pediatric vision impairment, including ophthalmia neonatorum, retinopathy of prematurity (ROP), vitamin A deficiency, amblyopia, and trauma. From studies addressing pediatric blindness, we know that the causes of these disorders are very different in industrialized nations than they are in developing countries. The chapters on ophthalmia neonatorum and vitamin A deficiency address two of the preventable causes of childhood blindness in developing countries. Amblyopia and ROP, on the other hand, are more of a factor in developed countries. However, it is crucial to understand how to prevent and treat the latter two because these will surely become more of an issue as developing countries become more advanced.

In Dr Isenberg's chapter on ophthalmia neonatorum, the sobering spectrum of this devastating condition is presented. Because of the lack of preventive medicine in some developing countries, neonatal conjunctivitis has a much greater impact than in countries where prophylaxis is the standard of care.

As prevention and treatment efforts progress worldwide, the predominant causes of pediatric blindness are in flux. In a recent study of worldwide pediatric blindness, Steinkuller and colleagues report that the leading conditions are cataract, ROP, and glaucoma. In this next chapter, Dr John Flynn reviews ROP as a significant cause of blindness in the pediatric population. In the United States, ROP is now second only to cortical blindness as a cause of vision loss in students in schools for the blind and visually impaired. ROP was once thought to be a disease limited to fully industrialized countries. However, it is now an important blinding disorder in emerging economies as well and will continue to grow as a cause of pediatric visual loss as new technologies become more available in developing nations.

Next, Drs James Tielsch and Alfred Sommer detail their extraordinary epidemiologic investigation into vitamin A deficiency around the world. In addition to the clinical presentation and findings associated with xerophthalmia, they give an interesting historical account and also discuss prevention and treatment.

Any discussion of pediatric blindness must include amblyopia, even though the vision loss is usually monocular. Amblyopia as a cause of severe vision impairment is given much more attention in developed countries, which have the luxury of being able to worry about monocular vision loss. Despite this, there are few data on the epidemiology, economic impact, prevention efforts, and treatment of amblyopia. In this chapter, Dr Flynn uses a pooled data set of published studies that is likely to comprise the most comprehensive data available to present his recent analysis of the results of amblyopia therapy.

Ocular trauma is a global health problem. A majority of these injuries affect young people. Prevention of injury is an opportunity to reduce morbidity and disability. Although great strides have been made in lowering the number of ocular injuries due to industrial accidents and sports in the Western world, prevention in developing countries needs to be addressed. In this final chapter of the section, Drs Mylan VanNewkirk and Paul Vinger present the state of ocular trauma worldwide, discuss successful strategies for prevention, and look to future possibilities for intervention.

The goals of this section include reporting the state of pediatric vision impairment around the world at the beginning of the 21st century; describing the social, geographic, and environmental factors that contribute to the differences in pediatric ophthalmic disease in different regions; and promoting the prevention of childhood blindness worldwide. We hope to begin by making the reader aware of the impact these blinding diseases have on an international scale. This may be the first step toward future eradication of avoidable causes of pediatric blindness.

> Gilbert C, Rahi J, Eckstein M, et al. Retinopathy of prematurity in middle-income countries. *Lancet.* 1997;350:12–14.
> Steinkuller PG, Du L, Gilbert C, et al. Childhood blindness. *JAAPOS.* 1999;3:26–32.
> World Health Organization. Blindness and visual disability. Part IV: Socioeconomic aspects. [Section on retinopathy of prematurity (ROP).] WHO Fact Sheet 145; February 1997.
> World Health Organization. Blindness and visual disability. Part V: Seeing ahead—projections into the next century. WHO Fact Sheet 146; February 1997.

Mary Louise Z. Collins, MD

CHAPTER 6

Pediatric Blindness

Background

Blindness in children is tragic but not hopeless. It offers the medical community an opportunity to score a major victory over a true scourge of humanity. Blindness is defined by the World Health Organization as category 3 or worse, indicating corrected visual acuity in the better eye of 20/400 (3/60) or worse. Worldwide, as many as 1.5 million children are blind. Of these, 48% live in Asia and 24% in Africa. It is estimated that up to 400,000 children in Africa, 270,000 in India, and 200,000 in China are blind. About half of the world's cases of avoidable pediatric blindness (corneal scar, cataract, and ROP) occur in India and Africa. The three main causes of pediatric blindness are retinal diseases (29%), corneal scarring (21%), and disorders of the entire globe (14%). The prevalence of childhood blindness varies from estimates of 100 per 100,000 in Kenya to 9 per 100,000 in the United Kingdom and the United States. Every year, a half million children become blind (Fig 6-1).

> Foster A. How can blind children be helped? *Community Eye Health*. 1998;11:33–34.

Although more adults than children are blind worldwide, the total number of years of blindness endured by all blind children challenges the total number of years of blindness suffered by all blind adults. Unlike most adults, blind children often have other disabilities such as intellectual impairment, seizure disorder, and hearing and speech impediments.

An ordered approach to dealing with world pediatric blindness would be

- Prevention
- Treatment of existing cases of blindness
- Dealing with children whose blindness cannot be improved with medical or surgical techniques

It is somewhat comforting to know that about half of all blind children can have their vision, including the ability to read normal-sized print, improved with proper optical means.

> Ager L. Optical services for visually impaired children. *Community Eye Health*. 1998;11:38–40.

To decrease the incidence of pediatric blindness, we must investigate the causes of blindness in children and then decide which techniques can be employed to carry this

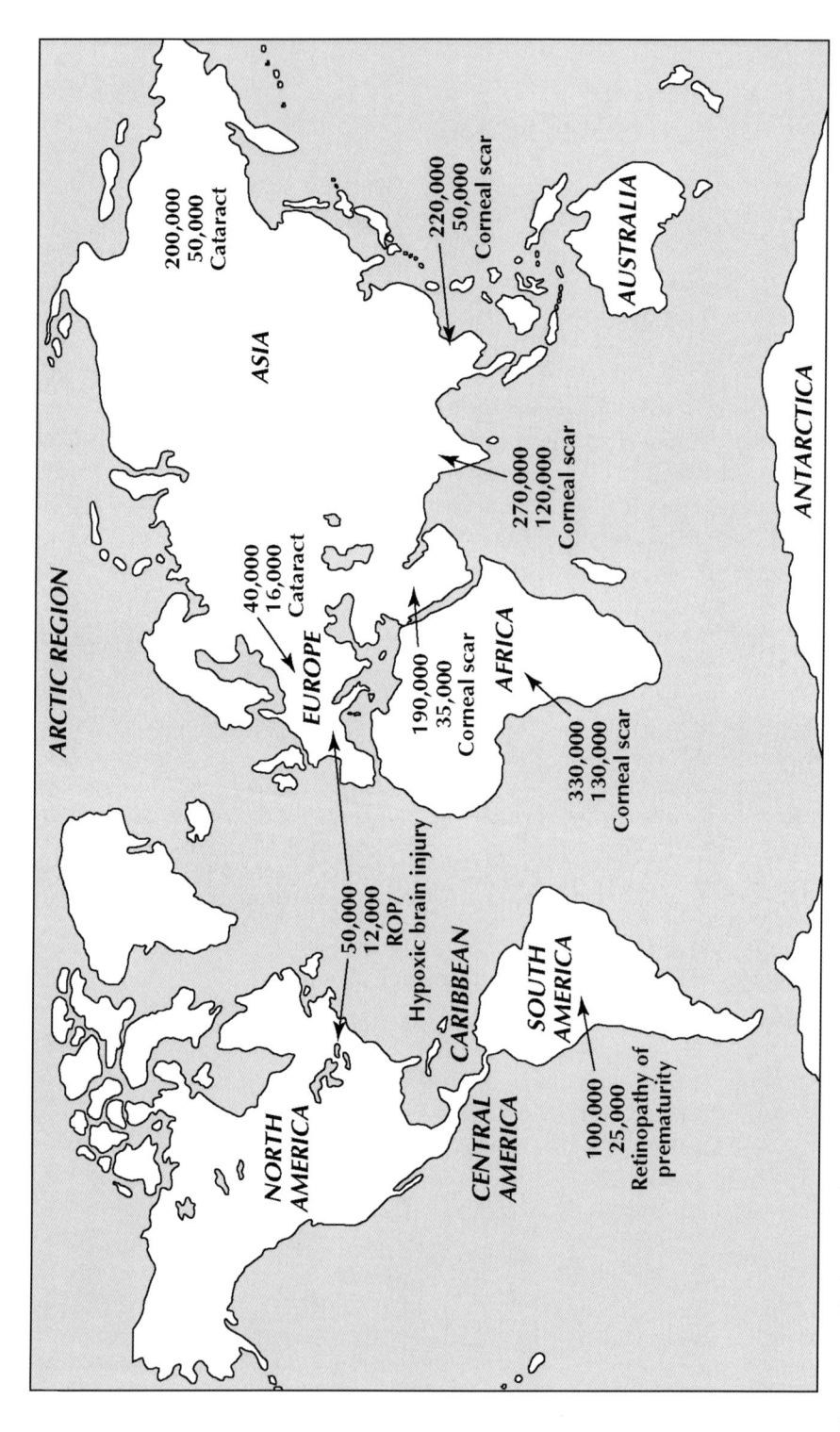

Figure 6-1 Estimates of pediatric blindness by region. Top number = total number of blind children; bottom number = number blind from avoidable causes. Below each set of numbers is the major cause of childhood blindness the numbers represent. *(Illustration by Jeanne Koelling.)*

out. The techniques will differ by location, socioeconomic group, local custom, endogenous and exogenous factors, sanitation, and many other factors.

> Gilbert CE, Anderton L, Dandona L, et al. Prevalence of visual impairment in children: a review of available data. *Ophthalmic Epidemiol.* 1999;6:73–82.

Methods for Assessing Childhood Blindness in a Population

Evaluating a large population to count the number of blind children would be expensive. Most investigations obtain data by surveying the local schools for blind children. However, there are two problems with this approach: Only school-age children are considered, and, in some cultures, not all children attend school (especially if it is perceived that they have no future). Despite these reservations, school surveys have provided most of the information available in the literature. More reliable data collection is often too costly.

Causes of Blindness

The causes of childhood blindness vary greatly throughout the world. If the world is divided into developed and developing countries, the differences in the causes of pediatric blindness are stark. In general, in developed countries childhood blindness arises from problems with premature care (retinopathy of prematurity), genetic diseases (cataract and retinal dystrophies), central nervous system problems (anoxia/hypoxia of visual pathways), congenital malformations (microphthalmos, anophthalmos, and optic nerve hypoplasia), and nystagmus. In developing countries, the major causes of blindness include corneal scarring resulting from vitamin A deficiency, often associated with measles or other illnesses; trachoma; genetic diseases; cataract; and ophthalmia neonatorum. The lists are quite different. More advanced developing countries, such as India, have etiologies encompassing parts of both lists. A recent Indian survey found the four major causes of pediatric blindness to be vitamin A deficiency, congenital abnormalities such as microphthalmos, inherited retinal dystrophies, and cataract.

> Rahi JS, Sripathi S, Gilbert CE, et al. The importance of prenatal factors in childhood blindness in India. *Dev Med Child Neurol.* 1997:39:449–455.

Factors Affecting Blindness in Particular Regions

Affluence
The difference between developed and developing societies has been mentioned. Even within one country, more affluent children are less likely to suffer from the infectious diseases or malnutrition that plague the less affluent.

Availability of neonatal intensive care units
In developing countries, as demonstrated in surveys conducted in parts of Africa, the frequency of ROP approaches zero because few low-weight neonates survive. In contrast, up to 38% of Asian children born in South Africa were blinded by ROP. As countries

become more developed, the prevalence of ROP increases because the technology to save the lives of low-weight premature infants becomes more available (see BCSC Section 12, *Retina and Vitreous*).

> Gilbert C, Rahi J, Eckstein M, et al. Retinopathy of prematurity in middle-income countries. *Lancet.* 1997;350:12–14.

Rural vs. city setting

In rural areas of the Philippines, the major cause of blindness was found to be corneal disease (49%) from vitamin A deficiency combined with infection such as that from measles. In urban Manila, the same study found, ROP was the major cause of blindness; in the rural areas no blindness from ROP was reported. In some developed countries (Sweden, for example), the incidence of blindness from ROP has been noted to be decreasing, as better screening and treatment methods are utilized.

> Gilbert C, Foster A. Causes of blindness in children attending four schools for the blind in Thailand and the Philippines: a comparison between urban and rural blind school populations. *Int Ophthalmol.* 1993;17:229–234.

Endogenous infections

In Brazil, the most frequent cause of pediatric blindness, toxoplasmosis macular scarring, causes 44% of all childhood blindness. This finding clearly points to a need for a focused attack on reducing exposure to the parasite by pregnant women by having them avoid raw meat and limit their association with cats (see BCSC Section 9, *Intraocular Inflammation and Uveitis*).

> de Carvalho KM, Minguini J, Moreira Filho DC, et al. Characteristics of a pediatric low-vision population. *J Pediatr Ophthalmol Strabismus.* 1998;35:162–165.

Cataract

It has been estimated that 200,000 children throughout the world are blind from cataract, although it is not usually the most frequent cause of blindness in any particular country. In Uganda, however, cataract was found to be the most frequent cause of pediatric blindness. This was attributed to genetic influences as well as to the common occurrence of rubella. Corneal scarring was the second most frequent cause.

Consanguinity

In some countries, the practice of consanguineous marriages, frequently between first cousins or uncle and niece, increases the frequency of genetic causes of blindness. In Sri Lanka, where about 25% of marriages are consanguineous, hereditary diseases account for at least 35% of pediatric blindness, including etiologies such as the retinal dystrophies Leber amaurosis and Usher syndrome, cataract, optic atrophy, and microphthalmia. Similarly, in the West Bank and Gaza, consanguinity was responsible for 62% of cases of blind children, and a positive family history was found in 57% of cases. Leber amaurosis, cone dystrophy, retinitis pigmentosa, and albinism were frequently encountered.

> Elder MJ, De Cock R. Childhood blindness in the West Bank and Gaza strip: prevalence, etiology, and hereditary factors. *Eye.* 1993;7(Pt 4):580–583.

Perinatal factors

Ophthalmia neonatorum and birth trauma have been identified as frequent causes of visual impairment in many countries. The former is frequently found in areas where gonorrhea and chlamydia are prevalent in the adult population and neonatal ocular prophylaxis is not used (Fig 6-2). The latter may result from inadequate obstetric care.

Migration patterns

Immigrants to a new country can present with diseases that are new or not frequently present in the host country. For example, immigrants from a generally nonsanitary environment may continue habits that lead to infections even after moving to a new region where better sanitation is the custom.

Reports published in the United Kingdom note that diseases previously unrecognized in Britain are now being reported. One involved population is an immigrant group from a region of Pakistan. Unusual disorders such as LOGIC syndrome (granulation tissue affecting the larynx, eye, skin, nails, and teeth) have been reported.

These disorders are largely autosomal recessive. It is believed that the high frequency of consanguineous marriages practiced in this particular population has led to this and other syndromes that often affect the eye. Compared with other ethnic groups, children of consanguineous Pakistani parents are 16 times more likely to have chronic illnesses and disabilities, have a 10% chance of death or serious illness in childhood, and have a high frequency of mental retardation. Similar phenomena have been reported in other countries, including Australia.

> Ainsworth JR, Shabbir G, Spencer AF, et al. Multisystem disorder of Punjabi children exhibiting spontaneous dermal and submucosal granulation tissue formation: LOGIC syndrome. *Clin Dysmorphol.* 1992;1:3–15.
> Bundey S, Alam H. A five-year prospective study of the health of children in different ethnic groups, with particular reference to the effect of inbreeding. *Eur J Hum Genet.* 1993;1: 206–219.

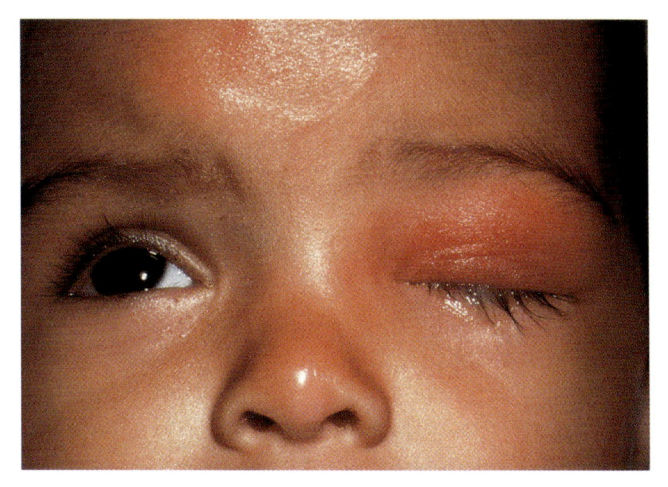

Figure 6-2 Conjunctivitis presenting within 30 days of birth is diagnosed as ophthalmia neonatorum. *(Photograph courtesy of Sherwin J. Isenberg, MD.)*

Nelson J, Smith M, Bittles AH. Consanguineous marriage and its clinical consequences in migrants to Australia. *Clin Genet.* 1997;52:142–146.

Suggestions for Reducing Childhood Blindness

Although the challenge to reduce blindness in children worldwide may at times look impossible to overcome, there are ways in which we can make a difference.

Some causes of childhood blindness are preventable. As known for more than 100 years, a drop of an appropriate antimicrobial agent delivered to the eye within 1 hour of birth can effectively reduce the incidence of ophthalmia neonatorum. Although this is a practice throughout most of the developed world, many countries still do not administer ophthalmic prophylaxis to newborns. Physicians should insist that an antimicrobial (povidone-iodine, erythromycin, or silver nitrate) be used universally (Fig 6-3). Povidone-iodine may be preferable in developing areas due to its effectiveness and very low cost.

Isenberg SJ, Apt L, Wood M. A controlled trial of povidone-iodine as prophylaxis against ophthalmia neonatorum. *N Engl J Med.* 1995;332:562–566.

Other disorders can also be prevented. Vitamin A oral supplements should be administered in areas of poverty and vitamin deficiency. Immunization against rubella and other conditions should be given as appropriate to mothers and children.

Advice from health professionals can be helpful. Education regarding nutrition and sanitation should be provided to families in areas of need. Genetic counseling should be available for families at risk.

Once a disease is present, early detection may be not only curative, but worsening of the final visual acuity may be prevented by amblyopia therapy. Glaucoma and cataract should be recognized and treated as soon as possible. Retinopathy of prematurity should also be recognized early by proper screening and treated, when appropriate. Optimal

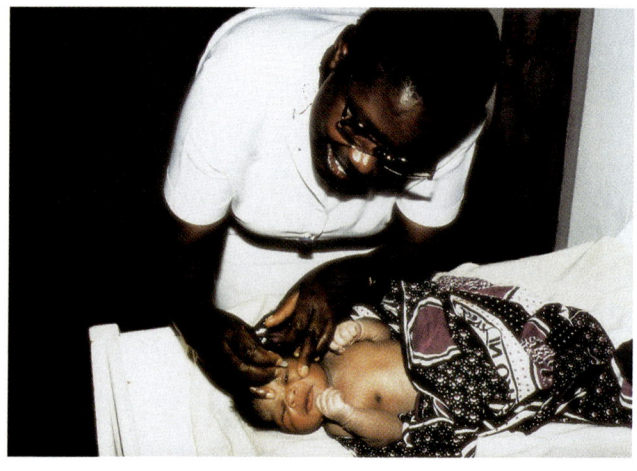

Figure 6-3 Within a few minutes of the infant's birth, this nurse in Kenya is applying a prophylactic eyedrop. *(Photograph courtesy of Sherwin J. Isenberg, MD.)*

care, including the option of surgery, as with cataract extraction and keratoplasty, should be available to the patient. Unfortunately, in some places many surgical alternatives are not available.

Ophthalmologists from industrialized countries can volunteer their time to less fortunate countries to provide services to patients and teaching to physicians, nurses, and technicians. Interested ophthalmologists can contact the Foundation of the American Academy of Ophthalmology (International Public Service section) at 415/447-0281. Lobbying officials from developing countries to provide better eye services may also be beneficial.

CHAPTER 7

Ophthalmia Neonatorum

Background

History

Among the causes of pediatric blindness, *ophthalmia neonatorum*, or congenital conjunctivitis, is particularly dangerous because it can blind babies before they reach 1 month of age. It has been recognized for centuries. In 19th-century Europe, it was the single greatest cause of blindness in children, as documented from records from schools for the blind.

> Credé CSR. Die verhutung der augenentzudung der neugebornen. *Arck Gynaekol*. 1881;18: 367–370.

Context

Although childbirth is usually a joyous time, a newborn developing an eye infection within the first postnatal month is distressing to new parents. More ominously, it can lead to blindness or reduced vision that can last a lifetime. Because the infection is acquired by the pathogenic organism entering the baby's eye from an infected birth canal, the mother is the direct cause. The infected child usually presents within the first few postnatal days, as may occur with gonococcus, or, if later, with other organisms.

> Holland GN. Infectious diseases. In: Isenberg SJ, ed. *The Eye in Infancy*. 2nd ed. St. Louis: Mosby; 1994.

Economic Impact

Cost of treatment

Because most of these infections are treated in an outpatient setting with standard antibiotics, the cost is quite low. Only if the cornea is thinning, as may result from gonococcal or other causes of keratitis, might the infant be admitted for careful monitoring and treated surgically at the first indication of corneal perforation.

Cost of lost productivity

No disease causes a greater loss of productivity than a disease that blinds a newborn baby. One must not only consider the immediate loss but also ponder the effect on the child's entire lifespan.

Pathogenesis

If a pathogenic organism occurs in the birth canal, the child's eye may acquire it if the delivery is vaginal. The organisms can be bacterial, such as gonococcus, *Staphylococcus aureus*, or a *Streptococcus* species, or viral, such as herpes simplex. Although HIV is usually acquired hematogenously, there have been suggestions from the literature that direct inoculation of the eye may be another portal of entry.

When the infection is acquired postnatally, as from contact with an infected parent's hands, but presents within 30 days of birth, it is still called ophthalmia neonatorum by convention.

Epidemiology

Risk Factors

The recognized risk factors involve the mother. The child is more likely to develop this infection if the mother is of a lower socioeconomic status, has a history of sexually transmitted diseases, or has an active vaginitis.

Geographic, Environmental, Social Factors

Although found worldwide, the disease is more prevalent in geographic areas with a higher incidence of sexually transmitted diseases. Prominent among these areas are East Africa and Southeast Asia. It is found more frequently in areas with little or no access to maternal prenatal care and in less affluent populations.

Ethnic Differences

Ethnic identity has no bearing on the incidence of ophthalmia neonatorum. Sexually transmitted diseases cross all ethnic groups. If, in a particular country, a certain ethnic group has a lower socioeconomic level, the disorder may occur more frequently among that group.

Surveys to Determine Prevalence/Incidence

The prevalence of this infection varies widely around the world. In developed countries, the incidence is in the range of 0.1% to 1.0% of all births. In developing countries, such as in East Africa, however, the incidence increases to more than 10% of all births. The latter high incidence rate reflects not only the aforementioned factors but also the general lack of prophylactic measures.

Clinical Presentation and Findings

This form of conjunctivitis, as noted by conjunctival injection, eyelid edema, and frequent conjunctival discharge, arises within 28–30 days of birth. It can be unilateral or bilateral. Because neonates do not develop follicles, the cellular morphology of the conjunctival reaction is not as important as in other forms of conjunctivitis. A conjunctival reaction within 24 hours of birth may result from a toxic reaction to the prophylactic topical agent and not be a true infection.

The postnatal timing of the infection has etiologic significance. The most common etiologic agent, *Chlamydia trachomatis*, can cause conjunctivitis any time after postnatal day 4 to 7. An infection arising within the first postnatal week raises the strong possibility of gonococcus, whereas an infection occurring from week 2 to 4 suggests gram-positive organisms such as staphylococcal and streptococcal species. If the child has a gram-negative septicemia, the same organism may cause the conjunctivitis.

Neisseria gonorrhoeae, the most feared organism for this disease, can perforate a cornea and cause endophthalmitis within a few days after birth. It causes a severe inflammatory reaction with extreme conjunctival injection, edema, and purulence. When severe purulence is found on the eye of a newborn, the diagnosis should be gonorrheal conjunctivitis until proven otherwise (Fig 7-1).

C trachomatis is the etiologic agent found most frequently in most countries. It causes a low level of chronic conjunctivitis but, unlike what happens to adults, does not produce follicles in infants. Over time, it causes corneal scarring. Chlamydial conjunctivitis may precede or follow chlamydial pneumonitis.

A number of different bacterial species may be causative, including *S aureus* and other staphylococcal species, pneumococcus, and *Haemophilus*. Infections can be from a few organisms simultaneously. Herpes simplex virus can produce corneal dendrites in newborns either alone or as part of a generalized herpetic infection, which can also cause encephalitis.

Chandler JW, Rapoza PA. Ophthalmia neonatorum. *Int Ophthalmol Clin.* 1990;30:36–38.

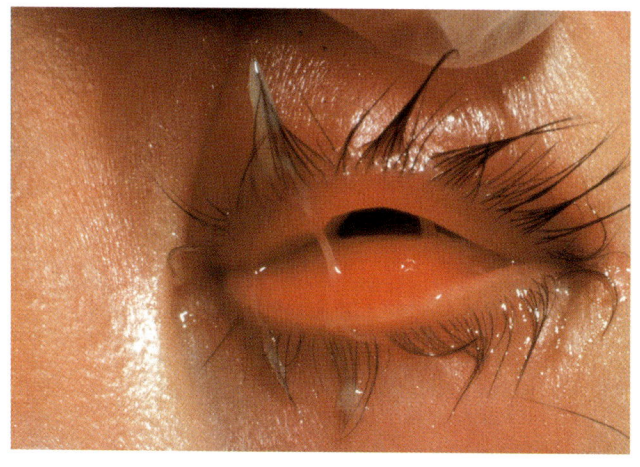

Figure 7-1 After the purulence was cleaned from these eyelids, additional pus continued to present. The culture was positive for gonococcus. *(Photograph courtesy of Sherwin J. Isenberg, MD.)*

Prevention

Prevention is paramount with this disease. There are two layers of prevention. The first is directed toward the mother. Proper prenatal care will reveal any vaginitis and lead to treatment of the mother before delivery. Studies in the United States and abroad have shown a decreased incidence of ophthalmia neonatorum in areas of widespread prenatal care. The mother should also be educated to present for treatment if signs of vaginitis appear.

The second layer of prevention is directed to the child. Since the 1880s, it has been recognized that an appropriate antimicrobial eyedrop applied to the eye shortly after birth will dramatically reduce the incidence of this disease. Silver nitrate ophthalmic solution was the first such medication used but is no longer available in the United States and many other countries. Erythromycin 0.5% ophthalmic ointment is now the most widely used agent, but it is not always effective. Other countries have been noted to use ophthalmic preparations of tetracycline, gentamicin, or other medications. The choice of medications should be carefully considered because such medications must, at a minimum, have strong activity against gonorrhea and chlamydia. For example, many cases of gonorrhea are now resistant to tetracycline. Povidone-iodine ophthalmic solution may become the agent of choice in the future.

Workup

A workup includes both a history and laboratory work (Table 7-1). A history from the parents may reveal a recent history or signs of an acquired sexually transmitted disease. The mother's obstetric history should be reviewed for any vaginal infections.

Specimens of conjunctival exudate and cells should be obtained, preferably with a spatula. Preparations for Gram and Giemsa stains should be examined for bacteria and

Table 7-1 Workup of Ophthalmia Neonatorum

History
1. From both parents (histories should be obtained separately)
   - Urethral or vaginal discharge?
   - Genital vesicles?
   - History of any sexually transmitted diseases?

Laboratory
1. Scrape the conjunctiva to obtain epithelial cells.
2. Perform the following tests immediately:
   - Gram stain (gonococcus and other bacteria)
   - Giemsa stain
     - Herpes: Multinucleated giant cells and intranuclear inclusions
     - Chlamydia: Purple intracytoplasmic inclusions
   - Direct immunofluorescent or PCR for chlamydia
3. Send culture specimens for
   - Gonococcus (Thayer-Martin)
   - Other bacteria (blood agar, and so on)
   - Chlamydia (optional)
   - Anaerobes (optional)

chlamydia, respectively. Bacterial cultures should be sent on a number of media: blood agar, chocolate agar, Thayer-Martin, and thioglycolate broth. If herpes is suspected, viral cultures may be sent. Chlamydia can be investigated with McCoy cell culture, direct immunofluorescent monoclonal antibody stains, or ELISA (enzyme-linked immunosorbent assay) stain. In less developed areas, it is important to at least perform a Gram stain and, if possible, appropriate cultures to detect gonococcus while the child is treated with less specific medication.

Current Treatment Programs

Screening

Screening is generally performed as part of the usual examination of the newborn. Any redness or discharge should be evaluated.

Specific Recommendations in the Presence of Infection

The following recommendations are optimal and may not be available in all areas (Table 7-2). Gonococcal conjunctivitis is most frequently treated with ceftriaxone 50 mg/kg IM or IV or cefotaxime 120 mg IM. The usual dose is about 120 mg in a term infant and 80 mg in a preterm. Conjunctival adhesions (symblepharon) should be broken. Topical bacitracin may also be applied.

Chlamydial conjunctivitis is treated with topical erythromycin or sulfacetamide ointment at least four times per day. In addition, oral erythromycin syrup should be given four times a day for 2 weeks at a dose of 50 mg/kg/day for the eye, as well as to prevent or treat systemic infections, particularly pneumonitis.

For other bacteria, an ointment preparation of gentamicin or erythromycin may be given four times per day for a week. Topical antiviral medications may be used for herpetic infections.

Success of Povidone-Iodine Prophylaxis

Povidone-iodine has many potential benefits compared with the commonly used prophylactic eyedrops (Fig 7-2). Among these are broad antimicrobial spectrum, lack of toxic reactions, turning the eye brown for 2 minutes (thus making the application evident to the health professional), and, very importantly, a very low cost with wide availability.

Table 7-2 **Treatment**

Organism	Systemic	Topical
Gonococcus	Ceftriaxone 50 mg/kg IM or IV	Bacitracin ointment and lid hygiene
Chlamydia	Erythromycin 12.5 mg/kg PO or IV qid for 14 days	Sulfacetamide 10% ointment qid
Other organisms		Neosporin ointment (or equivalent broad-spectrum) qid for a week

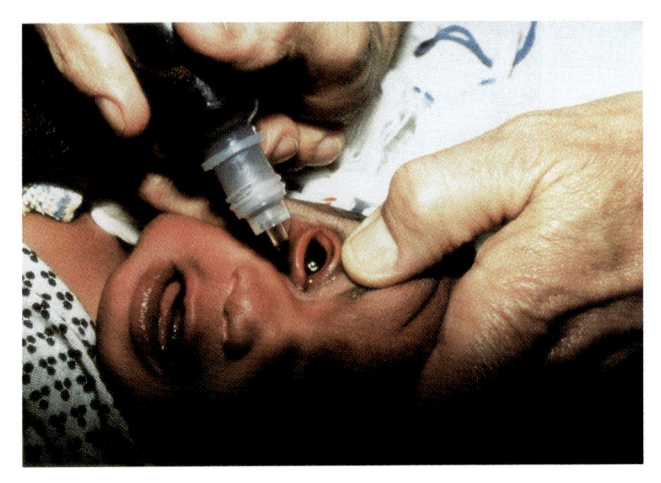

Figure 7-2 Povidone-iodine ophthalmic solution was applied to the eye of this newborn a few minutes after birth. The brown color on the eye, which persists for a few minutes, confirms that the drop has been properly administered. *(Photograph courtesy of Sherwin J. Isenberg, MD.)*

In a clinical trial of more than 3000 babies in Kenya, povidone-iodine ophthalmic solution was studied compared with two control groups that received either silver nitrate ophthalmic solution or erythromycin ophthalmic ointment. Povidone-iodine proved to be more effective than the other two agents while being less toxic. It should be considered for prophylaxis, especially in developing countries. (See Chapter 22 of this volume.)

Isenberg SJ, Apt L, Wood M. A controlled trial of povidone-iodine as prophylaxis against ophthalmia neonatorum. *N Engl J Med.* 1995;332:562–566.

CHAPTER 8

Retinopathy of Prematurity

Background

The disease we know today as *retinopathy of prematurity (ROP)* is a paradox of modern medical progress. It was known as *retrolental fibroplasia* during the 1940s and 1950s, when it was first described, and the role of excessive oxygen in its pathogenesis was demonstrated by the 1956 Kinsey study, the first application of the randomized clinical trial methodology in ophthalmology.

> Kinsey VE. Retrolental fibroplasia. Cooperative study of retrolental fibroplasia and the use of oxygen. *Arch Ophthalmol*. 1956;56:481.

During that era, every premature infant (<2500 grams birth weight) was given supplemental oxygen at 50% concentration whether it was medically indicated or not. The result was an epidemic of infant blindness. An estimated 10,000 infants born prematurely in the United States in the decade 1945 to 1955, and many more worldwide, developed the disease. With the curtailment of oxygen to under 40%, and then only as needed, the disease disappeared.

With the decade of the 1960s came a technological revolution in the care of premature newborns. Infants who would have died a decade before survived at birth weights of 1500 grams (very low birth weight: VLBW) and under. As time passed, the birth weight of survivability dropped from 1500 to 1000 grams and lower, until today it is not at all unusual to find infants surviving at 500 grams. Retinopathy of prematurity has reappeared with a vengeance in these extremely low weight infants. But the disease of today occurs in a completely different infant than the infant of the 1940s and 1950s. Back then, it was the healthiest, most robust premature infants who got the disease from toxic overexposure to oxygen. Today, it is the smallest, most gestationally immature, sickest infant who gets the disease in its worst form. But today, treatment with cryotherapy or laser is available, whereas none was available previously. And although far from a complete answer, treatment does arrest the disease in most cases prior to irreparable damage to the infant's visual system.

> Ben-Sira I, Nissenkorn I, Grunwald E, et al. Treatment of acute retrolental fibroplasia by cryopexy. *Br J Ophthalmol*. 1980:64:758–762.
> Multicenter trial of cryotherapy for retinopathy of prematurity: preliminary results. Cryotherapy for Retinopathy of Prematurity Cooperative Group. *Arch Ophthalmol*. 1988;106: 471–479.

Wachtmeister L, Algvere P, Gjotterberg M. Efficacy of cryotherapy for retinopathy of prematurity. *Acta Ophthalmol (Copenh)*. 1992;70:389–394.

Yamashita Y. Studies of retinopathy of prematurity: III. Cryocautery for retinopathy of prematurity. *Jpn J Clin Ophthalmol*. 1972;26:385–393.

Economic Impact

Each year 4 million infant births occur in the United States. Eight percent of these are premature by definition: <2500 grams birth weight and 36 weeks gestational age. Of these, upwards of 30,000 are extremely low birth weight (ELBW) (<1000 grams), less than 32 weeks gestational age infants. It is this pool of infants that is at highest risk for developing the most severe, sight-threatening forms of the disease. In a recent study, 49% of infants ≤1251 grams developed ROP in some form, and of these, approximately 7% reached threshold requiring treatment. Despite this intervention, one child developed bilateral stage 5 ROP with bilateral blindness. Without intervention, and sometimes despite it, ROP leading to blindness has staggering costs:

- The lifetime costs of blindness to an individual and immediate family
- Lost economic opportunities to the individual and to society
- The costs associated with providing the mobility, skills training, and education to fit the individual into a useful societal role
- The costs of providing the infrastructure to meet the needs of the visually handicapped for special educational benefits, social security, transportation, and other living needs

Onofrey CB, Feuer WJ, Flynn JT. The outcome of retinopathy of prematurity: screening for retinopathy of prematurity using an outcome predictive program. *Ophthalmology*. 2001; 108:27–34.

Siatkowski RM. Retinopathy of prematurity. In: Parrish RK II, ed. *Bascom Palmer Eye Institute Atlas of Ophthalmology*. Boston: Butterworth Heinemann; 1999:530–535.

Pathogenesis

Normal retinal vascularization is a finite process. It begins at 16 weeks of gestation when mesenchyme, the precursor tissue, pours out of the optic disc and migrates across the retina in the nerve fiber layer (the so-called vanguard of Ashton). On its trailing edge, it gives rise to primitive capillary tubes (the "rearguard") that form a "chickenwire" meshwork first described by Cogan. That primitive capillary network is the substrate from which the entire retinal vasculature, arteries and veins, develops by a process of remodeling, absorption of some capillaries, and enlargement of others in the major vessels, with surviving capillary meshwork between. The process is complete by 36 weeks nasally and 40 weeks temporally.

Ashton N, Ward B, Serpell G. Effect of oxygen on developing retinal vessels with particular reference to the problem of retrolental fibroplasia. *Br J Ophthalmol*. 1954;38:397.

Cogan DG. Development and senescence of the human retinal vasculature. *Trans Ophthalmol Soc UK*. 1963;83:465–489.

In the retina of a premature infant, an injury, as yet largely unspecified during this time period, destroys the vulnerable tissue, the newly formed capillaries in situ, leaving two tissues surviving. These two, the mesenchyme and the mature arterioles and venules, unite as a response to the injury to form a shunt. Where that shunt is located determines in large part the rest of the history of the disease. When the shunt is located far posterior, just beyond the disc and macula, the outlook for the eye is questionable, even with adequate treatment. If the injury occurs later, when the vessels are developed further peripherally in the retina, the prognosis is much better. Finally, if the injury does not occur until very late, the outlook is very good, and the vast majority of these eyes do well with no treatment at all.

> Flynn JT, O'Grady GE, Herrera J, et al. Retrolental fibroplasia. I. Clinical observations. *Arch Ophthalmol.* 1977;95:217–223.

Regression, spontaneous healing of the lesion, occurs in over 90% of eyes afflicted with ROP by 48 weeks gestational age. It occurs almost always in very anterior disease, often in midretinal disease, and almost never in posterior disease. Thus, the examining ophthalmologist is in a critical position to judge from the location and extent of the disease in the eye the likelihood that the disease will require treatment. One other clue is the presence of "plus disease." This is the presence of dilated and tortuous retinal vessels in the posterior pole. Plus disease, in combination with significant advanced ROP in the periphery, carries an ominous prognosis. The pathogenesis of plus disease is thought to be a very active, large-volume, high-velocity shunting mechanism at the site of abnormal vasculogenesis. Once the disease has reached this stage, there is little to be done except to treat it, as the likelihood of spontaneous regression is slim.

Progression of the disease from this point causes traction and detachment of the retina from its pigment epithelial bed. This can be partial, remaining chiefly peripheral (where it invariably starts), or progressing to involve the posterior retina, either partially or totally, where it becomes a serious threat to vision. The retinal detachment in these later stages of the disease is primarily tractional, accompanied at times by an exudative component. Needless to say, all efforts are directed at preventing the disease from reaching these advanced stages.

This information on ROP has been compressed into a classification system that has been adopted worldwide and has united the clinical observations of the disease at all its stages of evolution. (See BCSC Section 12, *Retina and Vitreous.*)

> An international classification of retinopathy of prematurity. The Committee for the Classification of Retinopathy of Prematurity. *Arch Ophthalmol.* 1984;102:1130–1134.

Epidemiology

Retinopathy of prematurity, as we know it, is worldwide in its distribution (see Table 8-1). It is clear that, using the standard epidemiologic tool for expressing incidence of diseases of infancy per 100,000 live births, ROP has a high rank. This is especially true considering the fact that ROP is almost exclusively a disease of the very lowest birth weight strata. As the art and science of modern tertiary care neonatology diffuses from

Table 8-1 Retinopathy of Prematurity: Outcome of the Disease by Country

Country	Time Period	Type of Study	Outcome #/100,000 Live Births	Outcome Other	Comment
Taiwan	1993–1996	Retrospective		Stages 3–5 = 73/13,835 live births	Acute disease only; no long-term follow-up
Australia	1986–1987 vs 1992	Retrospective		1986–1987 = 4.1% 1992 = 1.3%	Diminished in prevalence; little change in most severe forms
England	January 1984–December 1987	Retrospective	Blindness or SVL* 12.5/100,000		5.4% due to ROP
Second and third world countries*	1991–1996	Retrospective	Blindness in Africa secondary to ROP = 0.0%	Blindness in Cuba secondary to ROP = 38.6%	Infant mortality in African countries probably biases these results.
Norway	1989–1993	Population-based retrospective		Stage 3 ROP = 2.9% for infants <1500 grams	
Sweden	1990–1992	Population-based prospective	ELBW ≤1000 grams 10% stage 3 = 26/100,000		Acute ROP only
The Netherlands	1975–1987 vs 1986–1994	Population retrospective	1975–1987 = 1986–1994	4.2/100,000 5.1/100,000	Greater survival of ELBW in 1986–1994?
Denmark	1990–1993	Population retrospective	14/100,000 severe visual impairment		Probably most accurate estimate
Nordic	0–17 years	3.8M of 17M population	8/100,000 mean; severe visual impairment	12/100,000 Denmark; 5/100,000 Finland, Norway; 4/100,000 Iceland	Third most common cause of visual impairment
United States[†]	January 1, 1986–November 30, 1987	Best estimate only (no systematic study done)	17.6/100,000	Contact John T. Flynn, MD, Harkness Eye Institute, Columbia University.	A real need for the United States is valid statistics.

Blindness = NLP or barely LP; SVL = severe visual loss (<20/200 visual acuity)
ELBW = extremely low birth weight
* These are guarded estimates only.
[†] No countrywide data are available for the United States.

the more developed countries to those seeking to improve their development in medical care, smaller and smaller premature babies (VLBW and ELBW) will survive and ROP will inevitably follow. Efforts to reduce the incidence of pregnancies resulting in these latter two classes of premature babies at risk for ROP have thus far been singularly unsuccessful. Even the value of prenatal care as it is now practiced has been questioned in this regard. Although more black infants are born prematurely in the United States than their percentage of the population would indicate, they seem to possess a relative immunity from the ravages of the most serious forms of the disease. No satisfactory explanation of this exists at present.

> An international classification of retinopathy of prematurity. II. The classification for retinal detachment. The International Committee for the Classification of the Late Stages of Retinopathy of Prematurity. *Arch Ophthalmol.* 1987;105:906–912.
> Saunders RA, Donahue ML, Christmann LM, et al. Racial variation in retinopathy of prematurity. The Cryotherapy for Retinopathy of Prematurity Cooperative Group. *Arch Ophthalmol.* 1997;115:604–608.

Clinical Presentation

The disease is diagnosed on retinal examination by an ophthalmologist trained to examine a premature fundus. Ninety-five percent of ROP will first appear in the retina at 32 to 34 weeks postconception. Once diagnosed as present in the retina, the behavior of the disease follows a predictable pattern based on its location and extent in the retina. The vast majority ($\geq$75%) of ROP today is seen in zone II. Its further progress will be determined by the extent of the disease. When involvement is less than 5 clock hours, the disease usually follows a benign course and terminates in regression in 8 to 12 weeks following its appearance. When involvement is greater than 5 clock hours—and particularly when it is in double digits—careful observation is crucial. If signs of extraretinal proliferation of neovascular tissue (stage 3 ICROP [International Classification of ROP]) develop, generally accompanied by plus disease, then prompt laser treatment should be carried out to prevent traction retinal detachment.

> Palmer EA, Flynn JT, Hardy RJ, et al. Incidence and early course of retinopathy of prematurity. The Cryotherapy for Retinopathy of Prematurity Cooperative Group. *Ophthalmology.* 1991;98:1628–1640.

Prevention

At this time—and pending the development of a better method for preventing high-risk pregnancies—no method of effective prevention is available for these at-risk ELBW premature infants (<1000 grams).

Current Treatment

The current treatment for ROP begins with a thorough examination by an ophthalmologist skilled in diagnosing the disease. Guidelines concerning who should be examined and when are given in BCSC Section 6, *Pediatric Ophthalmology and Strabismus*. If the disease reaches threshold, the standard of care today calls for ablation by indirect laser or cryotherapy to the avascular retina anterior to the shunt, sparing that structure and the developing vasculature unaffected by ROP posterior to it. The entire avascular retina should be treated. How aggressive the treatment with ablative modalities should be is still a matter of some discussion.

Once treatment is completed, these eyes must be watched carefully for recrudescence of the disease, signalled by the persistence or increase in plus disease in the posterior pole. This calls for additional laser treatment or cryotherapy. If the disease progresses to the point where the retina is detached, the evidence is far less clear and compelling that surgical therapy, such as scleral buckling, vitrectomy, delamination, silicone, or air–fluid exchange, are of any benefit in terms of visual outcome although clearly retinal reattachments do occur as a result of these surgical maneuvers.

It is clear that every premature infant who develops anything more than the mildest form of ROP should be followed indefinitely for the occurrence of retinal breaks and detachments, as well as for high refractive error, particularly myopia, astigmatism, and anisometropia. The incidence of strabismus and amblyopia is higher than in normal birth weight infants. Retinopathy of prematurity can be looked upon in this light as a chronic disease needing a lifetime of ophthalmic care.

Clinical Research

Since the Cryotherapy for ROP Trial, a systematic approach has developed to the questions surrounding the best treatment available for this disease. The randomized trial instrument has been used to explore the possibility that ambient light in the neonatal intensive care unit might be a factor in the causation or intensification of ROP. A randomized trial has also examined the hypothesis that hypoxia plays a role in determining the severity of ROP. Neither was found to play a role in the incidence or severity of the disease. However, negative results are as important as positive results, as they allow clinical research to move forward.

> Reynolds JD, Hardy RJ, Kennedy KA, et al. Lack of efficacy of light reduction in preventing retinopathy of prematurity. Light Reduction in Retinopathy of Prematurity (LIGHT-ROP) Cooperative Group. *N Engl J Med.* 1998;338:1572–1576.
> Supplemental Therapeutic Oxygen for Prethreshold ROP (STOP-ROP), a randomized, controlled trial. I: primary outcomes. *Pediatrics.* 2000;105:295–310.

The Early Treatment for ROP Trial will test the hypothesis that treatment at the prethreshold stage for eyes at high risk for unfavorable outcomes in spite of adequate laser therapy might nevertheless benefit from such therapy, again using the randomized trial methodology.

Finally, technical advances in wide-angle digital fundus photography have introduced the possibility that infants in remote or underserved nurseries can also be screened. Neonatal nurses trained in the photographic techniques and using high-speed modem technology can transmit the images to reading centers where staff members have the expertise to interpret them.

> Roth DB, Morales D, Feuer WJ, et al. Screening for retinopathy of prematurity employing the RetCam 120: sensitivity and specificity. *Arch Ophthalmol.* 2001;119:268–272.
>
> Schwartz SD, Harrison SA, Ferrone PJ, et al. Telemedical evaluation and management of retinopathy of prematurity using a fiberoptic digital fundus camera. *Ophthalmology.* 2000;107:25–28.
>
> Yen KG, Hess D, Burke B, et al. The optimum time to employ telephotoscreening to detect retinopathy of prematurity. *Trans Am Ophthalmol Soc.* 2000;98:145–151.

A coherent picture of the basic phenomenon of vasculogenesis is emerging in laboratories that study the molecular biology of cytokines, such as vascular endothelial growth factor and insulin growth factor-1. These are bound to play a role in our advancing understanding of the abnormal vasculogenesis of ROP.

CHAPTER 9

Vitamin A Deficiency Disorders

Background

History

Although vitamin A was first identified as a required nutrient for growth in animals by E.V. McCollum in 1915, the clinical syndrome and appropriate treatment with animal liver was known to the ancient Egyptians over 3500 years ago. By the 1800s, the ocular signs and symptoms of xerophthalmia were recognized in Europe, and the efficacy of cod liver oil as a treatment was well documented. Following McCollum's work in animals, a Danish pediatrician, C.E. Bloch, published a classic series of papers in which he described the full clinical spectrum of disease: its epidemiology, etiology, and approaches to prevention and treatment.

From the early 1900s through the late 1970s, the importance of vitamin A deficiency in systemic health was overshadowed by its association with blinding xerophthalmia. At this time, Dr Alfred Sommer moved to Indonesia to conduct a series of large epidemiologic and clinical studies designed to complete the picture on the epidemiology, natural history, and clinical outcomes of xerophthalmia in pre–school-age children. These investigations resulted in a large series of publications and the design of a major, population-based trial to determine the efficacy of routine, high-dose vitamin A supplementation (200,000 IU) on the incidence of blinding (corneal) xerophthalmia in Aceh Province.

In the early 1980s, after Sommer had returned to an academic position in the United States and the Aceh trial was ready to begin, he conducted a longitudinal analysis on risk factors for the appearance and disappearance of ocular signs of xerophthalmia. He noticed that it was difficult to follow many children who had "mild" xerophthalmia (night blindness and/or conjunctival signs) over time, as they kept dropping out of his database. They were dying at a rate four times that of children who had normal eyes. This was the first time that "mild" xerophthalmia, previously thought to be important only as a predictor of populations at high risk for the blinding form of the disease, was associated with an increased risk of mortality. He and his colleagues quickly converted the Aceh trial to a study of mortality and demonstrated for the first time that routine high-dose supplementation could significantly reduce mortality, even among children without clinical signs of vitamin A deficiency. Since then, numerous community and hospital-based trials have confirmed the role of vitamin A in protecting young children from early death.

Context

The most severe clinical forms of vitamin A deficiency (corneal xerophthalmia) are usually associated with severe protein-energy malnutrition and acute febrile illnesses such as measles. Conjunctival forms of xerophthalmia and subclinical vitamin A deficiency are also associated with malnutrition and infectious diseases of childhood, such as diarrhea and acute respiratory illness, that are common in developing countries. Inadequate dietary intake of vitamin A or beta-carotene (its biological precursor) plays an important role as well. Evidence is accumulating that a minimal contribution of vitamin A from animal sources in the diet (dairy products, liver, fish oils, and so on) may be necessary for optimal vitamin A status. In most developing countries, such sources are expensive and out of reach for most families. These populations rely almost exclusively on plant sources of beta-carotene to supply their daily requirements. Plant sources vary widely in their bioavailability, and their vitamin A value depends on the species and strain, the growing conditions, the method of preparation, and whether they are consumed concurrently with a dietary source of fat.

Economic Impact

The economic impact of vitamin A deficiency is large, as it is a major cause of both blindness and increased mortality among pre–school-age children in the developing world. The World Bank, in collaboration with the World Health Organization, has developed a new measure of disease burden that combines both mortality and disability into a measure called a "disability-adjusted life-year" (defined as the loss of 1 year of healthy life to disease), or DALY. These organizations estimate the preventable fraction of DALYs attributable to vitamin A deficiency at 39–74 million each year. They also note that high-dose vitamin A supplementation of populations with known clinical and subclinical vitamin A deficiency is one of the most cost-effective health interventions available, at approximately $50 per death averted and $1 per DALY saved.

Cost of treatment and prevention

Treatment for children with clinical xerophthalmia is extremely inexpensive. Typical costs for high-dose vitamin A capsules are in the range of US$0.03/dose—less than US$0.10 for a treatment regimen of three doses. Clearly, the costs of diagnosis and delivery of care are much higher than the cost of vitamin A, but this will vary greatly depending on the system of care delivery and on the strategy used to distribute the vitamin A supplements. A number of countries have dramatically increased their coverage of the at-risk population in a cost-efficient fashion by linking vitamin A capsule distribution to national immunization days used in the polio eradication program. Whether such efforts will be sustainable once the polio eradication program in a country winds down is not clear. The most important message remains that vitamin A supplementation is one of the most cost-effective preventive strategies that can be used to reduce mortality in young children in developing areas of the world.

Pathogenesis

Since the 1920s, there has been a recognized association of vitamin A deficiency and alterations in immune system function. These changes include alterations in barrier function such as squamous metaplasia and keratinization of normal mucus-secreting epithelial tissue in the conjunctiva and in the respiratory and genitourinary systems. In addition, vitamin A deficiency is associated with compromise in the development of antibody response to some, but not all, antigens. Specifically, vitamin A deficiency is related to deficiencies in T-cell–dependent and T-cell–independent type 2 antibody response. Vitamin A deficiency also affects a variety of subclasses of cell-mediated immune response, including cytotoxicity as mediated by NK (natural killer) cells and blastogenic transformation of lymphocytes.

These limitations in immune function are likely responsible for the more recent emphasis on the role of vitamin A deficiency in increased risk of mortality among young children. That the association of vitamin A deficiency and mortality is causal is well supported by a number of both treatment and prevention trials conducted over the past 15 years in a variety of developing countries, such as Indonesia, India, Nepal, Tanzania, Ghana, and South Africa. A variety of meta-analyses of these trials demonstrates that vitamin A supplementation to young children in an environment with endemic subclinical deficiency can reduce total mortality by 20%–50%. The absolute magnitude of the reduction depends on the distribution of causes of death among young children and the degree of vitamin A deficiency in the population.

In addition to reducing mortality in young children, a recent community-based trial in Nepal suggests that a similar impact may be observed on maternal mortality in countries with endemic vitamin A deficiency. Vitamin A also plays a key role in iron metabolism, and supplementation can significantly improve hemoglobin levels in populations where vitamin A deficiency is endemic and anemia is an important problem.

Epidemiology

Surveys to Determine Prevalence/Incidence

Many prevalence surveys have been conducted in different countries over the past 25 years suggesting that 5–10 million children develop xerophthalmia every year and that 500,000 of them lose their sight. The best estimate from the early 1990s on the prevalence of subclinical deficiency among young children is in the range of 125 million, of whom 1–2.5 million die each year. These sobering numbers are tempered by the fact that the prevalence of clinical xerophthalmia is clearly declining in many countries. This has been best documented in Indonesia, where the prevalence of eye signs declined by 75% between 1977 and 1992. How much of this decline is attributable to vitamin A deficiency control programs is unclear, but most evidence suggests that control program activity is responsible for a large proportion. Whether these observed declines in prevalence apply to subclinical vitamin A deficiency is not known, but with a recent expansion of vitamin A supplementation programs in many countries around the world, it is reasonable to assume that the prevalence of subclinical deficiency, and hence the risk of mortality, has declined as well. For example, the national vitamin A deficiency control program in Nepal reached full, nationwide expansion in 2001, with coverage rates of over 90%. This resulted in an annual saving of over 39,000 lives in this small south Asian country alone.

Risk Factors

Geographic

The global distribution of vitamin A deficiency is characterized by high prevalence in Africa and south and Southeast Asia, with moderate prevalence found in selected countries of Central and South America (Fig 9-1). China and other less developed countries in northeast Asia may have significant subclinical deficiency as well. The map reflects our understanding of the geographic distribution of risk of vitamin A deficiency at the country level. Major vitamin A deficiency control programs have been mounted over the past few years in many countries such that the actual levels of vitamin A deficiency have declined dramatically. Without continued intervention, however, these countries would likely revert to the situation as depicted in the map. In addition to geographic variation in prevalence at the country level, xerophthalmia and subclinical vitamin A deficiency cluster at the provincial, district, village, and household level. The household and village clustering of xerophthalmia offers the possibility of targeting interventions to those villages or households at highest risk. However, such an approach has not been tried in any major country program to date.

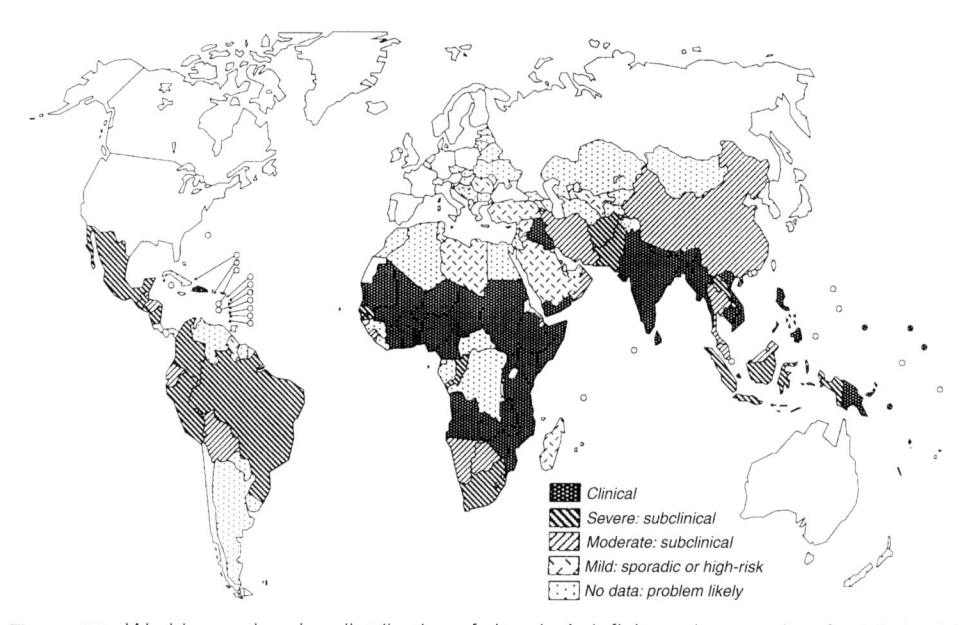

Figure 9-1 World map showing distribution of vitamin A deficiency by severity of public health problem. *(From World Health Organization, 1995. The designations employed and the presentation of material on this map do not imply the expression of any opinion whatsoever on the part of the World Health Organization concerning the legal status of any country, territory, city or area, or of its authorities, or concerning the delimitation of its frontiers or boundaries. Dotted lines represent approximate border lines for which there may not yet be full agreement.)*

Social factors

Vitamin A deficiency is concentrated among the poorer socioeconomic classes in the developing world. Households of children with xerophthalmia are poorer and have fewer high-status possessions than households without xerophthalmic children. Although poor countries with effective vitamin A supplementation programs have dramatically reduced the burden of clinical and subclinical deficiency in their populations, in most cases the underlying factors associated with vitamin A deficiency, such as poverty, poor diet, and so on, have not changed. This suggests that continued political will and resources are needed to keep the burden of vitamin A deficiency under control in these settings.

Ethnic difference

There is no evidence that ethnic variation plays a causative role in the susceptibility to either vitamin A deficiency or its clinical expression. Variations in the prevalence and/or severity of vitamin A deficiency by ethnicity are best explained by cultural variations in dietary practices and socioeconomic status.

Clinical Presentation and Findings

Xerophthalmia is a set of ocular signs and symptoms that are regarded as pathognomonic for vitamin A deficiency. The clinical classification of xerophthalmia is divided into four basic stages: night blindness (stage XN), conjunctival signs (stages X1A and X1B), corneal signs (stages X2, X3A, and X3B), and sequelae of active corneal lesions and corneal scars (stage XS) (see Table 9-1 and Figs 9-2A–9-2H). Night blindness, the earliest and most prevalent form of xerophthalmia, is commonly assessed by asking a mother about the behavior of her child at dusk or in darker, interior locations in the house, or, during pregnancy, about the behavior of the woman herself. In settings where vitamin A deficiency is endemic, local terms that are specific for this condition are often used. Objective measures of dark adaptation can also be used in conjunction with a history of clinical symptoms to reinforce the diagnosis. More recently, consensual pupillometry has been developed as a less time-consuming approach to assessing retinal scotopic sensitivity.

Conjunctival signs of xerosis almost always precede the more severe, blinding form with corneal involvement. Vitamin A deficiency causes a widespread keratinizing metaplasia of mucus-secreting epithelial tissues. This occurs throughout the body and is especially prominent on the conjunctiva and in the respiratory and urinary tracts. A xerotic plaque on the conjunctiva overlaid by a white foamy material is known as a *Bitôt spot*, despite the fact that Hubbenet was the first to describe it. Conjunctival xerosis without a Bitôt spot (stage X1A) is often overdiagnosed, especially in dry or arid climates, where one often finds similar-looking corrugated, pigmented lesions in the interpalpebral zone (upon closer examination, however, these lesions do not shed tears and are therefore not truly xerotic plaques; see Fig 9-2A). For this reason, the clinical stage X1A is a nonspecific sign and should not be used for diagnosis.

Corneal involvement in xerophthalmia is divided into stages that can heal without sequelae (stage X2; see Fig 9-2C) and those that will, at a minimum, leave a small corneal scar but can also include total corneal melting and discharge of intraocular contents

Table 9-1 Clinical Classification of Xerophthalmia

Clinical Grade	Clinical Description
Night blindness (XN)	Limitation in scotopic retinal sensitivity, a result of the inability of the retina to regenerate rhodopsin, leading to increased rod thresholds and subsequent clinical symptoms.
Conjunctival xerosis (X1A)	An isolated, dry, wrinkled lesion that sheds tears (Fig 9-2A). It consists of a thickened layer of keratinized superficial epithelium without evidence of goblet cells. Evidence of mild, chronic inflammation is often associated with these lesions.
Bitôt spots (X1B)	Conjunctival xerotic lesions accompanied by an overlay of white, foamy material consisting of desquamated keratinized epithelium and bacteria (Fig 9-2B).
Corneal xerosis (X2)	The earliest sign of corneal xerosis is a superficial punctate keratopathy beginning inferiorly and involving a larger proportion of the corneal surface as the disease progresses (Fig 9-2C). A totally involved cornea has a ground glass or orange peel appearance as a result of confluent SPK and an anterior stromal edema.
Corneal ulceration/ keratomalacia (less than one third of corneal surface) (X3A)	Corneal ulceration is characterized by the presence of one or more corneal ulcers of varying depth (Fig 9-2D). In their most common presentation, they appear as small, round, punched-out ulcers. Often there is little local inflammation, and they are usually located in the periphery, 1–2 mm from the limbus. These ulcers can be of any depth, including full perforation or descemetocele formation. Ulcers that perforate often form scars, with iris incarcerated in the wound. All ulcers that resolve, usually through treatment, result in corneal scarring. Keratomalacia (stromal necrosis) can be focal, and, if it involves less than one third of the cornea, is classified as X3A.
Corneal ulceration/ keratomalacia (one third or more of corneal surface) (X3B)	This stage involves one third or more of the total corneal surface and can include (although rarely) large ulcers (Fig 9-2E). Most often at this stage of severity, stromal necrosis is the primary mechanism of damage. Focal or complete corneal melting can be observed with full-thickness necrosis, resulting in an anterior staphyloma or phthisis (Fig 9-2F).
Corneal scar (XS)	All cases of corneal stromal damage result in scarring (Fig 9-2G). These can range from small, isolated peripheral scars that do not affect central vision to full-thickness scars with iris incarceration. As many types of injury to the cornea can cause scarring, attributing corneal scars to xerophthalmia is difficult using a retrospective history.
Xerophthalmic fundus (XF)	These lesions appear as small, discrete, yellowish dots deep within the retina, generally located peripherally to the temporal vascular arcade (Fig 9-2H). They most likely represent focal depigmentation of the retinal pigment epithelium.

(From Sommer A. *Vitamin A Deficiency and Its Consequences: A Field Guide to Detection and Control.* 3rd ed. Geneva: WHO; 1995).

(stages X3A and X3B; see Figs 9-2D–9-2F). In general, corneal xerosis is accompanied by severe conjunctival involvement where there is a corrugated, skinlike appearance to the conjunctiva. The most severe stages of xerophthalmia involve loss of corneal stromal structure through one of two potential pathophysiologic mechanisms. The first mechanism is corneal ulceration, most often without associated inflammation. At this stage, ulcers often appear as small, punched-out ulcerations in the periphery of the cornea;

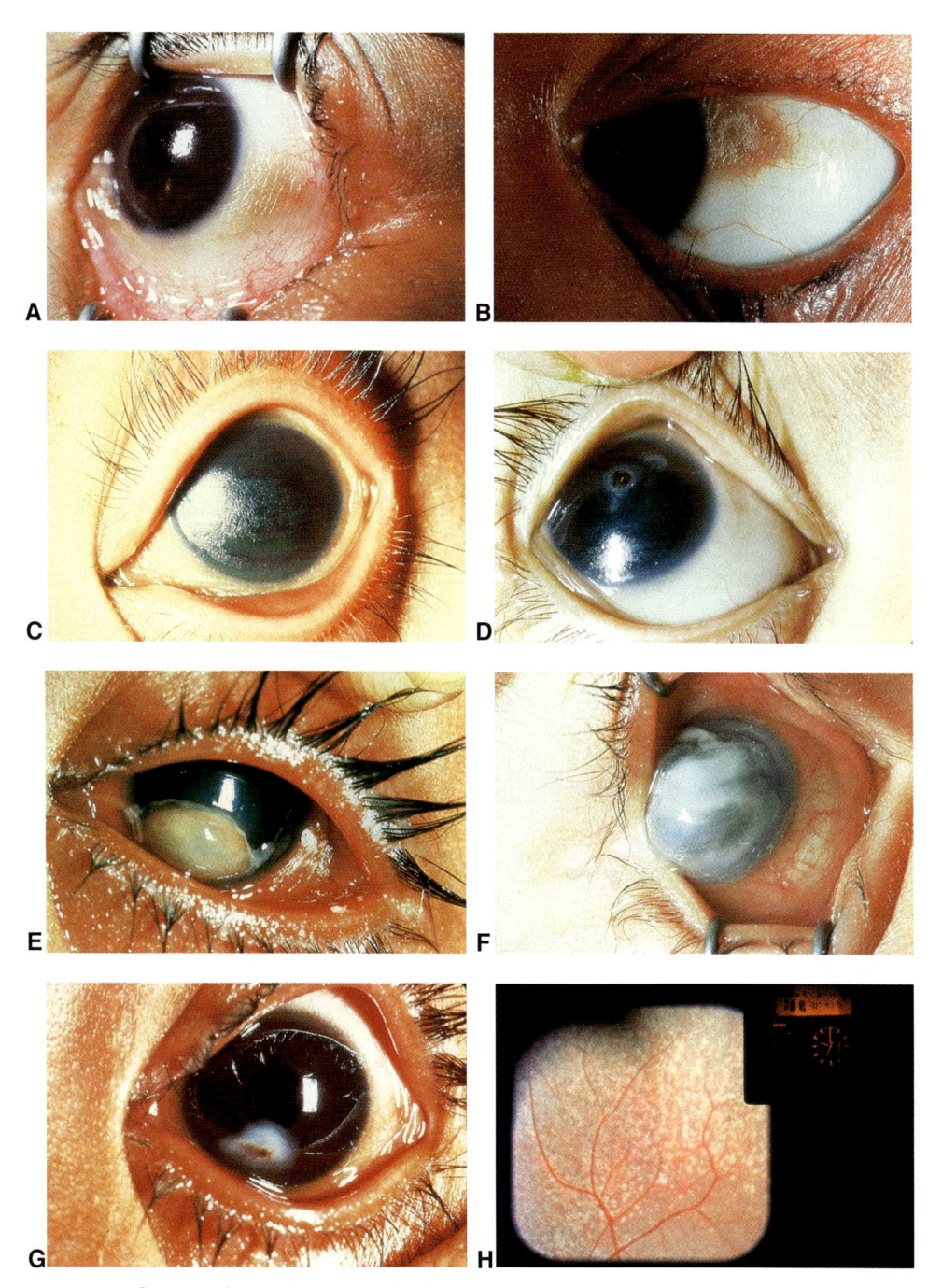

Figure 9-2 Stages of xerophthalmia. **A,** Severe temporal conjunctival xerosis in a 1-year-old boy from Indonesia; stage X1A. **B,** Classic foamy Bitôt spot overlying conjunctival xerosis in a 3-year-old girl from India; stage X1B. **C,** Extensive corneal and conjunctival xerosis in a 3-year-old boy from Indonesia; stage X2. **D,** Typical round, punched-out corneal ulcer (depth to Descemet's membrane) in a 4-year-old boy from Indonesia; stage X3A. **E,** Focal corneal stromal necrosis in a 2-year-old boy from Indonesia; stage X3B. **F,** Full corneal necrosis in a 10-month-old boy from Indonesia; stage X3B. **G,** Inferior adherent leukoma 1 month after treatment in the same eye of the 2-year-old Indonesian boy depicted in **E;** stage XS. Note that the scar has healed without compromising the visual axis in the central cornea. **H,** Small, yellow-white lesions in the fundus of a 24-year-old woman from Indonesia. She also had night blindness and severe conjunctival and corneal xerosis; stage XF. *(From* Vitamin A Deficiency: Health, Survival, and Vision *by Alfred Sommer and Keith P. West. Copyright © 1996 by Oxford University Press, Inc. Used by permission of Oxford University Press, Inc.)*

they can range in size from superficial to full thickness with perforation. The second type of stromal damage is characterized by necrosis of the stroma. This can be isolated to a small section of the cornea or involve the entire cornea. Complete corneal melting is a rare but dramatic expression of this process of keratomalacia.

In almost all of these cases, the structure of the eye is lost, resulting in a protuberant staphyloma or phthisis. The presentation of corneal ulceration or keratomalacia can occur in the absence of conjunctival signs of xerophthalmia. This situation occurs most often in a severely malnourished child who acquires a severe, acute, febrile illness such as measles or pneumonia. In this circumstance, the child can progress from a normal ocular appearance to full, bilateral corneal melting in 2–3 days. As these children are often photophobic, especially in the case of measles, this process can occur completely hidden from view behind closed lids.

Damage to the corneal stroma results in corneal scarring or, with perforation, loss of intraocular contents and a disorganized or phthisical eye. When the precipitating process of corneal scarring is attributable to a previous episode of active xerophthalmia, it is classified as stage XS (see Fig 9-2G). As a variety of injuries to the cornea can cause scarring, attributing the scar to xerophthalmia is often difficult and influenced by clinical judgment based on the history. Xerophthalmic corneal scars are usually quite rare, even in high-risk populations, because the mortality rate of children with corneal involvement is extremely high.

The most recent clinical sign attributed to xerophthalmia is fundus specks (stage XF; see Fig 9-2H). The pathophysiologic significance of these specks is not well understood.

Measles Comorbidity

Vitamin A deficiency is an important risk factor for severity and ocular complications of measles. In vitamin A–deficient populations, the tremendous demand on vitamin A stores caused by the catabolism associated with measles infection can precipitate severe corneal xerophthalmia. Vitamin A status is also strongly associated with other systemic complications of measles. The causal nature of this association is well supported by the vitamin A treatment trials conducted among children with clinical measles and the prevention trials conducted in vitamin A–deficient populations. In both situations, treatment with vitamin A was associated with a 50% reduction in measles-related mortality. The evidence suggests that the incidence of measles is unaffected by vitamin A supplementation, but the case fatality is lowered dramatically. Similarly, measles has a profound effect on vitamin A status and is an important risk factor for all stages of xerophthalmia. During the acute phase of measles infection, circulating vitamin A levels drop significantly, most likely due to a combination of increased demand generated by the catabolic response to measles infection and disturbances in the release and transport of vitamin A stores from the liver. These two associations, vitamin A deficiency with measles and measles with vitamin A deficiency, can be synergistic, as vitamin A deficiency increases the severity of measles complications such as diarrhea, which in turn reduces the intake and absorption of vitamin A in the diet.

Prevention

There are three primary strategies for preventing xerophthalmia and subclinical vitamin A deficiency:

- Periodic supplementation with high-dose vitamin A
- Fortification of foodstuffs with vitamin A
- Increasing dietary intake and absorption of vitamin A–rich foods

These approaches are not mutually exclusive and, in most programs, various combinations of these strategies are employed. The most common approach used in vitamin A deficiency control programs is periodic high-dose supplementation. With this approach, 200,000 IU oil-based capsules are given every 4–6 months to children over 12 months of age and one half this dose to those 6–12 months of age. Vitamin A is stored in the liver and released gradually, as body demands require. High-dose supplementation is often linked to other health care delivery opportunities, such as well-baby visits and national immunization days. Although this approach is intended as a short- to medium-term strategy for preventing vitamin A deficiency until adequate and sustainable food-based programs are put in place, in practice it has been difficult to withdraw these efforts because dietary improvement strategies have not, as yet, proven effective.

Fortification of commonly consumed foods is a central strategy used around the world to improve vitamin A status. This includes most Western countries, where milk and margarine are two examples of commonly fortified foods. To be effective, however, the appropriate food vehicle must be chosen. Such a vehicle must be consumed in adequate quantities by the target population (usually the poorest segments of the population), it should be centrally processed so quality-control measures are relatively easy to implement, and the addition of vitamin A must not alter the taste, color, or organoleptic qualities of the food product nor raise the cost to unacceptable levels. This approach has been tried in a number of developing countries, and a variety of products fortified with vitamin A is now available. However, fortification has yet to become a central component of the vitamin A deficiency control program in any country, primarily because a food product purchased in adequate quantities by the very poor has yet to be found and proven to satisfy the technical criteria for fortification.

Increasing the dietary intake of preformed retinol or beta-carotene, which is converted to retinol in the body, is the preferred long-term, sustainable approach to controlling vitamin A deficiency. However, numerous barriers to dietary behavior change have proven difficult to overcome. These include basic cultural perspectives on proper food for young children, the fact that sources of preformed retinol in the diet are expensive and thus out of reach for those at highest risk, and the seasonal lack of available foods rich in vitamin A activity. Although this approach remains the goal of most development agencies, there is growing acceptance that supplementation will serve as the primary control strategy for the foreseeable future.

Current Treatment Recommendations

The currently recommended treatment schedule for xerophthalmia is based on vitamin A in oil that is administered orally. Oil-miscible vitamin A preparations should never be given as injections, as the oil-based form is not easily released. Water-miscible preparations are available and acceptable for use in treatment, but they are expensive and no more effective than orally delivered oil-based treatment. The World Health Organization currently recommends the following treatment schedule for people with clinical xerophthalmia:

- **For children less than 12 months age:** 100,000 IU immediately, again the following day, and repeated again 2–4 weeks later.
- **For children 12 months or older:** 200,000 IU immediately, again the following day, and repeated again 2–4 weeks later.
- **For women of childbearing age:** Those with only night blindness or Bitôt spots should be treated with daily doses of 10,000 IU for 2 weeks or weekly doses of 25,000 IU for at least 4 weeks. This reduction in dose is due to concerns about the teratogenic effects of large vitamin A doses in the first trimester. However, if corneal lesions are present, the full therapeutic regimen of 200,000 IU in three doses should be used.

In addition to treating children with xerophthalmia, the WHO recommends that children with severe protein-energy malnutrition be treated monthly with the age-appropriate doses (as in the schedule just given) until the protein-energy malnutrition resolves. Because of the strong relationship of vitamin A deficiency and measles, it is also recommended that children with measles who reside in communities where vitamin A deficiency is a recognized problem or where measles case fatality is over 1% receive a single age-appropriate large dose of oral vitamin A. However, all the measles treatment trials have used two doses, and this more prudent strategy should be followed until there is evidence that one dose is equally protective.

Clinical Research Currently Under Way

Two major topics in vitamin A deficiency are in active clinical investigation. The first involves examining the role of vitamin A supplementation in reducing maternal mortality in developing countries. A recently conducted community-based clinical trial from Nepal has demonstrated that weekly, low-dose supplementation of women of reproductive age with vitamin A or beta-carotene can reduce maternal mortality by over 40%. Follow-up trials using an antenatal supplementation approach are currently under way in Bangladesh, Ghana, and Indonesia. The second topic addresses the potential benefit of supplementing newborn infants with a large dose of vitamin A soon after delivery. In the early 1990s, a small hospital-based clinical trial in Indonesia showed a marked reduction in infant mortality associated with newborn dosing. This intriguing result is being addressed currently in a larger community-based clinical trial in southern India and in a large hospital-based trial in Zimbabwe.

Bloch CE. Clinical investigation of xerophthalmia and dystrophy in infants and young children (xerophthalmia et dystropia alipogenetica). *J Hygiene.* (Cambridge) 1921; 19:283–301.

Bloch CE. Further clinical investigations in the diseases arising in consequence of a deficiency in the fat-soluble A factor. *Am J Dis Child.* 1924;28:659–667.

Humphrey JH, West KP Jr, Sommer A. Vitamin A deficiency and attributable mortality among under-5-year-olds. *Bull World Health Organ.* 1992;70:225–232.

McCollum EV, Davis M. The essential factors in the diet during growth. *J Biol Chem.* 1915; 23:231–254.

Muhilal, Tarwotjo I, Kodyat B, et al. Changing prevalence of xerophthalmia in Indonesia, 1977–1992. *Europ J Clin Nutr.* 1994;48:708–714.

Semba RD. Vitamin A as "anti-infective" therapy, 1920–1940. *J Nutr.* 1999;129:783–791.

Semba RD. Vitamin A and immunity to viral, bacterial and protozoan infections. *Proc Nutr Soc.* 1999;58:719–727.

Snell S. On nyctalopia with peculiar appearances on the conjunctiva. *Trans Ophthalmol Soc UK.* 1880– 1881;1:207–215.

Sommer A, West KP Jr. *Vitamin A Deficiency: Health, Survival, and Vision.* New York: Oxford University Press; 1996.

West KP Jr, Katz J, Khatry SK, et al. Double blind, cluster randomised trial of low dose supplementation with vitamin A or beta carotene on mortality related to pregnancy in Nepal. The NNIPS-2 Study Group. *BMJ.* 1999;318:570–575.

World Bank. *World Development Report 1993: Investing in Health.* New York: Oxford University Press; 1993.

CHAPTER 10

Amblyopia

Background

History

Probably the first known description of amblyopia and its treatment was given during the Dark Ages by Paulus Sextineus in AD 783. Its more modern description by Comte de Buffon in 1743 included the first description of the use of occlusion therapy. It is important to note that even during that primitive era the value of occlusion was recognized as being helpful in overcoming or ameliorating the condition, clearly separating it from other forms of visual impairment for which no treatment existed. In 1803, Erasmus Darwin, the grandfather of Charles, recommended the use of differing forms of occluders on the sound eye for differing levels of amblyopia. Its first mention in the English language literature displayed a clear indication of the level of sophistication of clinical thinking about the condition at that time:

> If the squinting has not been confirmed by long habit, and one eye be not much worse than the other, a piece of gauze stretched on a circle of whalebone, to cover the best eye in such a manner as to reduce the distinctness of vision of this eye to a similar degree of imperfection with the other, should be worn some hours every day, or the better eye should be totally darkened by a tin cup covered with black silk for some hours daily.

Buffon GL. Dissertation sur la Cause du Strabisme. Mem Acad Sciences pour 1743; 1748.
 Cited by Wilkenson O. *Strabismus: Its Etiology and Treatment.* St Louis: Mosby; 1927.
Darwin E. *Zoonomia, or the Laws of Organic Life.* 3rd ed. London: J Johnson; 1801.

Context

In the specialty of ophthalmology, practically none of the therapeutic modalities used to treat common eye conditions are the same as those in use 3 or even 2 decades ago. An almost unique exception to this is the use of occlusion therapy for the treatment of amblyopia. This might suggest that occlusion is a fully satisfactory therapy requiring no change or critical analysis. Clinicians who treat amblyopia in children (where it is most commonly detected), parents, and children themselves know otherwise. The truth is that there is no common agreement among clinicians as to the best way to treat amblyopia—even to the extent of questioning whether patching of the sound eye is the best way to treat the condition. A significant minority of clinicians eschew the patch and opt instead for the use of some form of blurring, optical or pharmacologic, to treat amblyopia. The situation presents a unique opportunity to determine the answer to the question in a systematic way by carrying out a randomized clinical trial, much as was done with diabetic retinopathy in the 1970s and 1980s and retinopathy of prematurity in the 1980s and 1990s.

The central theme of this chapter is to determine, based on available data, the answer to certain basic questions concerning our concepts of amblyopia and its treatment:

- What is the effect of occlusion of the dominant eye on the resolution of amblyopia in the nondominant eye?
- What risk factors influence that outcome?
- What can be said about the compliance with occlusion therapy of patients with amblyopia?
- What can be said about recidivism following successful occlusion therapy?

In providing answers to these questions, even approximate ones based on available hard data, it is hoped that, in addition to serving the fundamental purposes of this volume, a useful agenda for future research will emerge from the unanswered questions.

Epidemiology

Estimates of the incidence and prevalence of amblyopia vary in the range of 1%–2.5% in children. However, few are based on true prevalence and incidence studies. Many are institution-based, use small samples, and suffer from the biases inherent in such studies. Perhaps among the best today are four studies (Attebo et al, Chew et al, Dana et al, Krueger et al) of the causes of monocular vision deficit and blindness in true population-based studies.

>   Attebo K, Mitchell P, Smith W. Visual acuity and the causes of visual loss in Australia. The Blue Mountains Eye Study. *Ophthalmology.* 1996;103:357–364.
>   Chew E, Remaley NA, Tamboli A, et al. Risk factors for esotropia and exotropia. *Arch Ophthalmol.* 1994;112:1349–1355.
>   Dana MR, Tielsch JM, Enger C. Visual impairment in a rural Appalachian community: prevalence and causes. *JAMA.* 1990;264:2400–2405.
>   Dowling A. Ocular defects in sixty thousand selectees. *Arch Ophthalmol.* 1945;33:137–143.
>   Krueger D, Ederer F. Report on the National Eye Institute Visual Impairment Survey Pilot Study. Office of Biometry and Epidemiology. Bethesda: NIH/HHS; 1984.
>   Lennerstrand G, Jakobsson P, Kvarnstrom G. Screening for ocular dysfunction in children: approaching a common program. *Acta Ophthalmol Scand Suppl.* 1995:26–38.
>   Vereecken E, Feron A, Evens L. The importance of early detection of strabismus and amblyopia. [Article in French.] *Bull Soc Belge Ophtalmol.* 1966;143:729–739.
>   Vinding T, Gregerson E, Jensen A, et al. Prevalence of amblyopia in old people without previous screening and treatment: an evaluation of the present prophylactic procedures among children in Denmark. *Acta Ophthalmol (Copenh).* 1991;69:796–798.
>   Woodruf M. Vision and refractive error among grade 1 children of the province of New Brunswick. *Am J Optom Physiol Optics.* 1986;63:545–552.

Amblyopia is among the top three causes of monocular visual loss in the adult age group from 18 to 85 years. This is a disconcerting finding, as these are the ages where the bilateral diseases of the older ages—cataract, macular degeneration, diabetic retinopathy, glaucoma—take their toll. It suggests that the condition persists well beyond the childhood years, resistant to therapy and leaving its victims vulnerable to the abovementioned diseases in later life. It was this persistence of amblyopia despite treatment that led two British researchers to conclude that visual screening for amblyogenic factors (such as high refractive error, anisometropia, strabismus) was of little use, as the incidence of amblyopia was the same in a nonscreened school population as in a screened (and treated) one. Although this study, commissioned by the National Health Service of Great Britain, recommended that all current childhood screening programs for these amblyogenic factors be discontinued and new ones not undertaken, the policies have not been adopted in Great Britain. In the United States, a consensus conference on the value of preschool visual screening was held in 1998 under the combined auspices of the National Eye Institute and the Division of Maternal and Child Health of the US Public Health Service. Its recommendations included a qualified endorsement of an initiative to encourage vision screening of preschool children, with the caution that research and field trials of new and unproven screening technology be carried out before committing to countrywide screening.

>Hartmann EE, Dobson V, Hainline L, et al. Preschool vision screening: summary of a Task Force report. Behalf of the Maternal and Child Health Bureau and the National Eye Institute Task Force on Vision Screening in the Preschool Child. *Pediatrics.* 2000;106:1105–1116.
>Snowden S, Stewart-Brown S. Preschool vision screening. Health Technology Assessment. Vol 1(8). Oxford University Press; 1997.

Notable at this conference was the accord reached by representatives of the vision science community; the academies of ophthalmology, pediatrics, and optometry; organizations that support voluntary screenings, such as Prevent Blindness America; as well as commercial interests. It is hoped that careful field testing of newer technologies before wholesale adoption will lead to a more balanced outcome than either that suggested by the British initiative or the commercial huckstering that has accompanied the introduction of some new technologies with decidedly mixed results.

>Cooper CD, Bowling FG, Hall JE, et al. Evaluation of photoscreener instruments in a childhood population. 1. Otago photoscreener and Dortmans videophotorefractor. *Aust N Z J Ophthalmol.* 1996;24:347–355.
>Lee J, Adams G, Sloper J, et al. Future of preschool visual screening. Cost effectiveness of screening for amblyopia is a public health issue. *BMJ.* 1998;316:937–938.
>Rahi JS, Dezateux C. The future of preschool vision screening services in Britain [editorial]. *BMJ.* 1997;315:1247–1248.
>Simons BD, Siatkowski RM, Schiffman JC, et al. Pediatric photoscreening for strabismus and refractive error in a high-risk population. *Ophthalmology.* 1999;106:1073–1080.
>Tong PY, Enke-Miyazaki E, Bassin RE, et al. Screening for amblyopia in preverbal children with photoscreening photographs. National Children's Eye Care Foundation Vision Screening Study Group. *Ophthalmology.* 1998;105:856–863.
>Weinand F, Graf M, Demming K. Sensitivity of the MTI photoscreener for amblyogenic factors in infancy and early childhood. *Graefes Arch Clin Exp Ophthalmol.* 1998;236:801–805.

Economic Impact

There are few reliable data on the cost of treating amblyopia. A surrogate might be to identify the cost of screening for and detecting a single case of amblyopia in a child. Assuming that a screening test costs US$2 per child, a test with a sensitivity of 0.95 and a specificity of 0.90 (high for amblyopia screening tests), an incidence of 4%, and a cost of an eye examination by an eye professional at $100, the cost per correct referral would be $385. Such data indicate that although the cost is high compared with some of the costs of screening for less common afflictions (newborn phenylketonuria, for instance, where the cost of a positive case detected by screening is more than $10,000 per patient), it does not seem unreasonable.

Data on the duration of amblyopia therapy, although scant, suggest a median duration of 23 weeks.

> Flynn JT, Schiffman J, Feuer W, et al. The therapy of amblyopia: an analysis of the results of amblyopia therapy utilizing the pooled data of published studies. *Trans Am Ophthalmol Soc.* 1998;96:431–450.
>
> Gold MR, Siegel JE, Russell LB, et al, eds. *Cost-Effectiveness in Health and Medicine.* New York: Oxford University Press; 1996.
>
> Katz J, Tielsch J. Visual function and visual acuity in the Baltimore Eye Survey. *J Vis Impairment & Blindness.* 1996;90:367–377.
>
> Klein D. Spatial vision in amblyopia. In: Cronly-Dillon JR, ed. *Vision and Visual Dysfunction.* Vol 10B. Boca Raton, FL: CRC Press; 1991.

Success is inversely related to the duration of therapy: The shorter the duration, the more likely it is to be successful. Longer duration is associated with a less successful result, but that is often confounded with poor compliance and factors not related to the validity of the therapy. At the present time, it is impossible to determine reliably the cost–benefit or cost-effectiveness of amblyopia treatment. Clearly such a project is worth the effort in this cost-conscious era.

Some argue that it is not worth the effort and time to detect amblyopia, for, after all, we have two eyes. Would such an argument be given credence if applied to an acquired and treatable condition affecting the development of, for example, an arm? Suffice it to say that adults with amblyopia are well aware of the loss they have suffered, the burden they carry of having only one eye, and the regret of having very often been the agent of failure as a child to the therapy that might have restored a level of functional vision, had it been successful.

Pathogenesis

Perhaps the best definition of amblyopia available is that of Levi: "Amblyopia is a developmental defect of spatial vision, the chief symptom of which is loss of visual acuity." It is almost always associated with the presence of strabismus, anisometropia, a combination of both, or from deprivation early in life. The loss may be monocular or binocular. The emphasis in this definition is on "developmental defect," for the condition occurs during the cascade of events recent neuroscience and psychophysical studies have described as "visual development."

In contrast to the auditory system, where sound acuity thresholds are adult level at birth (after the external canals have been cleared of amniotic fluid), the visual system thresholds in a newborn are several log units below adult levels, in spite of optics that have 20/20 clarity. The auditory system is "hard wired" at birth. The visual system, although hard wired in its basic plan at birth, requires visual experience and especially the competitive interaction between the visual pathways of the two eyes in the visual cortex to develop adult levels of vision. As the study of the development of the visual nervous system has progressed in the last 2 decades, it has become clear that there are many critical periods. The concept of plasticity and continuing visual development over a long span of time has arisen to challenge the old orthodoxies. The best evidence is that a severe insult is required to produce a level of deprivation, such as that of a dense axial monocular cataract or corneal leukoma, that will lead to an irremediable defect in an eye's visual thresholds.

> Flynn J, Woodruff G, Thompson J, et al. The therapy of amblyopia; an analysis comparing the results of amblyopia therapy utilizing two pooled data sets. *Trans Am Ophthalmol Soc.* 1999;97:373–390.
>
> Hubel DH. *Eye, Brain, and Vision.* New York: Scientific American Library; 1988.

Clinical Presentation and Findings

Although a number of risk factors are associated with the development of amblyopia, three factors are by far the most common: strabismus, anisometropia, or both in an infant or child. Although the level of amblyopia may be difficult to quantitate in the nonverbal or preverbal child, the inability to hold fixation under binocular conditions, disproportionate resistance to the covering of one eye, and asymmetry of Teller acuity thresholds (not their absolute values) are good clues to its existence. In the verbal child, the task becomes easier, for acuity test objects such as picture naming, and beyond that, simple letter charts are available. Determining the vision of the amblyopic eye of the child is the most important part of the examination. It can give rise to confusing and often confounded findings. Determining visual acuity, which is central to the diagnosis, prognosis, and response to therapy, should not be relegated to an office assistant.

Several simple tests are worth doing as part of the examination of the visual function of the amblyopic eye. The first of these is testing the effect of "crowding" on visual acuity. In the clinical setting, single symbol acuity is significantly better than linear (lines of) acuity. Often it is tempting to simplify the task for the child by presenting symbols singly. There is nothing wrong with that, provided it is not relied on as the real threshold for form vision potential, which is best determined by presenting linear or, better, logMAR acuity symbols.

> Bailey IL, Lovie JE. New design principles for visual acuity letter charts. *Am J Optom Physiol Opt.* 1976;53:740–745.

Another is using the Neutral Density Filter Test (NDF). An NDF filter of 3 log units is placed before the suspected amblyopic eye and the vision remeasured. If the visual acuity is considerably worse—for example, a vision of 20/100 falls to hand motions or counting fingers—the likely cause is organic visual loss and not amblyopia. With amblyopia, the vision with the NDF stays the same (20/100 in the example) or even improves slightly. Hence, this simple office test is useful in differentiating organic visual loss from the functional visual loss characteristic of amblyopia.

> Ammann E. Einige beobachtung bei den funksprufing in der sprechstunde: "Zentrales" sehen–sehender glaukomatosen, sehen der amblyopie. *Klin Monatsbl Augenheilkd.* 1921; 67:564–573.
>
> Von Noorden G, Burian H. Visual acuity in normal and amblyopic patients under reduced illumination. *Am J Ophthalmol.* 1958;46:63.

Finally, the direct ophthalmoscope can be used to determine fixation in the amblyopic eye (most direct scopes come equipped with a fixation device built into the optics), particularly eccentric fixation in an older patient. It is a simple and useful test of prognostic significance, particularly if the fixation does not improve with patching.

Prevention

The literature on prevention of amblyopia is sparse and confusing. Ingram has published on the early detection of high refractive errors, particularly hyperopia and anisometropia, in children through school screening programs. He has reached the conclusion that it does not prevent amblyopia.

Others, however, with a smaller study group of children, have come to the conclusion that the early detection and treatment of high hyperopic (>3 D) refractive errors can prevent accommodative strabismus, one of the precursor conditions of amblyopia.

> Atkinson J, Braddick O, Robier B, et al. Two infant screening programmes: prediction and prevention of strabismus and amblyopia from photo- and videorefractive screening. *Eye.* 1996;10(Pt 2):189–198.
>
> Ingram RM. The problem of screening children for visual defects. *Br J Ophthalmol.* 1977; 61:4–7.
>
> Ingram RM, Walker C, Wilson JM, et al. A first attempt to prevent amblyopia and squint by spectacle correction of abnormal refractions from age 1 year. *Br J Ophthalmol.* 1985;69: 851–853.

Current Treatment Programs

Screening

Although population studies seem to raise questions about the utility of screening to reduce the prevalence of amblyopia, it is probably true that in our current state of knowledge we have no better way to detect children with one or more risk factors for amblyopia, on a population-wide basis. We do know that high-risk groups such as premature infants and the developmentally delayed are at high risk for amblyopia. To really advance our abilities in the area of preventive ophthalmology, photo screening and other technologies must prove themselves able to detect refractive risk factors and micro-misalignments prior to the onset of frank strabismus and amblyopia (if indeed they do precede them). The field today is limited by gaps in our current knowledge of the natural history of these proto-conditions prior to the onset of the conditions themselves. Such are the real constraints today on the prophylactic potential of early screening programs. Screening for the strabismic, refractive, and ocular diseases associated with amblyopia is on firmer empirical grounds. However, the lack of rigorous study of these methodologies' sensitivity and specificity in the diverse populations studied, as well as the lack of follow-up studies of compliance with referral, makes it difficult to draw precise conclusions as to the worth of these methods. Debate continues on the value of screening for amblyopia.

Treatment

No true randomized clinical trials of therapy with occlusion are reported in the literature. Although occulsion therapy is the accepted method of treatment for amblyopia, there is no agreement in the literature as to the type, total or partial; the extent; the duration; or the rules for stopping. Most current literature consists of reports of case series with well-recognized selection, publication, and other biases. A recent compilation pooling of data from 23 studies published over the last 30 years from seven different countries where the raw patient data were available was compared with a single study of a similar number of patients gathered in a single year from one country. It identified risk factors such as the age of the child at the start of treatment and the depth of amblyopia as strong predictors of the outcome of therapy. First-time occlusion therapy resulted in a successful outcome (success being defined as a visual acuity of 20/40, as it is in most studies) in about 65%–75% of these patients, independent of the type of amblyopia.

The probability of a successful outcome with occlusion therapy is given in Table 10-1. From the clinical standpoint, it was the large size of this sample ($n = 987$) that allowed the table to be developed. It employs the two major risk factors as parameters: anisometropia and strabismus. This had not been possible with the smaller sample sizes of previous published studies.

More recently, there has been investigation into the use of penalization therapy by optical or pharmacologic means, or combinations of these, to treat amblyopia. Several studies have found that penalization of the nonamblyopic eye with either atropine drops

Table 10-1 **Probability of Success of Amblyopia Therapy ($n = 987$)**

Pretherapy Acuity	Age Group 0–3	4–5	6–7	8–10
≥20/50	0.96	0.92	0.88	0.83
20/60	0.91	0.85	0.78	0.69
20/70	0.88	0.79	0.71	0.61
20/80	0.86	0.76	0.67	0.57
20/100	0.80	0.67	0.56	0.45
20/200	0.72	0.57	0.46	0.35
20/320	0.73	0.58	0.47	0.36
20/640	0.62	0.46	0.35	0.25
<20/640	0.64	0.47	0.36	0.27

or high plus or minus lenses is as effective as occlusion for moderate amblyopia (acuity ≥20/100). This may be related to the enhanced compliance when these methods are used. In the United States, a multicenter, randomized trial comparing atropine penalization with occlusion therapy for the treatment of moderate amblyopia has recently been completed. This study found that the modalities produced equivalent improvement in visual acuity in children with amblyopia with onset visual acuity of 20/40 to 20/100.

> A randomized trial of atropine vs. patching for treatment of moderate amblyopia in children. The Pediatric Eye Disease Investigator Group. *Arch Ophthalmol.* 2002;120:268–278.

Although studies on the outcome of amblyopia therapy by occlusion or penalization are legion, most do not address the issue of compliance with occlusion therapy in any meaningful way. This remains one of the most difficult problems in amblyopia management. Among the issues that need addressing is a definition of the term. What do we mean when we say a child has been compliant with therapy? Often we confuse the issue with success of therapy, but they are not the same. Conversely, the child who fails to respond to therapy is, ipso facto, felt to be noncompliant. Is that really the case? One of the real needs in this field is to apply modern technology to monitor time and appropriate application of occlusion. Such an approach will yield useful information on the whole series of interrelated questions revolving around the issue of compliance; it will enable us to separate true treatment failures from failures due to lack of compliance with therapy.

Recidivism

The data from the study comparing atropine penalization with occlusion therapy, cited in the previous section, suggest that the results of amblyopia therapy endure, particularly if a successful result has been attained. At the conclusion of therapy, when results have been successful (vision ≥20/40), 73% retained that vision for 1 year, 61% for 2 years, and 53% for 3 years (Fig 10-1) using Kaplan-Meier analysis, which adjusts for the length of follow-up after cessation of treatment. Although the numbers of individuals in the cohort diminishes at each of these dates, this method of analysis nevertheless provides the best estimate of how acuity diminishes over time in the cohort of successful results. The challenge for the future is to ensure that the results of the therapy remain durable over decades or the lifetime of the individual, rather than 1, 2, or 3 years.

Conclusion

Where should the field of clinical and basic research in amblyopia go in the future? A great deal of work needs to be done on the clinical side. A group of pediatric ophthalmologists has recently been organized in the United States to perform randomized clinical trials to determine which forms of occlusion work best in which type of amblyopia. Clearly one size does not fit all. Numerous questions deserving evidence-based answers around the topic of amblyopia easily lend themselves to clinical trials. For compliance and its monitoring, the work of Fielder and his colleagues points the way toward a better approach than we have now. Finally, on a more speculative level, the recent work of Tsien with gene insertion in a knockout mouse to enhance the function of Hebbian (learning)

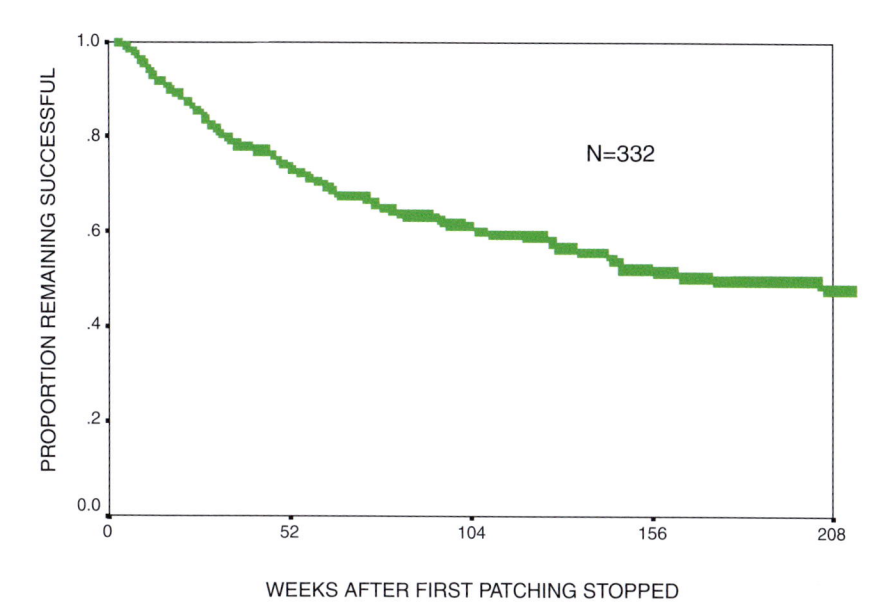

Figure 10-1 Recidivism after first patching. *(Courtesy of John T. Flynn, MD.)*

synapses in the central nervous system may provide, at some future date, a way to prevent the recidivism that occurs over time after successful patching.

Moseley MJ, Fielder AR. Future directions in treatment of amblyopia. *Lancet.* 1997;349: 1917–1918.

Tang YP, Shimizu E, Dube GR, et al. Genetic enhancement of learning and memory in mice. *Nature.* 1999;401:63–69.

CHAPTER 11

Ocular Trauma Epidemiology and Prevention

Background

Ocular trauma is a global health problem. Although preventable, trauma causes mortality, morbidity, and disability. In fact, ocular trauma is a leading cause of unilateral blindness worldwide. It is defined as the result of mechanical, electrical, thermal, or chemical energy damage to the eye. Unfortunately, greater effort and resources are being invested in the clinical and surgical management of ocular trauma than in its prevention. Too often, injury is considered to be an accident beyond the individual's control and not a public health problem. However, a growing number of physicians practice as if injury prevention is a realistic goal of health care. The possibilities for preventing trauma are numerous.

> Thylefors B. Epidemiological patterns of ocular trauma. *Aust N Z J Ophthalmol.* 1992;20: 95–98.

Compared to injury restoration and rehabilitation, prevention of injury is an opportunity to reduce morbidity, disability, and mortality, with significant savings in both financial and human terms. A prevention of injury strategy begins with collecting data and identifying risk factors to define the problem. Then a consensus is reached among those involved in the activity at all levels as to what that prevention strategy is. The strategy is then implemented. Changing behavior and adopting preventive measures often requires expanded community and government involvement. The media, newspapers, radio, and television are extremely important in creating awareness of the problem in the community and building demand for action. The final step is assessing the outcomes of measures adopted.

Context

The World Health Organization (WHO) Program for the Prevention of Blindness estimates that 55 million eye injuries occur globally each year. Of these, 750,000 require hospitalization and approximately 200,000 are open-globe injuries. The prevalence of blindness (<3/60 or <20/400) as a result of injury is about 1.6 million. There are 19 million with vision impairment.

> Négrel AD, Thylefors B. The global impact of eye injuries. *Ophthalmic Epidemiol.* 1998;5: 143–169.

Economic Impact

International cost estimates regarding eye injuries are rare, but in a 1989–1991 study in the state of Victoria, Australia, it was estimated that 31,000 eye injuries occurred at a cost of US$30.25 million and work-time totaling 147 work-years was lost at a cost of US$3.7 million. The social cost of eye trauma, the most common ophthalmic indication for hospitalization, is enormous. National projections estimate annual US hospital charges of US$175 million to $200 million for 227,000 eye trauma hospital-days. In the late 1980s, the eye injuries seen in 6 months in one emergency department were responsible for direct and indirect costs totaling US$5 million and a loss of 60 work-years.

> Fong LP, Taouk Y. The role of eye protection in work-related eye injuries. *Aust N Z J Ophthalmol.* 1995;23:101–106.
> Schein OD, Hibberd PL, Shingleton BJ, et al. The spectrum and burden of ocular injury. *Ophthalmology.* 1988;95:300–305.
> Tielsch JM, Parver LM. Determinants of hospital charges and length of stay for ocular trauma. *Ophthalmology.* 1990;97:231–237.

Over 1.2 million North American hockey players now wear face protectors when they play. They suffer 70,000 fewer eye and facial injuries than they would have were they not protected, with a savings to society of over US$10 million in medical bills yearly in 1980 US dollars.

> Vinger PF. Sports eye injuries: a preventable disease. *Ophthalmology.* 1981;88:108–113.

Ocular Trauma Terminology

Research and publication in international ocular trauma has been hampered by a lack of a common terminology. This problem has been addressed with a proposed international classification and terminology that has been widely endorsed (Fig 11-1 and Table 11-1).

> Kuhn F, Morris R, Witherspoon CD, et al. A standardized classification of ocular trauma. *Ophthalmology.* 1996;103:240–243.

Classification System for Mechanical Injuries of the Eye

The Ocular Trauma Classification Group has designed a standardized system for reporting mechanical injury characteristics of open- and closed-globe injuries. The purpose of this system is to aid in evaluating new treatment modalities and assessing patient outcomes. The system is based on four specific variables that influence the prognosis of final vision outcome:

- Type of injury
- Grade of injury based on visual acuity at initial examination
- Presence or absence of a relative afferent pupillary defect in the involved eye
- Zone of the injury

(See Tables 11-2 and 11-3.)

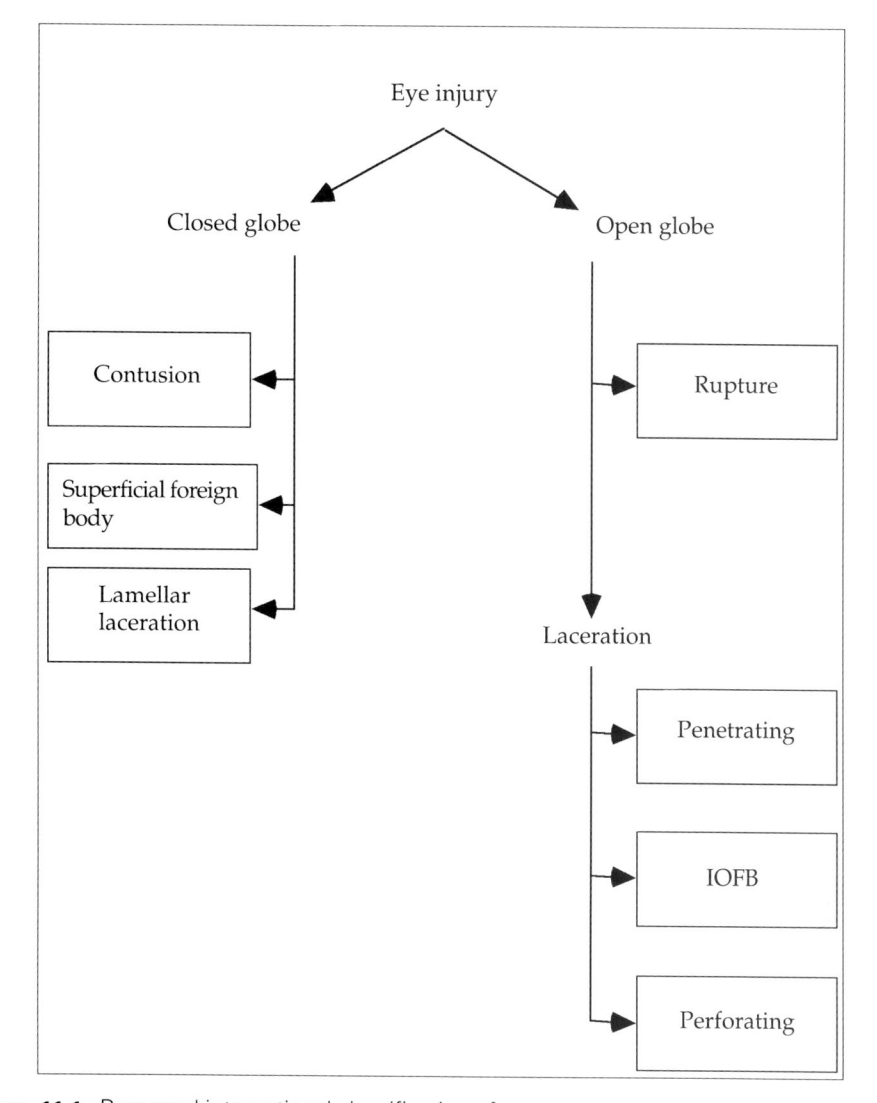

```
                              Eye injury
                           ↙           ↘
                   Closed globe       Open globe
                        │                 │
                   ┌─────────┐       ┌─────────┐
                   │Contusion│←      →│ Rupture │
                   └─────────┘       └─────────┘
                   ┌──────────────┐       │
                   │Superficial   │←      ↓
                   │foreign body  │   Laceration
                   └──────────────┘       │
                   ┌──────────┐           │
                   │Lamellar  │←      →┌────────────┐
                   │laceration│        │Penetrating │
                   └──────────┘        └────────────┘
                                       ┌────────────┐
                                      →│   IOFB     │
                                       └────────────┘
                                       ┌────────────┐
                                      →│Perforating │
                                       └────────────┘
```

Figure 11-1 Proposed international classification of eye trauma. *(Courtesy of Mylan VanNewkirk, MD.)*

Kuhn F, Morris R, Witherspoon CD, et al. A standardized classification of ocular trauma. *Graefes Arch Clin Exp Ophthalmol.* 1996;234:399–403.

Pieramici DJ, Sternberg P Jr, Aaberg TM Sr, et al. A system for classifying mechanical injuries of the eye (globe). The Ocular Trauma Classification Group. *Am J Ophthalmol.* 1997;123: 820–831.

The system divides the eye into three zones because of the differences in prognosis of full-thickness or open-globe injuries (Fig 11-2). Zone I injuries involve the cornea and/or the limbus. Zone II injuries involve the sclera posterior from the limbus to the pars plana, approximately 5 mm posterior to the limbus. Zone III injuries involve full-thickness scleral injuries more than 5 mm posterior to the limbus.

Table 11-1 Definitions of the Proposed Ocular Trauma Terms

Term	Definition	Remarks
Eyewall	Sclera and cornea	Though technically the wall of the eye has not one but three tunics (coats) posterior to the limbus, for clinical purposes it is best to restrict the term *eyewall* to the rigid structures of the sclera and cornea.
Closed-globe injury	The eyewall does not have a full-thickness wound.	Injury caused by blunt force (contusion), superficial foreign body, and partial-thickness sharp force (lamellar laceration)
Contusion	Closed-globe injury resulting from a blunt object	Injury can occur at the impact site, even though they eyewall remains intact, or at a distant site caused by deformity of the globe.
Superficial foreign body	Closed-globe injury usually caused by a projectile lodging in the conjunctiva or eyewall	The force of the impact may be blunt, sharp, or both.
Lamellar laceration	Closed-globe injury at the site of impact, usually caused by a sharp object	Partial-thickness defect of bulbar conjunctiva or eyewall
Open-globe injury	The eyewall has a full-thickness wound.	The cornea and/or sclera sustained a through-through injury. Depending on the inciting object's characteristics and the injury's circumstances, ruptures and lacerations are distinguished. The choroid and the retina may be intact, prolapsed, or damaged.
Rupture	Full-thickness wound of the eyewall caused by a blunt object. The impact results in momentary increase of the IOP (intraocular pressure) and an inside-out injury mechanism.	The eyewall gives way under blunt force at its weakest point, which may or may not be at the impact site. The actual wound is produced by an inside-out force; consequently, tissue is frequently herniated, often substantially.
Laceration	Full-thickness corneal and/or scleral wound caused by a sharp object	The wound (globe opening) occurs at the site of impact; pellet and BB injuries are included here although significant contusion damage coexists.
Penetrating injury	Single full-thickness laceration of the eyewall, usually caused by a sharp object	No exit wound has occurred.
Intraocular foreign-body (IOFB) injury	Retained foreign object/s causing entrance laceration/s	An IOFB is technically a penetrating injury but is grouped separately because of different clinical implications (treatment, prognosis).
Perforating injury	Two full-thickness lacerations	The two wounds (entrance and exit) of the eyewall are caused by the same agent (sharp object or missile).

Other important variables include the size or length of the wound, the presence of vitreous hemorrhage, involvement of the lens, and the presence of endophthalmitis. The size of the wound may not be as important as the location, so it is not included in the

Table 11-2 Open-Globe Injury Classification

Type or Mechanism of Injury	A. Rupture B. Penetrating C. Intraocular foreign body D. Perforating E. Mixed
Grade Based on Presenting Visual Acuity	1. ≥20/40 2. 20/50 to 20/100 3. 19/100 to 5/200 4. 4/200 to light perception 5. No light perception of bright light
Pupil	*Positive:* relative afferent pupillary defect present in injured eye *Negative:* relative afferent papillary defect absent in injured eye
Zone	I: Isolated to cornea; may include the limbus II: Corneoscleral limbus and up to 5 mm posterior in sclera III: Posterior sclera more than 5 mm posterior to limbus

(Reproduced with permission from Elsevier Science Inc. From Pieramici DJ, Sternberg P Jr, Aaberg TM Sr, et al. A system for classifying mechanical injuries of the eye (globe). The Ocular Trauma Classification Group. *Am J Ophthalmol.* 1997;123:829.)

Table 11-3 Closed-Globe Injury Classification

Type or Mechanism of Injury	A. Contusion B. Superficial foreign body C. Lamellar laceration D. Mixed
Grade Based on Presenting Visual Acuity	1. ≥20/40 2. 20/50 20/100 3. 19/100 to 5/200 4. 4/200 to light perception 5. No light perception of bright light
Pupil	*Positive:* relative afferent pupillary defect present in injured eye *Negative:* relative afferent pupillary defect absent in injured eye
Zone	I: External, bulbar conjunctiva, cornea, sclera II: Anterior segment, including posterior lens capsule and pars plicata III: Posterior segment past posterior lens capsule

(Reproduced with permission from Elsevier Science Inc. From Pieramici DJ, Sternberg P Jr, Aaberg TM Sr, et al. A system for classifying mechanical injuries of the eye (globe). The Ocular Trauma Classification Group. *Am J Ophthalmol.* 1997;123:830.)

classification. The presence of vitreous hemorrhage and involvement of the lens may not be easily assessed initially, so these variables are also not included. Endophthalmitis is a poor prognosticator but is rare at initial assessment.

Figure 11-2 Zones of injury in open-globe trauma. Zone I (yellow): wound involvement is isolated to the cornea. Zone II (red): full-thickness wound involves the sclera no more posteriorly than 5 mm from the corneoscleral limbus. Zone III (blue): full-thickness wound is posterior to zone II. *(Reproduced with permission from Elsevier Science Inc. From Pieramici DJ, Sternberg P Jr, Aaberg TM Sr, et al. A system for classifying mechanical injuries of the eye (globe). The Ocular Trauma Classification Group. Am J Ophthalmol. 1997;123:824.)*

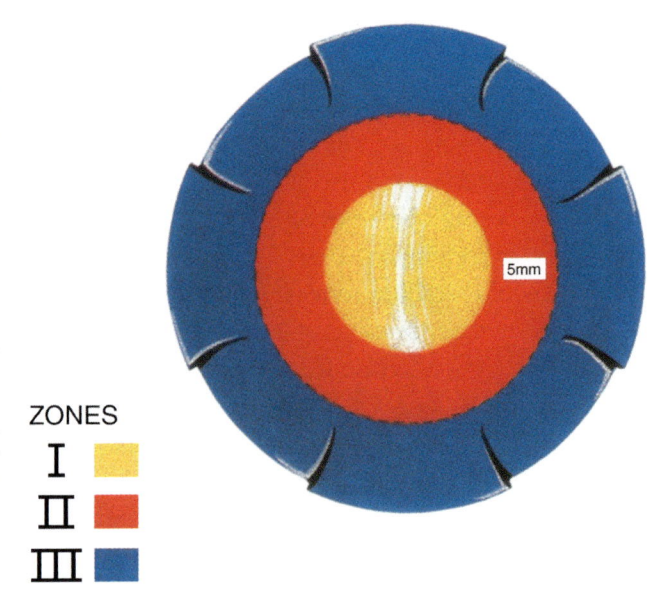

Refer to BCSC Section 12, *Retina and Vitreous,* for a discussion of open- and closed-globe injuries.

Ocular Trauma Epidemiology

Prevalence and Incidence

Although few truly comparable studies of the prevalence and incidence of ocular trauma exist, there are many reports of ocular trauma in the scientific literature that describe hospital data. These usually underestimate the number of minor injuries. Population-based data are infrequent but provide a better estimate of the occurrence of ocular trauma in communities and reduce the bias toward more serious ocular trauma that comes from hospital reports.

According to reports in the past decade, it is estimated that of the 1.6–2.4 million Americans who sustain eye injuries each year, 40,000 will be legally blinded in the injured eye. About one third of these injuries result from sports. Data from hospital discharge studies estimate the annual incidence of ocular injury in the United States to be 13.2 per 100,000 discharges. Similar observational studies of hospital data from four other continents are summarized in Table 11-4. An annual incidence rate is calculated using the number of eye injuries as the numerator and the defined local population during that period of time as the denominator. Although the studies summarized in Table 11-4 show a variety of rates, causes, and outcomes, each study found men to have a much higher risk of eye injuries than women.

Klopfer J, Tielsch JM, Vitale S, et al. Ocular trauma in the United States: eye injuries resulting in hospitalization, 1984 through 1987. *Arch Ophthalmol.* 1992;110:838–842.

Table 11-4 Hospital Ocular Trauma Studies

Location	Type of Study (n)	Annual Rate of Injury (per 100,000)	#1 Cause of Injury (%)	Gender, Age Group of Highest Rate	Gender Ratio M:W	Outcomes/ Comments
Dodoma, Tanzania[1]	Retrospective (157)	8.3	Sticks (67%)	Men, 60 years and older (52.2/100,000)	2.6:1	More than two thirds presented with >3/60 (>20/400) vision
Singapore[2]	Retrospective (2506)	12.6	Globe penetration	Men 20–29 years of age	4:1	Indian men affected at twice the rate of Chinese and Malayan men
Melbourne, Australia[3]	Prospective (9390)	15.2	Pounding metal on metal	Male auto workers		52 penetrating injuries occurred at work
Scotland[4]	Prospective (415)	8.14	Home (52%)	Men ages 15–34	9:1	9.1% were <3/60 (<20/400), and more than 66% were NLP

[1] Abraham DI, Vitale SI, West SI, et al. Epidemiology of eye injuries in rural Tanzania. *Ophthalmic Epidemiol.* 1999;6:85–94.
[2] Wong TY, Tielsch, JM. A.population-based study on the incidence of severe ocular trama in Singapore. *Am J Ophthalmol.*1999;128:345–351.
[3] Fong LP, Taouk Y. The role of eye protection in work-related injuries. *Aust N Z J Ophthalmol.* 1995;23:101–106.
[4] Desai P, MacEwen CJ, Baines P, et al. Incidence of cases of ocular trauma admitted to hospital and incidence of blinding outcome. *Br J Ophthalmol.* 1996;80:592–596.

Surveys usually provide a better estimate of minor eye injuries (Table 11-5). Comparable self-reporting methods were used to collect data on ocular injuries in the Baltimore Eye Survey (BES) and Visual Impairment Project (VIP), whereas the Nepal Survey required that signs of ocular trauma exist along with a history of eye injury. Extreme caution must be used when attempting to compare studies with major differences in methodology. In the VIP study, men in rural areas were more likely (42%) to have a history of eye injury than men in urban areas (31%). The rate of injury in white males was higher in the VIP study (34%) than it was among white males in the BES study (20%).

> Brilliant LB, Pokhrel RP, Grasset NC, et al. Epidemiology of blindness in Nepal. *Bull World Health Organ.* 1985;63:375–386.
>
> Katz J, Tielsch JM. Lifetime prevalence of ocular injuries from the Baltimore Eye Survey. *Arch Ophthalmol.* 1993;111:1564–1568.
>
> McCarty CA, Fu CL, Taylor HR. Epidemiology of ocular trauma in Australia. *Ophthalmology.* 1999;106:1847–1852.

Table 11-5 Population-Based Studies of Ocular Trauma

Location	Type of Study (n)	Annual Rate of Injury (per 100,000)	#1 Cause of Injury (%)	Gender, Age Group of Highest Rate	Gender Ratio M:W	Outcomes/ Comments
Nepal	Survey (39,887) all ages	860		55 years to 59 years		91 of 336 (27%) monocular blindness
VIP (Australia)	Survey (4735) ≥40 years	21,000	60% work-related	Rural men	3.4:1	12 (0.25%) monocular vision impairment
BES (USA)	Survey (5308) ≥40 years	14,400		22,000/ 100,000 black males		

Risk Factors

Childhood eye injuries are frequently serious penetrating injuries. A study of penetrating eye injuries in southern Turkey over a 5-year period included 242 children (175 boys and 67 girls). Most penetrating injuries occurred during unsupervised play on the streets. Metal caused one third of the penetrating injuries. No light perception was the outcome in over 20% of these injuries.

In a study of 33 monocular young people under 21 years of age, polycarbonate safety glasses were used following enucleation. One third of the sample wore protective eyewear all waking hours; 61% wore protective eyewear more than 80% of the time; and 85% of the sample wore protective eyewear more than 50% of the time. Nearly half of the participants in the study, 15 of 33, reported having at least one potentially serious eye injury prevented by the protective eyewear.

> Drack A, Kutschke PJ, Stair S, et al. Compliance with safety glasses wear in monocular children. *J Pediatr Ophthalmol Strabismus.* 1993;30:249–252.

The prognosis of ocular trauma is frequently related to the type of trauma and the location in the eye of the injury. In the 205 ocular trauma patients studied at the University of Nigeria, visual outcome was best in patients with mild nonpenetrating injuries and worst in those with penetrating injuries that involved the posterior segment.

> Soylu M, Demircan N, Yalaz M, et al. Etiology of pediatric perforating eye injuries in southern Turkey. *Ophthalmic Epidemiol.* 1998;5:7–12.
> Umeh RE, Umeh OC. Causes and visual outcome of childhood eye injuries in Nigeria. *Eye.* 1997;11(Pt 4):489–495.

Bilateral Ocular Injuries

Although most injuries affect one eye, certain types of eye injuries, such as chemical and blast injuries, are commonly bilateral. In an Ethiopian study of 94 patients with blast injuries, 30% involved both eyes, and 6 of these patients were blinded in both eyes.

> Zerihun N. Blast injuries of the eye. *Trop Doct.* 1993;23:76–78.

In a hospital-based study of blindness in northwestern Cambodia, bilateral trauma accounted for 17 of 453 cases of blindness (4%). Land-mine explosions blinded 14 of these patients, including 13 men between the ages of 15 and 35 years.

In a referral hospital study of ocular chemical injuries, two thirds occurred in young people working in laboratories and factories. Forty-three patients (42%) suffered bilateral injuries. Fifty-two eyes (35.9%) suffered severe (grade 3/4) injuries. Visual outcome correlated with severity of injury at initial presentation.

> Jackson H. Bilateral blindness due to trauma in Cambodia. *Eye.* 1996;10(Pt 4):517–520.
> Saini JS, Sharma A. Ocular chemical burns—clinical and demographic profile. *Burns.* 1993; 19:67–69.

Occupation

An important complication of corneal trauma is corneal infection caused by organisms from vegetative material. This is so common in warm agricultural areas of Southeast Asia and Africa (Madagascar) that this complication is known as rice-harvesting keratitis. Corneal scarring is second only to cataract as the major cause of blindness in many of the developing nations of Asia, Africa, and the Middle East. Rice, sugar cane, and bamboo are most commonly associated with the corneal trauma that precedes these secondary infections. Inadequate injury prevention and poor access to eye care are important factors in this problem. In 1994, a 3-month study of all infectious corneal ulcers seen at Aravind Eye Hospital (India) involved 434 patients. A more recent study revealed injury in 284 patients (65%). The majority of these patients were farm workers (56%) involved in rice or sugar cane farming. Cultures were positive in 297 patients (68%); bacteria and fungi were grown separately in nearly 33% and a mixed growth occurred in 3%. Thus corneal trauma is an important risk factor of corneal ulcers.

> Srinivasan M, Gonzales CA, George C, et al. Epidemiology and aetiological diagnosis of corneal ulceration in Madurai, south India. *Br J Ophthalmol.* 1997;81:965–971.
> Thylefors B, Négrel AD, Pararajasegaram R, et al. Available data on blindness (update 1994). *Ophthalmic Epidemiol.* 1995;2:5–39.

In Finland, a review of 662 hospital records was used to calculate a retrospective annual incidence of eye injuries by occupation: construction (5.28/10,000), agriculture (3.46/10,000), industry (1.9/10,000). Unilateral blindness was seen in 17 cases (17.7%), of which 6 occurred in agriculture from penetrating injuries and 5 in lumber. Alkali chemicals were the most frequent cause of eye injury in farming (6/10) and the most common cause of all chemical eye burns (6/7).

> Saari KM, Aine E. Eye injuries in agriculture. *Acta Ophthalmol Suppl.* 1984;161:42–51.

Cultural

A factor that may complicate treatment of eye injuries in Africa is the use of traditional medicines. Topically applied traditional medicines of plant juices, milk mixed with black powder, and/or pounded roots were used by 49% of the patients studied in Dar es Salaam.

Use of traditional medicines was found to be associated with more inflammation and a worse visual outcome.

> Mselle J. Visual impact of using traditional medicine on the injured eye in Africa. *Acta Trop.* 1998;70:185–192.

A case-control study design looking at socioeconomic status was used to identify the risk factors associated with presumed microbial keratitis in children. Fifty cases of fresh corneal ulceration in children aged 12 years or younger were compared with 50 controls. The study variables were age, gender, immunization status, nutritional status (weight for height), and socioeconomic status. Lower socioeconomic status was significantly associated with the occurrence of corneal ulceration. Corneal trauma (38%) and systemic illness (24%) were the most common predisposing factors.

> Vajpayee RB, Ray M, Panda A, et al. Risk factors for pediatric presumed microbial keratitis: a case-control study. *Cornea.* 1999;18:565–569.

Sport

Unfortunately, a significant number of athletes do not wear protective eyewear. In one study, warning information and placement of protective eyewear in close proximity to the players' court entrance improved the compliance and use of such eyewear.

> Hathaway JA, Dingus TA. The effects of compliance cost and specific consequence information on the use of safety equipment. *Accid Anal Prev.* 1992;24:577–584.

Protective eyewear does not interfere with visual function in sport. A study shows no significant difference in the results of visual field testing when standard kinetic visual fields were measured with and without protective eyewear in normal adult volunteers.

> Miller BA, Miller SJ. Visual fields with protective eyewear. *J Orthop Sports Phys Ther.* 1993; 18:470–472.

Data Collection

The Canadian Ophthalmological Society (COS) has collected data on ocular trauma since 1974 in a national prospective database.

The United States Eye Injury Registry, formed in 1988, is a federation of state registries that collects data, in a standardized manner, involving injuries resulting in a permanent and significant structural or functional ocular change. This type of eye injury registry is expanding internationally.

> Chisholm L, Crawford J. Letter: Eye injuries in hockey. *Can Med Assoc J.* 1974;111:501–502.
> Kuhn F, Mester V, Berta A, et al. Epidemiology of severe eye injuries. United States Eye Injury Registry (USEIR) and Hungarian Eye Injury Registry (HEIR). [Article in German.] *Ophthalmologe.* 1998;95:332–343.

Pathogenesis

Due to the complex nature of ocular trauma, pathogenesis and outcomes vary considerably, in part depending on the type of injury and the anatomical involvement. A Turkish military review of 228 eyes in 212 patients with open-globe ocular injuries applied the Ocular Trauma Classification Group's system to estimate visual outcome. The best predictors for a favorable visual outcome are injuries that fit the following criteria: type B (penetrating); grade 1, ≥20/40; negative afferent pupillary defect; zone I (open wound of the cornea or limbus). Of the 10 injuries graded type D (perforating), 77% resulted in an unfavorable outcome. All of the 25 injuries with grade 5 (NLP) had an unfavorable outcome. When the zone of injury was III (posterior to pars plana), 73% of the results were unfavorable.

> Sobaci G, Mutlu FM, Bayer A, et al. Deadly weapon-related open-globe injuries: outcome assessment by the ocular trauma classification system. *Am J Ophthalmol.* 2000;129:47–53.

Sport is an important cause of eye injuries. Badminton is played seriously in Southeast Asia and accounts for two thirds of all ocular injury from sports in Malaysia, including over 50% of hyphemas.

Boxing has long been associated with eye injuries. A case-control study of amateur boxers in Vienna found that 25 boxers and 25 age-matched controls had 20/20 visual acuity. Signs of contusion injury were observed in 19 (76%) of the boxers. These injuries most commonly involved the retina. The control group revealed only one participant (4%) with an atrophic retinal hole.

> Chandran S. Hyphaema and badminton eye injuries. *Med J Malaya.* 1972;26:207–210.
> Wedrich A, Velikay M, Binder S, et al. Ocular findings in asymptomatic amateur boxers. *Retina.* 1993;13:114–119.

Prevention Standards

The American Society for Testing and Materials is the jurisdictional body overseeing a majority of sports eyewear standards. The best sports standards are performance standards that specify how a protector must perform (eg, visual fields, impact resistance, distribution of forces) rather than design standards that contain certain design elements that may or may not relate to performance.

Little is known about the efficacy of protective eyewear in shotgun injuries. Shotguns can easily propel pellets with enough energy to penetrate the human eye at ranges exceeding 40 yd. Although polycarbonate is known to be the best lens material for shotgun eye protection, little is known about the most effective design parameters of the protective system that keeps the polycarbonate securely over the eye. The most protective eyewear design includes side shields and a headband with polycarbonate lenses.

> Varr WF 3d, Cook RA. Shotgun eye injuries: ocular risk and eye protection efficacy. *Ophthalmology.* 1992;99:867–872.

An excellent example of identifying an ocular trauma problem and developing a prevention strategy in sports comes from youth ice hockey in Canada. Dr. T.J. Pashby, a Canadian ophthalmologist, has been intimately involved in this success story and was motivated to prevent ice hockey eye injuries by the success of the compulsory industrial safety eyewear program reported by Dr Novak in steel plants in Pittsburgh, Pennsylvania (Table 11-6).

Table 11-7 describes the eye injuries recorded by members of the Canadian Ophthalmological Society.

These data clearly define a problem. During the 1974 ice hockey season, the Canadian Amateur Hockey Association (CAHA) rescinded a rule prohibiting use of a face protector without a physician's order and enacted a rule allowing face protectors to be worn. The use of face protectors attached to helmets increased and demand exceeded supply. In another significant step to safeguard vision, the CAHA ruled to exclude participation of players or officials having vision in only one eye.

In January 1976, questionnaires were sent to the 12 districts of the CAHA regarding the use and type of face protectors in each district. Responses came from 20,026 players, who revealed that 26% wore helmets with face protectors (15% polycarbonate and 11% wire mesh). The next action by the Canadian Ophthalmological Society committee concerning eye injuries in hockey was encouraging the CAHA to adopt a high-sticking penalty. Additional data regarding the serious nature of eye injuries was published, revealing that 33 of 250 retinal detachments secondary to contusion of the globe (13.2%) were secondary to hockey. Despite surgery, 42.4% of these eyes became legally blind.

> Antaki S, Labelle P, Dumas J. Retinal detachment following hockey injury. *Can Med Assoc J.* 1977;117:245–246.

During the 1977–1978 hockey season, 51 eye injuries occurred among players, with 8 eyes becoming legally blind. The next season, 42 eye injuries occurred, with 12 eyes becoming legally blind. Only 1 of the 20 eyes severely injured during these two seasons occurred in players wearing face protectors, and that one was a goalie using a molded mask. Today, all goal-tenders must wear CSA (Canadian Standards Association)-approved wire mesh protectors. In 1979, the CSA-approved face protectors attached to CSA-approved helmets were made mandatory in the CAHA and in minor youth league hockey in the United States. In the 1991–1992 Canadian ice hockey season, 28 eye injuries

Table 11-6 Chronology of Eye Protection Success

Year	Eye Protection Worn	Number of Disabling Eye Injuries/Million Working Hours
1953	None	17.8
1954	Voluntary	9.2
1958	Voluntary	7.0
1960	Compulsory	0.26
1975	Compulsory	0.5
1980	Compulsory	0

(Data from Dr Novak adapted from Pashby TJ. Eye protection. *Can Fam Physician.* 1986;32:1491–1496.)

Table 11-7 Eye Injuries in Hockey

	1972–1973	1974–1975	1977–1979
Total	287	253	93
Due to stick		63%	
Due to puck	19%	29%	
Total days in hospital	996	899	
Resulting in ≤20/200	39 (14%)	42 (16%)	20 (22%), but only 1 where player wore face protection

(From Pashby TJ, Pashby RC, Chisholm LD, et al. Eye injuries in Canadian hockey. *Can Med Assoc J.* 1975;113:663–674.)

occurred, with 7 resulting in vision that was less than 20/200. These blinding injuries occurred in older players with an age range of 29 to 45 years. None occurred in a player wearing a CSA-approved face protector or visor.

Eye and face injuries accounted for two thirds of all injuries in ice hockey before the introduction of mandatory eye and face protection in play sponsored by schools, colleges, and amateur hockey associations. The widespread use of these protective devices has virtually eliminated eye and face injuries to protected players, while keeping fun and appeal in the game. Dr Pashby has remained an advocate of protective eye wear in sport and has worked diligently to prevent avoidable ocular injury. It is hoped that the Pittsburgh steel plant and Canadian hockey models can be applied to eye injuries in other sports and occupations, with rapid adoption and increasing safety.

Pashby TJ. Eye injuries in Canadian amateur hockey. *Am J Sports Med.* 1979;7:254–257.
Pashby TJ. Eye injuries in Canadian hockey. Phase III: older players now most at risk. *Can Med Assoc J.* 1979;121:643–644.
Pashby TJ. Eye injuries in Canadian sports and recreational activities. *Can J Ophthalmol.* 1992;27:226–229.

Prevention of Eye Injuries in Auto Accidents

Seat belt legislation may have resulted in prevention of eye injuries in Japan and Germany. In Japan, a 12% reduction in the rate of ocular injuries in traffic accidents occurred after the 1986 introduction of seat belt legislation. A German study compared hospital data of 384 people with perforating ocular injuries during the years 1981–1983 and 1987–1989. The number of occupational injuries were unchanged, but of 39 injuries to women, 17 (43%) were related to traffic accidents in 1981–1983 as opposed to only 1 of 16 injuries (6%) in 1987–1989. Perforations during traffic accidents declined from 26% (52 of 199) to 11% (19 of 170), and this decline may be related to seat belt legislation that passed in 1984, as well as to the requirement that auto manufacturers use impact-resistant windscreen glass.

Schrader W. Perforating injuries: causes and risks are changing. A retrospective study. *Ger J Ophthalmol.* 1993;2:76–82.
Yamamoto M, Uchio E, Kohno T, et al. Statistical study of ocular injuries—effect of the seat belt legislation in traffic ocular injuries. *Nippon Ganka Gakkai Zasshi.* 1993;97:122–126.

Data are accumulating on the spectrum of airbag ocular injuries; these range from minor trauma with complete resolution to severe injuries resulting in total loss of vision. Early estimates indicate that one quarter of ocular injuries are bilateral.

> Lee WB, O'Halloran HS, Pearson PA, et al. Airbags and bilateral eye injury: five case reports and a review of the literature. *J Emerg Med.* 2001;20:129–134.

Prevention Educators

The most effective health and injury prevention educators may be peers of the target audience. In a study measuring significant change in cognitive aspects of eye health relating to vitamin A deficiency and ocular trauma among primary school students, the greatest cognitive change occurred when their peers functioned as health educators.

> Murthy GV, Verma L, Ahuja S. Evaluation of an innovative school eye health educational mode. *Indian Pediatr.* 1994;31:553–557.

Conclusion

Ocular trauma is a major cause of monocular vision impairment throughout the world. Comparative studies of ocular injury are limited, in part, by a failure to use common definitions and terminology. The epidemiology and important risk factors of ocular trauma provide valuable assistance in developing a preventive strategy. Essential principles of eye injury prevention include:

- Recognition of the problem
- Collection of data
- Development of performance standards for protective eyewear (visual fields, impact resistance, distribution of forces, comfort and style) and vehicular safety devices
- Quality control to ensure that products are manufactured to these standards
- Development of public support and education to ensure widespread use of eyewear protection
- Collection of outcome data to measure the effect

Application of these strategies can prevent eye injuries and the morbidity and economic losses associated with them. An excellent illustration is the successful campaign engineered by the Canadian Ophthalmological Society to prevent ocular injuries in ice hockey.

PART III

The Prevalence, Causes, and Prevention of Adult Vision Impairment

Introduction

Allen Foster of the International Agency for the Prevention of Blindness (IAPB) estimates that the number of people in the world who are vision impaired (<20/400) has increased from 30 million in 1980 to approximately 50 million today and projects that the total could be 75 million by 2020. Age is associated with an increase in the prevalence of adult blindness; in the developing world, where over 80% of the blind reside, vision impairment is observed at an earlier age than in the developed world.

In Part III, we present details on the magnitude and leading causes of preventable vision impairment in adults. Although comparable worldwide data on prevalence and the leading causes of vision impairment are limited, Dr R. Klein and I make an attempt at a global view of the subject. Dr Dandona addresses uncorrected refractive error, the leading cause of vision impairment in the developed as well as the developing world. Dr West describes the epidemiology of cataract and suggests that as much as a quarter of all cataract surgery could be avoided if smoking and diabetes were eliminated. Drs Nemesure and Leske and Ms Wu review the epidemiology and emphasize the ethnic differences observed in primary open-angle glaucoma (POAG), including data from their excellent studies in Barbados. Mr Foster addresses the important problem of primary angle-closure glaucoma (PACG) and shares research data on diagnosis and prevention. PACG is a significant disease in Asia. Finally, Drs Blankenship and Stefánsson join with me in reporting Iceland's success in applying the findings from published clinical diabetes trials and surveys.

Although the management of POAG is somewhat controversial, the management and potential favorable outcome are quite good for the other diseases discussed in Part III. In most parts of the world with accessible technology, success can be achieved in the ophthalmic treatment of uncorrected refractive error, cataract, PACG, and diabetic retinopathy. Economic and social rewards await efforts to screen for and treat these diseases.

Mylan VanNewkirk, MD

CHAPTER 12

Prevalence and Common Causes of Vision Impairment in Adults

Background

History

The study of eye diseases that cause vision impairment is an evolving science. Sorsby used a registry to compile and report the incidence and causes of blindness in England and Wales for the period of 1948 through 1962. However, a registry tends to underestimate the true prevalence in the population because it represents only those members of the population on the list.

> Sorsby A. The incidence and causes of blindness in England and Wales 1948–1962. Report on public health and medical subjects. No. 114. London: HMSO; 1966.

In 1978, the World Health Organization (WHO) established the Programme for the Prevention of Blindness, and its task force developed an epidemiologic model for estimating blindness using a simplified, low-cost field survey methodology. The major weakness in such an approach is that it does not include refraction, indirect ophthalmoscopy, photography, and visual fields. In 1987, the WHO, using surveys, estimated that 27–35 million people in the world had profound vision impairment (<20/400) and that approximately 75%–80% of those resided in Asia and Africa. A conservative estimate of worldwide childhood blindness was estimated to be 1 million children.

Using that estimate, the prevalence of adult blindness in the world would have been approximately 26–34 million. More recently, the WHO estimated that 135 million people worldwide are vision impaired (<20/60) and nearly 45 million persons have profound vision impairment (<20/400). The numbers are increasing as world population and the average life expectancy increase.

> Foster A, Johnson GJ. Magnitude and causes of blindness in the developing world. *Int Ophthalmol.* 1990;14:135–140.
>
> Thylefors B, Négrel AD, Pararajasegaram R, et al. Global data on blindness. *Bull World Health Organ.* 1995;73:115–121.

Context

Because it is impractical if not impossible to examine every member of a population, epidemiologic tools have been developed to examine a representative sample of a population. Refer to Chapter 4 of this volume and to BCSC Section 1, *Update on General Medicine*.

Surveys measure the prevalence of disease in a specified population. The *prevalence* is the number of people who have the condition in a specific population at a point in time divided by the total number of that population at that specific time. Often prevalence is presented as a rate within the study population and is not extrapolated to the population as a whole. Knowledge of the distribution and prevalence of eye diseases, causes of vision impairment, and associated risk factors is essential to facilitate appropriate eye health care planning in both therapy and prevention.

Importance of Complete Eye Examinations in Eye Disease Surveys

In India, a 1992 report of an eye disease study by the National Programme for Control of Blindness (NPCB) stated that cataract caused 60.8% of blindness. However, this study did not include dilated detailed fundus examination or visual field testing in its methodology. Table 12-1 compares the causes of blindness in the national study with those in the Andhra Pradesh Eye Disease Study (APEDS), which included dilated detailed fundus examination, fundus photography, and visual field testing. The results differ dramatically and may underscore the importance of diagnostic accuracy in assigning causes of vision impairment.

Factors Influencing the Causes of Vision Impairment

Accessibility, utilization, and quality of eye-care services impact eye disease prevalence data in communities, especially in the area of preventable blindness caused by cataract, diabetic retinopathy, and glaucoma. In combination with these health care delivery issues, environmental, educational, and geographic factors influence infectious and nutritional causes of

Table 12-1 Comparing Causes of Blindness

Cause	NPCB Methods Percent of Vision Impairment <3/60	APEDS Methods Percent of Vision Impairment <3/60 or <10° Visual Field
Cataract	60.8	34.3
Retinal disease	6.3	22.4
Corneal disease	23.6	20.1
Glaucoma	0	15.2
Optic atrophy	7.4	6.4
Trauma	1.9	1.6

(From Dandona L, Dandona R, Naduvilath TJ, et al. Is current eye-care policy focus almost exclusively on cataract adequate to deal with blindness in India? *Lancet*. 1998;351:13112–1316; and Mohan M. Survey of blindness, India (1986–89): summary and results. In: Directorate General of Health Services, Ministry of Health and Family Welfare, Government of India. *Present Status of National Programme for Control of Blindness (NPCB) 1992*. New Delhi: Government of India; 1992:79–100.)

blindness. Onchocerciasis, trachoma, and vitamin A deficiency are significant causes of blindness in some parts of the world. Developed countries show a pattern of causes of visual loss due to eye disease primarily related to age, whereas the developing countries have a much higher rate of visual loss due to infectious and nutritional causes. Also, typically age-related cataract occurs at an earlier age in developing countries. Significant ethnic and racial patterns exist in ocular disease—for example, angle-closure glaucoma occurs most often in Mongolians, Chinese, Eskimo, and Inuit populations; primary open-angle glaucoma occurs often in blacks; and age-related macular degeneration is a common disease of both blacks and whites.

Comparison of Eye Disease Studies

Comparing eye diseases in different ethnic populations around the world using similar methodology is an important approach in expanding knowledge of these diseases. Unfortunately, few comparable studies of eye disease prevalence exist for the developing world.

As populations in various parts of the globe undergo shifts in socioeconomic status, physical activity, and age distribution, the problem of decreased vision imposes individual limitations and social needs because of loss of independence and increased health care costs. This has resulted in the need for epidemiologic information regarding the prevalence and incidence of common eye diseases and their associated risk factors. Because population-based data are costly and difficult to obtain, most of the earlier data collected on age-related macular degeneration and diabetic retinopathy were from clinical case series. Such studies are affected by selection processes, whether self-selection or based on sociodemographic factors. In the past 2 decades, data from a number of population-based studies have become available. Despite the availability of these new data describing the prevalence and incidence of diabetic retinopathy and age-related macular degeneration, however, precise comparable estimates of rates of these conditions in various ethnic groups remain limited for a number of reasons.

Comparisons of the prevalence of diabetic retinopathy among different ethnic groups, for example, may be limited by differences in time of and criteria used for diagnosing the diabetes, levels of glycemic control prior to study, and selective mortality. These concerns may differentially affect ethnic groups in the same study, leading to inaccurate rates and to possibly spurious differences in the rates and in associations of risk factors with the disease among the groups.

> Harris MI, Klein R, Cowie CC, et al. Is the risk of diabetic retinopathy greater in non-Hispanic blacks and Mexican Americans than in non-Hispanic whites with type 2 diabetes? A U.S. population study. *Diabetes Care.* 1998;21:1230–1235.
> Klein R. Epidemiology. In: Berger JW, Fine SL, Maguire MG, eds. *Age-related Macular Degeneration.* St. Louis: Mosby; 1999:31–55.
> Klein R, Klein BE, Cruickshanks KJ. The prevalence of age-related maculopathy by geographic region and ethnicity. *Prog Retin Eye Res.* 1999;18:371–389.
> Klein R, Klein BEK. Vision disorders in diabetes. In: Harris MI, Cowie CC, Stern MP, et al, eds. *Diabetes in America.* 2nd ed. NIH Publication No. 95–1468. Washington, DC: National Institutes of Health; 1995:chap 14, 293–338.

It has also been difficult to attain uniformity and precision of diagnostic procedures, especially prior to the advent of accepted classification schemes and severity scales. The presence of subtle and early lesions of macular degeneration may, for example, be difficult to define and to identify. Photography, although not flawless, permits standard images and protocols for evaluation to be applied uniformly, thus eliminating some of the concern about uniformity of diagnostic criteria.

> Bird AC, Bressler NM, Bressler SB, et al. An international classification and grading system for age-related maculopathy and age-related macular degeneration. The International ARM Epidemiological Study Group. *Surv Ophthalmol.* 1995;39:367–374.
>
> Fundus photographic risk factors for progression of diabetic retinopathy. ETDRS report number 10. Early Treatment of Diabetic Retinopathy Study Research Group. *Ophthalmology.* 1991;98(suppl 5):823–833.
>
> Klein R, Davis MD, Magli YL, et al. The Wisconsin age-related maculopathy grading system. *Ophthalmology.* 1991;98:1128–1134.

When comparing studies of eye disease, particularly studies of age-related macular degeneration and diabetic retinopathy, it is important to assess the following:

- Differences in any time period of data collection
- Participation rates and possible biases, resulting in varying participation by different racial/ethnic groups
- Differences in obtaining the data (eg, for fundus photography: type of film, whether stereoscopic images were obtained, number of fields, fluorescein angiography)
- Specifically defined classification systems used to determine the presence and severity of lesions

Examples of concerns that might arise in studies of various ethnic and racial groups of age-related maculopathy and diabetic retinopathy are described in several references.

> Cruickshanks KJ, Hamman RF, Klein R, et al. The prevalence of age-related maculopathy by geographic region and ethnicity. The Colorado-Wisconsin Study of Age-related Maculopathy. *Arch Ophthalmol.* 1997;115:242–250.
>
> Klein R, Clegg L, Cooper LS, et al. Prevalence of age-related maculopathy in the Atherosclerosis Risk in Communities Study. *Arch Ophthalmol.* 1999;117:1203–1210.
>
> Klein R, Klein BE, Jensen SC, et al. Age-related maculopathy in a multiracial United States population. The National Health and Nutrition Examination Survey III. *Ophthalmology.* 1999;106:1056–1065.
>
> Smith W, Assink J, Klein R, et al. Risk factors for age-related macular degeneration: pooled findings from three continents. *Ophthalmology.* 2001;108:697–704.

Economic Impact

The cost of vision impairment includes health care consumables and delivery costs, the loss of productivity caused by disability, and the cost to families and society in terms of time and support. All eye disease prevalence studies have demonstrated an increasing prevalence of eye diseases with age. Knowing the distribution and determinants of the prevalence and the associated risk factors are vitally important in health care planning.

In all countries, significant increases in health care infrastructure, consumable resources, and personnel will be required to deal with the increasing demand for eye care as populations age. Logic dictates that a balance be established between increasing therapeutic services and expanding the prevention of blindness. Prevention of blindness has been established to be cost-effective and a major socioeconomic benefit to the community.

Definitions of Blindness

It is difficult to compare many prevalence studies of vision impairment because of the many definitions of blindness that are used. The WHO encountered 67 different definitions for the term during an attempt to compare rates of blindness among different countries. Because vision impairment can be caused by a reduction of visual acuity and/or visual field, it is logical to include measures of both in its definitions. See Chapter 4 of this volume.

Comparable Studies

This chapter compares the prevalence of vision impairment in adults found in eye disease surveys that have used similar methodologies. Population-based studies depend on the methods of data collection and the accuracy of parameter measurement to reduce random and systematic errors. Comparability with other studies depends on common definitions and measurement methods. Selected surveys and participation rates are shown in Table 12-2. The validity and applicability of a population-based study depends on a high response rate. Even though these population-based surveys are usually planned with specified sampling fractions, participation rates have often ranged from 55% to 85%, making it difficult to define biases associated with nonparticipation, which may influence estimated rates.

Prevalence of Profound and Severe Vision Impairment

Table 12-3 shows a wide range in the prevalence of profound vision impairment (<20/400 visual acuity and/or <5° visual field), from 0.16% in the Visual Impairment Project to 2.23% in the Andhra Pradesh Eye Disease Study, in spite of the inclusion of younger participants and a small difference in visual field criteria in the latter. The Visual Impairment Project rate does not include the 403 participants from the institutional cohort, which had an age-standardized profound vision impairment rate of 5.2%. Although inclusion of this cohort increases the overall Visual Impairment Project rate slightly, to 0.18%, the data may reflect a difference in ocular disease among the people of the states of Victoria, Australia, and Andhra Pradesh, India. Ethnic differences in eye disease and resource utilization may be reflected by the differences in rates of profound vision impairment between the white populations and black populations studied in Maryland (Baltimore Eye Survey, Salisbury Eye Evaluation Study) and Barbados (Tables 12-3, 12-4).

The rate of severe visual impairment reported in the Andhra Pradesh study is higher than the rates found in all of the predominantly white populations studied—for example,

Table 12-2 Comparable Studies

Study	Region/Country	Participation Rate (%)
Baltimore Eye Survey[1]	Maryland, US	79
Salisbury Eye Evaluation Study[2]	Maryland, US	66
Beaver Dam Eye Study[3]	Wisconsin, US	83
Barbados Eye Study[4]	Barbados, West Indies	84
Rotterdam Eye Study[5]	The Netherlands	77
Oulu Study[6]	Finland	89
Casteldaccia Eye Study[7]	Sicily, Italy	67
Sofia Study[8]	Western Bulgaria	98
Andhra Pradesh Eye Disease Study[9]	Andhra Pradesh, India	85
Visual Impairment Project[10]	Victoria, Australia	86

[1] Sommer A, Tielsch JM, Katz J, et al. Racial differences in the cause-specific prevalence of blindness in east Baltimore. *N Engl J Med*. 1991;325:1412–1417.
[2] Muñoz B. West SK, Rubin GS, et al. Causes of blindness and visual impairment in a population of older Americans: The Salisbury Eye Evaluation Study. *Arch Ophthalmol*. 2000;118:819–825.
[3] Klein R, Klein BE, Linton KLP, et al. The Beaver Dam Eye Study: visual acuity. *Ophthalmology*. 1991;98:1310–1315.
[4] Hyman L, Wu SY, Connell AM, et al. Prevalence and causes of visual impairment in the Barbados Eye Study. *Ophthalmology*. 2001;108:1751–1756.
[5] Klaver CC, Wolfs RC, Vingerling JR, et al. Age-specific prevalence and causes of blindness and visual impairment in an older population: the Rotterdam Study. *Arch Ophthalmol*. 1998;1116:653–658.
[6] Hirvelä H, Laatikainen L. Visual acuity in a population aged 70 years or older; prevalence and causes of visual impairment. *Acta Ophthalmol Scand*. 1995;73:99–104.
[7] Ponte F, Giuffrè G, Giammanco R. Prevalence and causes of blindness and low vision in the Casteldaccia Eye Study. *Graefes Arch Clin Exp Ophthalmol*.1994;232:469–472.
[8] Vassileva P, Gieser SC, Vitale S, et al. Blindness and visual impairment in western Bulgaria. *Ophthalmic Epidemiol*. 1996;3:143–149.
[9] Dandona L, Dandona R, Naduvilath TJ, et al. Is current eye-care policy focus almost exclusively on cataract adequate to deal with blindness in India? *Lancet*. 1998;351:1312–1316.
[10] VanNewkirk MR, Weih L, McCarty CA, et al. Cause-specific prevalence of bilateral visual impairment in Victoria, Australia: the Visual Impairment Project. *Ophthalmology*. 2001;108:960–967.

Table 12-3 Prevalence of Profound Vision Impairment (<3/60 [6/120] and/or ≤5° Visual Field)

Study	Year	Age (Years)	n	Rate (%)	95% CI
Visual Impairment Project	1996	40–101	4744	0.16	(0.056, 0.26)
Casteldaccia Eye Study	1992	≥40	1068	0.47[†]	
Sofia Study	1994	≥40	6275	0.49	
Rotterdam Eye Study	1993	≥55	6775	0.5*	
Baltimore Eye Survey	1988	≥40	2395 blacks	1.02[†]	
			2913 whites	0.43[†]	
Barbados Eye Study	1992	40–84	4631	1.7[†]	
Oulu Study	1991	≥70	500	1.9[†]	
Andhra Pradesh Eye Disease Study	1997	≥30	1399	2.23*	(1.17, 3.29)

* = visual field criteria <10°, [†] = no visual field category

Table 12-4 Prevalence of Severe Vision Impairment (< 20/200 and/or <10° Visual Field)

Study	Year	Age (Years)	n	Rate (%)	95% CI
Beaver Dam Eye Study	1990	43–86	4926	0.5*	
Visual Impairment Project	1996	40–101	5147	0.53	(0.32, 0.74)
Rotterdam Eye Study	1993	≥55	6775	0.75	
Salisbury Eye Evaluation Study	1994	65–84	1853 whites	0.5*	(0.3, 1.0)
			666 blacks	1.7*	(0.8, 3.0)
Baltimore Eye Study	1988	≥40	2395 blacks	1.75*	
			2913 whites	0.76*	
Andhra Pradesh Eye Disease Study	1997	≥30	1399	3.5†	(1.95, 4.21)

* = ≤20/2200, † presenting visual acuity and visual field = <20°

the Baltimore Eye Survey and Salisbury Eye Evaluation Study white groups, the Rotterdam Eye Study, Beaver Dam Eye Study, and the Visual Impairment Project. Overlap probably occurs with the 95% confidence interval (CI) in the Andhra Pradesh study data and the prevalence observed in the black populations of the Barbados, Baltimore, and Salisbury eye studies (see Tables 12-3 and 12-4). The rate in the Oulu Study may appear high, but this study includes people 70 years of age and older, which is not different from age-specific rates of most other studies.

A difference in severe vision impairment is shown in Table 12-4, where only the black groups in the Baltimore and Salisbury studies appear to overlap with the Andhra Pradesh rates.

Age as a Major Risk Factor

The age-specific rates of profound vision impairment in all the major studies increase with age, with the exception of the Baltimore study's black rate (Fig 12-1). In Figure 12-1, the Casteldaccia Eye Study of Sicily reported rates of profound vision impairment in age groups 70 years and 75 years that were similar to rates observed in the other studies at age 80 years and older.

In addition to the higher rates of profound vision impairment observed in the Andhra Pradesh study, 17.8% of the impaired were in the 30–39 years' age group. Rates of severe vision impairment in this study showed an increase by age group beginning in the 50 years' age group: 30–39 years, 1.3%; 40–49 years, 1.3%; 50–59 years, 4.2%; 60–69 years, 6.5%; ≥70 years, 15.8%. Figure 12-2 illustrates the increase in age-specific rates of severe vision impairment in the US (Beaver Dam, Salisbury), European (Rotterdam), and Australian (Visual Impairment Project) studies.

Factors other than age may be involved in the rate of vision impairment. For example, the Beaver Dam study found the rate of legal blindness in the United States to be significantly higher in participants aged 75 years and older living in nursing homes (19.1%) compared with the same age group living at home (1.7%). The Visual Impairment Project age-adjusted rate of profound vision impairment was 5.2% (95% CI, 1.8–8.6) in its institutional cohort, which was significantly greater than in its urban and rural cohorts of 0.13% (95% CI, 0–0.25) and 0.29% (95% CI, 0–0.57), respectively.

146 • International Ophthalmology

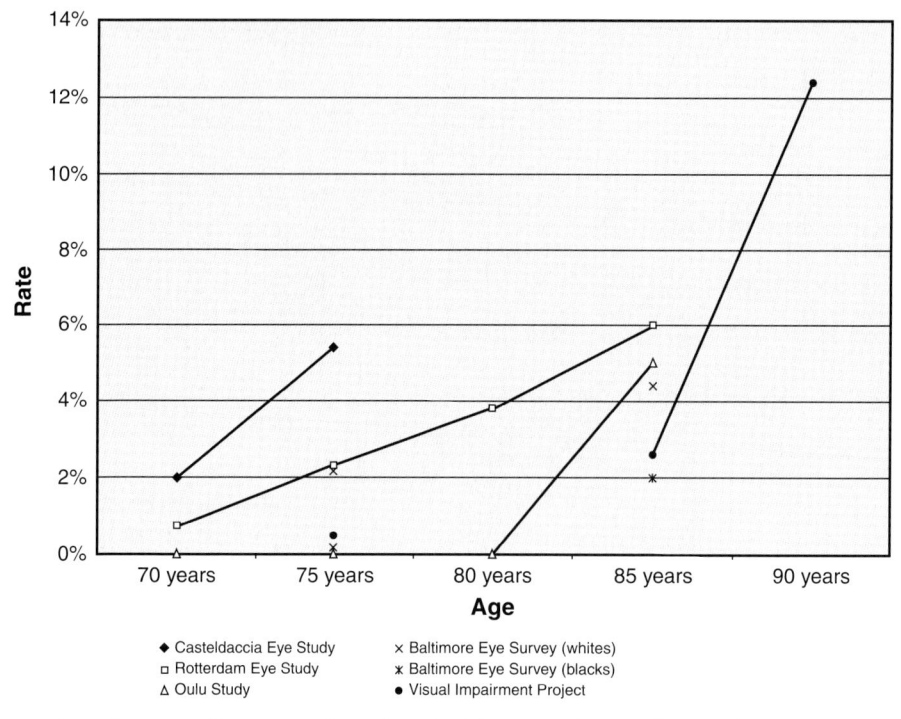

Figure 12-1 Age-specific rates of profound vision impairment by study. *(Courtesy of Mylan VanNewkirk, MD.)*

VanNewkirk MR, Weih L, McCarty CA, et al. Visual impairment and eye diseases in elderly institutionalized Australians. *Ophthalmology.* 2000;107:2203–2208.

Causes of Vision Impairment

The most common cause of vision impairment observed in comparable surveys is uncorrected refractive error; it most commonly involves mild and moderate vision impairment. (See Chapter 13 of this volume.) Diabetic retinopathy, optic neuropathy, and myopic choroidal degeneration are important causes of vision impairment in people under 70 years of age. Myopic choroidal degeneration was the most frequent cause of vision impairment ≤6/18 (20/60) in this age group in the Rotterdam study and the most common cause of vision impairment in the Hong Kong Vision Study, which used the same methodology as the Visual Impairment Project. Myopia was present in 41% of the Chinese population in the Hong Kong study, and extreme myopia, >10 diopters, was present in 2.5% (Chapter 26). A WHO protocol survey using pinhole vision testing, pupil dilation, and direct ophthalmoscopy in Shunyi County, China, reported 28.4% had vision impairment ≤6/18 (20/60) due to unspecified refractive error and 12.7% (258/2031) had vision impairment due to retinal abnormalities, which included 202 patients with macular degeneration; 34 with vascular abnormalities, including diabetic retinopathy; and 22 with optic atrophy. Interestingly, the text comments on refractive errors and retinal abnor-

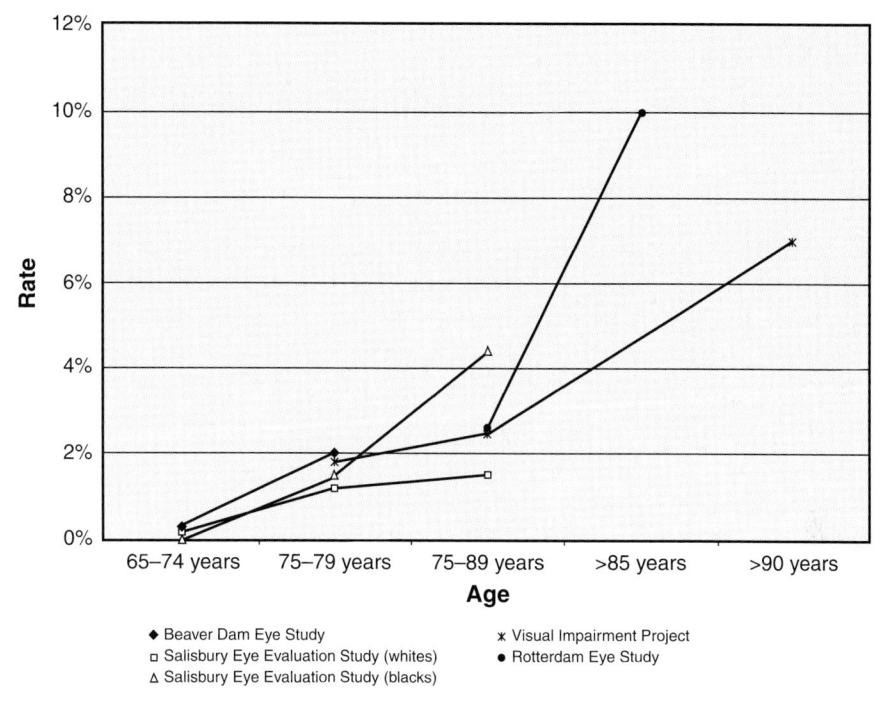

Figure 12-2 Age-specific rates of severe vision impairment by study. *(Courtesy of Mylan VanNewkirk, MD.)*

malities include no mention of myopia or myopic degeneration. No refraction, indirect ophthalmoscopy, or fundus photography was done.

> VanNewkirk MR. The Hong Kong Vision Study: a pilot assessment of visual impairment in adults. *Trans Am Ophthalmol Soc.* 1997;95:715–749.
> Zhao J, Jia L, Sui R, et al. Prevalence of blindness and cataract surgery in Shunyi County, China. *Am J Ophthalmol.* 1998;126:506–514.

Causes of Severe and Profound Vision Impairment

Age-related macular degeneration (AMD), followed by glaucoma and cataract, was found to be the leading cause of severe and profound vision impairment in studies of older white populations in the developed world: the Rotterdam study, Oulu study, Visual Impairment Project, the Salisbury Evaluation, Beaver Dam study, and Baltimore study. The black populations of the Barbados study with <3/60 vision and the Baltimore study with ≤20/200 were found most commonly to have cataract and glaucoma. Blacks in the Salisbury study (11/666) were observed to have equal prevalences of AMD, diabetic retinopathy, trauma, and optic atrophy as the leading causes.

The Andhra Pradesh and Sofia studies observed cataract, followed by retinal diseases, corneal diseases, and glaucoma, as the most common causes of severe and profound vision impairment.

Other Studies

A number of other studies also illustrate important ethnic and geographic influences on eye disease.

Asia

A survey conducted in three Mongolian regions *(aimaks)* included 4345 people aged 40 years or older with a participation rate of 96%. The prevalence of blindness was 1.5% (95% CI, 0.8–2.3); cataract and glaucoma were the most common causes, each at 35%. The prevalence of climatic droplet keratopathy was high (15% to 50%) in this population, which included a large number of semi-nomadic cattle breeders. Climatic droplet keratopathy caused blindness in 7.2% of the population and was more common in men. Trauma was the most common cause of monocular blindness.

> Baasanhu J, Johnson GJ, Burendei G, et al. Prevalence and causes of blindness and visual impairment in Mongolia: a survey of populations aged 40 years and older. *Bull World Health Organ.* 1994;72:771–776.

Central and South America

Few data are available on the prevalence of blindness in Central and South America. Prevalence of profound vision impairment in this region is estimated by the WHO database to be 0.5%.

> Thylefors B, Négrel AD, Pararajasegaram R, et al. Global data on blindness. *Bull World Health Organ.* 1995;73:115–121.

Africa

Although not comparable because of critical differences in methodology and inclusion criteria to the major studies mentioned earlier, the results of several surveys in Africa are presented in Table 12-5.

In Kenya, cataract was the leading cause of both blindness and visual impairment. Trachoma was the leading cause of corneal blindness and the second most common blinding disease observed. As in Mongolia, trauma was the most common cause of monocular blindness. The rate of blindness increased with each age cohort.

Table 12-5 **Prevalence and Principal Cause of Profound Vision Impairment in African Countries**

Country	n	Year	Percent <3/60	#1 Cause
Kenya	13,803	1980s	0.7	Cataract
Tanzania	1847	1990	1.26	Corneal disease
Mali	5871	1990	2.0	Cataract
Cameroon	10,647	1992	1.2	Cataract
Tunisia	3547	1993	0.8	Cataract
Ethiopia	7423	1994–1995	0.85	Cataract
Central African Republic	6086	1995	2.2	Onchocerciasis

The central Tanzanian survey examined individuals over the age of 7. Corneal opacities accounted for 44% of total blindness; the causes were trachoma, vitamin A deficiency, and the use of traditional eye medicines. The second most common cause of blindness was cataract (22%).

In rural Mali, 43% of the unilateral blindness was associated with trauma. Other major eye diseases accounting for high percentages of visual impairment were trachoma and glaucoma. Xerophthalmia appeared to be a major public health problem among children up to 5 years of age.

The survey in the Extreme North Province of Cameroon included participants 6 years and older. As in other developing countries, senile cataract was the most common diagnosis. The definition of blindness used was WHO Category 3, or less than counting fingers at 3 m.

The survey in Tunisia used WHO methodology and had a participation rate of 89%. Nearly 10% of the cataract blindness was due to uncorrected aphakia.

In Jimma Zone of southwestern Ethiopia, corneal opacity from trachoma was responsible for 20.6% of all blindness. Almost 25% of the study population had active trachoma, and 0.9% of preschool children had signs of vitamin A deficiency.

A study in the Central African Republic, where onchocerciasis is endemic, observed that the disease accounted for 73% of blindness.

There is some evidence to suggest that a 10-year national eye-care program in the Gambia is reducing cataract blindness. After 10 years, a resurvey using a different sample reported a 40% reduction in the crude prevalence of blindness—from 0.70% to 0.42%—largely due to a decrease in the prevalence of cataract blindness.

Ayed S, Négrel AD, Nabli M, et al. Prevalence and causes of blindness in the Tunisian Republic. Results of a national survey conducted in 1993. Tunisian Team on the Evaluation of Blindness. [Article in French.] *Santé.* 1998;8:275–282.

Faal H, Minassian DC, Dolin PJ, et al. Evaluation of a national eye care program: re-survey after 10 years. *Br J Ophthalmol.* 2000;84:948–951.

Kortlang C, Koster JC, Coulibaly S, et al. Prevalence of blindness and visual impairment in the region of Segou, Mali. A baseline survey for a primary eye care programme. *Trop Med Int Health.* 1996;1:314–319.

Rapoza PA, West SK, Katala SJ, et al. Prevalence and causes of vision loss in central Tanzania. *Int Ophthalmol.* 1991;15:123–129.

Schwartz EC, Huss R, Hopkins A, et al. Blindness and visual impairment in a region endemic for onchocerciasis in the Central African Republic. *Br J Ophthalmol.* 1997;81:443–447.

Whitfield R, Schwab L, Ross-Degnan D, et al. Blindness and eye disease in Kenya: ocular status survey results from the Kenya Rural Blindness Prevention Project. *Br J Ophthalmol.* 1990;74:333–340.

Wilson MR, Mansour M, Ross-Degnan D, et al. Prevalence and causes of low vision and blindness in the Extreme North Province of Cameroon, West Africa. *Ophthalmic Epidemiol.* 1996;3:23–33.

Zerihun N, Mabey D. Blindness and low vision in Jimma Zone, Ethiopia: results of a population-based survey. *Ophthalmic Epidemiol.* 1997;4:19–26.

Middle East

A population-based survey (2882 people) of the prevalence of major causes of blindness and visual impairment was conducted in the Bisha region of Saudi Arabia. The prevalence of <3/60 vision, best corrected in the better eye, was 0.7%. Cataracts were responsible for 52.6% of blindness.

> al Faran MF, al-Rajhi AA, al-Omar OM, et al. Prevalence and causes of visual impairment and blindness in the southwestern region of Saudi Arabia. *Int Ophthalmol.* 1993;17: 161–165.

South Pacific

Data on the prevalence and causes of blindness and visual impairment in Polynesians are very limited. In a survey designed to obtain an accurate estimate of blindness and its causes in Tonga, a sample of 4056 persons aged 20 years and over was selected by stratified cluster sampling. The prevalence of bilateral blindness in the study population was 0.47%, and all affected were over 50 years of age. Cataract was responsible for 68.4% of bilateral blindness.

> Newland HS, Woodward AJ, Taumoepeau LA, et al. Epidemiology of blindness and visual impairment in the kingdom of Tonga. *Br J Ophthalmol.* 1994;78:344–348.

Prevention

Although prevention of blindness is a laudable goal, many obstacles exist, and they are not confined to the usual explanations of maldistribution of doctors, nurses, medicine, and surgery. A study in rural Ethiopia concluded that ignorance about the causes of blindness is widespread, and this becomes a major barrier in blindness prevention.

> Alemayehu W, Tekle-Haimanot R, Forsgren L, et al. Perceptions of blindness. *World Health Forum.* 1996;17:379–381.

In the LVI Edward Jackson Memorial Lecture (1998), Sommer said, "Poverty is a powerful, multifaceted societal determinant of health. A country's wealth influences health, but only to a point. Costa Rica has one-tenth the wealth of the United States [per capita] but shares the same 75-year life expectancy." Costa Rica has a literacy rate much higher than that of most developing world countries. Because little research exists on the relationship of literacy and health, an association between the two is presumptive. International evidence consistently shows that groups with low socioeconomic status experience significantly higher mortality and morbidity rates. The main contributing factors include a higher rate of health-damaging behaviors, less utilization of and access to the health care system for preventive purposes, and a higher adverse risk factor profile. Further research in understanding and modifying these contributing factors is required.

> Sommer A. Health, medicine, and ophthalmology: facing the facts and paying the piper. LVI Edward Jackson Memorial Lecture. *Am J Ophthalmol.* 1999;128:673–679.
> Turrell G, Mathers CD. Socioeconomic status and health in Australia. *Med J Aust.* 2000;172: 434–438.

In the Andhra Pradesh study, blindness was more common in participants from the extreme lower socioeconomic strata. In the United States, poor people access eye care to a lesser extent than the nonpoor. It does appear that lifestyle and the effects of socioeconomic variables influence health status. Although an inverse correlation between the prevalence of global blindness and the level of economic development showed less correlation than expected using total country estimates of blindness per capita income, an indication of this relationship was demonstrated.

> Ho VH, Schwab IR. Social economic development in the prevention of global blindness. *Br J Ophthalmol.* 2001;85:653–657.

Public health education should be designed to fit within the local culture and include outcome assessments so that education methods can be studied efficiently and revised when necessary.

Conclusion

A truly accurate comparison of eye disease prevalence throughout the world is impossible because of methodologic, political, and/or cultural impediments. Comparable studies of eye disease indicate that significant differences may exist in eye diseases and prevalence of vision impairment among different ethnic and geographic communities in the world. These data agree that the rate of eye disease increases with age and that the rates are increasing as the world's population ages. Today, most studies of white populations in the developed world observe a prevalence of profound vision impairment of 0.5%, or 5 per 1000. The rate of profound vision impairment may be 2–4 times greater for blacks in Maryland and Barbados, as well as in Andhra Pradesh, than for whites in America or Europe. These differences may be due to genetic, socioeconomic, and cultural factors.

Because 80% of global blindness is avoidable or treatable, a challenge exists for the ophthalmologic community to apply current technology and human resources in appropriate ways to eliminate this problem. Prioritization has been a useful method for many developed countries to improve the cost-effectiveness of their health care systems. Several financially self-sustaining models of quality eye-care delivery in the developing world are described in Part VI of this volume. Although many communities consider access to health care a right, most governments have great difficulty funding a high-quality accessible health care program.

CHAPTER 13

Uncorrected Refractive Error

Background

History

Although indirect reference to refractive error has been made in various cultures worldwide for centuries, the first documented use of spectacles dates back to the 14th century AD in Europe. Early spectacles were convex lenses used by elderly people to help them read. Glasses for myopia are thought to have been first used in the 16th century and cylindrical lenses in the 19th century.

Context

A high prevalence of visual impairment due to uncorrected or inadequately corrected refractive error has been reported over the past decade from various population-based surveys, including the Baltimore Eye Survey, the Blue Mountains Eye Study, the Victoria Visual Impairment Project, and the Andhra Pradesh Eye Disease Study. Inadequately treated refractive error accounted for visual impairment (presenting distance visual acuity <20/40 in the better eye) in 2.5% of the population 40 or more years of age in Victoria, Australia. In the Indian state of Andhra Pradesh, 4.0% of the entire population had visual impairment (presenting distance visual acuity <20/60 in the better eye) due to refractive error (3.2% due to myopia and 0.8% due to hyperopia). Refractive error was responsible for blindness (presenting distance visual acuity <20/200 in the better eye) in 0.30% of the population in Andhra Pradesh. The prevalence of refractive error blindness in those 40 years of age or older was 1.06% in Andhra Pradesh and 0.11% in Victoria. Refractive error has also been reported to be a prominent cause of visual impairment in other parts of the world. The high prevalence of visual impairment due to refractive error, which is reported from many parts of the world, is avoidable, as the majority of it is easily correctable.

>Attebo K, Mitchell P, Smith W. Visual acuity and the causes of visual loss in Australia: the Blue Mountains Eye Study. *Ophthalmology*. 1996;103:357–364.
>Dandona R, Dandona L. Refractive error blindness. *Bull World Health Organ*. 2001;79: 237–243.
>Dandona L, Dandona R, Naduvilath TJ, et al. Is eye-care-policy focus almost exclusively on cataract adequate to deal with blindness in India? *Lancet*. 1998;351:1312–1316.
>Dandona L, Dandona R, Srinivas M, et al. Blindness in the Indian state of Andhra Pradesh. *Invest Ophthalmol Vis Sci*. 2001;42:908–916.

Tielsch JM, Sommer A, Witt K, et al. Blindness and visual impairment in an American urban population: the Baltimore Eye Survey. *Arch Ophthalmol.* 1990;108:286–290.

VanNewkirk MR, Weih L, McCarty CA, et al. The cause-specific prevalence of bilateral visual impairment in Victoria, Australia: the Visual Impairment Project. *Ophthalmology.* 2001; 108:960–967.

Economic Impact

Cost of treatment

In the developed countries, various options to correct refractive error are readily available, including spectacles, contact lenses, and refractive surgery. In these countries, spectacles and contact lenses are generally affordable to the majority of people who need them. If not, they are usually provided by governmental or social service agencies. Refractive surgery is expensive but is covered by insurance in some instances.

In developing countries, spectacles are, relatively speaking, the most easily available form of correction for refractive error. Often, the cost of obtaining spectacles is not high in absolute terms. For example, in India, an examination to detect refractive error may cost US$1–2.50 and simple myopic glasses can be bought for US$3–5. Because of many other competing demands on their meager earnings, however, poorer people may find it difficult to afford even these low prices. This difficulty can be better appreciated when annual incomes in various countries are compared. The annual per capita income in 1999 for the United States was US$31,910; Australia, US$20,950; Brazil, US$4350; Russia, US$2250; China, US$780; India, US$440; and Ethiopia, US$100.

Providing spectacles to those who need them is currently a challenge in many developing countries. Different strategies have been tried to increase the availability and affordability of glasses, with varying degrees of success. These include manufacturing low-cost spectacles in developing countries using trained staff, an approach that has been tried in Africa and Asia; using ready-made glasses with spherical correction for refractive errors; and providing spectacles at cost to the poor.

Another complicating factor that decreases access to refractive correction and keeps cost high in some countries—in Latin America, for example—is that legislation prohibits nonophthalmologists from prescribing spectacles.

Cost of lost productivity

The cost of lost productivity in developing countries due to visual impairment caused by refractive error has not been calculated. However, it would not be unreasonable to assume that this cost is huge, particularly because evidence suggests that a large proportion of those having visual impairment due to refractive error are in the economically productive age group.

Dandona L, Dandona R, Naduvilath TJ, et al. Burden of moderate visual impairment in an urban population in southern India. *Ophthalmology.* 1999;106:497–504.

Epidemiology

The majority of research on the epidemiology of refractive error has focused on myopia—probably because it is the most common refractive error responsible for visual impairment. It can be associated with other ocular conditions such as retinal detachment and myopic retinal degeneration, which may lead to vision loss.

Risk Factors

Evidence suggests that both environmental and genetic factors play a role in the onset and progression of myopia. These factors include higher levels of education, near work, intelligence, prematurity, low birth weight, and family history. Myopia has been reported to be higher in Chinese populations in East Asia compared with other populations.

Data from Australia, Hong Kong, Singapore, and Taiwan suggest that the prevalence of myopia has probably increased over the past few decades. This may be related to more education and a greater amount of near work in recent years, but the exact reasons for this trend are not fully understood. The trend could result in a higher prevalence of high and moderate myopia, which, if not adequately corrected, could result in an increase in the number of people who are blind or visually impaired due to refractive error.

Hyperopia has been reported to be more prevalent in females in some populations.

> Goh WS, Lam CS. Changes in refractive trends and optical components of Hong Kong Chinese aged 19–39 years. *Ophthalmic Physiol Opt.* 1994;14:378–382.
> Lin LL, Shih YF, Tsai CB, et al. Epidemiologic study of ocular refraction among school children in Taiwan in 1995. *Optom Vis Sci.* 1999;76:275–281.
> Saw SM, Katz J, Schein OD, et al. Epidemiology of myopia. *Epidemiol Rev.* 1996;18:175–187.
> Seet B, Wong TY, Tan DT, et al. Myopia in Singapore: taking a public health approach. *Br J Ophthalmol.* 2001;85:521–526.
> Wensor M, McCarty CA, Taylor HR. Prevalence and risk factors of myopia in Victoria, Australia. *Arch Ophthalmol.* 1999;117:658–663.

Geographic and ethnic differences

Geographic variation in the prevalence of myopia has been reported (Table 13-1). Certain ethnic groups—for example, the Chinese—have a higher prevalence of myopia, whereas Africans have a lower prevalence. In the United States, the prevalence of myopia has been reported to be higher in whites than in blacks.

> Attebo K, Ivers RQ, Mitchell P. Refractive errors in an older population: the Blue Mountains Eye Study. *Ophthalmology.* 1999;106:1066–1072.
> Dandona R, Dandona L, Srinivas M, et al. Population-based assessment of refractive error in India: the Andhra Pradesh eye disease study. *Clin Experiment Ophthalmol.* 2002;30:84–93.
> Katz J, Tielsch JM, Sommer A. Prevalence and risk factors for refractive errors in an adult inner city population. *Invest Ophthalmol Vis Sci.* 1997;38:334–340.
> Lewallen S, Lowdon R, Courtright P, et al. A population-based survey of the prevalence of refractive error in Malawi. *Ophthalmic Epidemiol.* 1995;2:145–149.
> Pokharel GP, Négrel AD, Munoz SR, et al. Refractive error study in children: results from Mechi zone, Nepal. *Am J Ophthalmol.* 2000;129:436–444.

Table 13-1 **Prevalence of Myopia in Various Populations**

Dates of Survey	Location of Survey	Age (Years)	Sample Size	Definition of Myopia	Percent Prevalence
1985–1988	Baltimore, United States	≥40	2659 (white) 2200 (black)	Worse than −0.5 D	28.1 19.4
1987–1992	Barbados, West Indies	40–84	4036	Worse than −0.5 D	21.9
1988–1990	Beaver Dam, United States	43–84	4533	Worse than −0.5 D	26.2
1992–1994	Blue Mountains, Australia	49–97	3174	Worse than −0.5 D	14.4
1992–1996	Victoria, Australia	≥40	4506	Worse than −0.5 D	16.9
1993	Southern Region, Malawi	18–35	648	−0.5 D or worse	2.5
1995	Taiwan	7–18	11,178	Worse than −0.25 D	53.9
1996–2000	Andhra Pradesh, India	≤15 16–39 ≥40	2603 3691 3588	Worse than −0.5 D	3.2 9.0 36.6
1997–1998	Tanjong Pagar, Singapore	40–79	1232	Worse than −0.5 D	38.7
1998	Shunyi, China	5–15	5882	−0.5 D or worse	16.2
1998	La Florida, Chile	5–15	5293	−0.5 D or worse	6.8
1998	Mechi, Nepal	5–15	4977	−0.5 D or worse	1.2

Wang Q, Klein BE, Klein R, et al. Refractive status in the Beaver Dam Eye Study. *Invest Ophthalmol Vis Sci.* 1994;35:4344–4347.

Wong TY, Foster PJ, Hee J, et al. Prevalence and risk factors for refractive errors in adult Chinese in Singapore. *Invest Ophthalmol Vis Sci.* 2000;41:2486–2494.

Wu SY, Nemesure B, Leske MC. Refractive errors in a black adult population: the Barbados Eye Study. *Invest Ophthalmol Vis Sci.* 1999;40:2179–2184.

Zhao J, Pan X, Sui R, et al. Refractive error study in children: results from Shunyi district, China. *Am J Ophthalmol.* 2000;129:427–435.

Surveys to Determine Prevalence/Incidence

Prevalence data for myopia from recent population-based eye surveys are summarized in Table 13-1.

In Victoria, Australia, myopia between −2.5 D and −5 D was found in 10.4% of those 40 years of age or older and worse than −5 D in 2.1%. In Hyderabad, India, myopia between −3 D and −5 D was reported in 3.8% of those older than 15 years of age and worse than −5 D in 2.8%. The prevalence of myopia greater than −0.5 D, as well as myopia of higher magnitude, increased with increasing age in Hyderabad. In Taiwan, myopia worse than −6 D increased markedly during the second decade of life, with an average prevalence of 4.3% in those 7–18 years of age. Myopia worse than −5 D was reported to be present in 9.1% of Chinese 40–79 years of age in Singapore.

The prevalence of hyperopia greater than −0.5 D has been reported to be more than that of myopia in populations 40 years of age or older in the United States, Australia, and the West Indies. In Hyderabad, India, the prevalence of this level of hyperopia has been reported to be similar to that of myopia in the 40 or more years' age group but about half that of myopia if all those older than 15 years of age are considered together.

Recent population-based longitudinal data on change in refractive error over 5 years in Beaver Dam, Wisconsin, revealed a small hyperopic shift in those aged 43–64 years and a small myopic shift after the age of 65 years.

> Dandona R, Dandona L, Naduvilath TJ, et al. Refractive errors in an urban population in southern India: the Andhra Pradesh Eye Disease Study. *Invest Ophthalmol Vis Sci.* 1999; 40:2810–2818.
>
> Lee KE, Klein BEK, Klein R. Changes in refractive error over a 5-year interval in the Beaver Dam Eye Study. *Invest Ophthalmol Vis Sci.* 1999;40:1645–1649.

Clinical Presentation and Findings

Defective vision is the dominant presenting symptom in cases of high refractive error; it is one of the symptoms in lower refractive error. The other symptoms of refractive error include eye strain, headache, and fatigue.

High myopia is associated with a higher likelihood of degenerative changes in the vitreous, peripheral retinal degeneration, macular degeneration, posterior staphyloma, and retinal detachment. Angle-closure glaucoma is more likely when hyperopia greater than 2 D is present.

In astigmatism, the motion with plane mirror retinoscopy has different magnitude and/or direction in different meridians. The most common form of astigmatism is due to different curvature of the cornea in different meridians, which can be confirmed with keratometry.

Cycloplegic refraction is essential in assessing refractive errors in children accurately because, without it, the significant accommodation power in young eyes can lead to erroneous refractive error assessment. For the dosage of cycloplegic agents needed in different age groups, see BCSC Section 6, *Pediatric Ophthalmology and Strabismus*.

Prevention

Although there is no proven method or treatment available to prevent refractive error per se, the visual impairment caused by refractive error can be corrected with spectacles and other devices. In some cases, particularly in those of high refractive error and anisometropia, amblyopia leading to permanent vision loss may develop if refractive errors are not corrected in early childhood.

Accommodation is considered to be associated with refractive error. Investigations are under way to determine if the use of cycloplegics or bifocals can reduce the onset and progression of myopia. However, at this stage, no method of preventing myopia has been proven.

Current Treatment Programs

Screening

Refractive error can be detected through vision screening. This can be a useful method of detecting and correcting visual impairment, particularly in developing countries, where awareness of and access to refractive error correction is limited. Vision screening is most commonly carried out in school children, where it helps to identify potentially treatable ocular abnormalities, including refractive error. School screening is performed in various ways, including simple visual acuity assessment by teachers or paramedical professionals; occasionally computers are used to assess vision. Children with visual impairment are referred for an eye examination, including refraction, and spectacles are prescribed if needed. In recent years, vision screening has also included preschool children in the developed countries (and infants as young as 6 months in some countries), but the prophylactic potential of early screening of preschool children is limited because the current understanding of the natural history of refractive error and amblyopia is not complete.

Community vision-screening programs are also conducted in developing countries because many children in these countries do not attend school. This approach is more useful than school screening alone, but it also requires more resources because it screens not only school-*going* children but also school-*aged* children, as well as young adults and the older population, in order to identify and treat uncorrected refractive error.

> Limburg H, Vaidyanathan K, Dalal HP. Cost-effective screening of schoolchildren for refractive errors. *World Health Forum.* 1995;16:173–178.

Strengths, Weaknesses, and Results of Treatment Programs

The treatment for refractive error is generally simple, as it can be easily corrected with spectacles. Worldwide, spectacles are the most common form of treatment for refractive error, and the success rate can be considered very high. Despite this, considerable visual impairment due to uncorrected or undercorrected refractive error remains in many parts of the world. Some sociodemographic variables associated with uncorrected or undercorrected refractive error have been identified. In those 40 years of age or older in Victoria, Australia, the risk of decreased vision due to uncorrected or undercorrected refractive error was higher in those who did not complete secondary school, did not have private insurance, lived alone, were born outside of Australia, and had lower income. It also increased with increasing age. In Andhra Pradesh, India, two thirds of those with refractive error of spherical equivalent ± 3.00 D or worse were not using spectacles. In this population, visual impairment due to uncorrected or undercorrected refractive error was higher in the rural than the urban population, was higher in females, and peaked in the 50- to 59-year-old age group, after which it declined somewhat. It had a tendency to be lower in the uppermost socioeconomic stratum.

Contact lenses are used by many people in developed countries, whereas in developing countries they are used by very few. Successful use of contact lenses requires regular and proper cleaning of the lenses. The most dreaded complication of contact lens wear is infectious keratitis. This occurs more commonly in contact lens wearers than in non-wearers, and among wearers, the risk is highest in those who wear their contact lenses while they sleep.

> Cheng KH, Leung SL, Hoekman HW, et al. Incidence of contact-lens-associated microbial keratitis and its related morbidity. *Lancet.* 1999;354:181–185.

Refractive surgery is the most recent option for the correction of refractive error. In the early stages of the development of this treatment, radial keratotomy (RK) was the only available technique. This has been replaced by photorefractive keratectomy (PRK) or laser in situ keratomileusis (LASIK). Although the risk of complications is reportedly becoming smaller in the United States as physicians gain experience, devastating complications such as keratitis leading to vision loss are still being encountered in developing countries. Refractive surgeries are being increasingly used in developed countries to correct refractive error, but they are unlikely to become a common method of treating refractive error in developing countries in the near future because of the high cost of the laser and the inability of the majority of the population to access expensive treatments. For example, many people in the United States may be able to afford a fee of US$1000 for LASIK on one eye, but very few in India can afford the same treatment at a fee of US$300–600. At the same time, an interesting phenomenon is taking place in China, where the number of refractive surgeries has been increasing very rapidly over the past few years, with some claiming that the number now exceeds the number of cataract surgeries in some areas. The benefit or harm of this phenomenon to the population at large will become evident only gradually.

A cost analysis of PRK versus soft contact lenses in the United States reported that the expenses for PRK and follow-up care were roughly equivalent to those for daily-wear soft contact lenses over a 10-year period and less for PRK when the comparison is extended to 20 years.

> Javitt JC, Chiang YP. The socioeconomic aspects of laser refractive surgery. *Arch Ophthalmol.* 1994;112:1526–1530.

The public health challenge in treating refractive error is that, even though a simple and highly successful treatment is known, a significant proportion of the population in the developing countries continues to suffer from visual impairment due to refractive error. This is also true to a lesser degree in developed countries. In India, for example, it is estimated that among the 1-billion-person population in the year 2000, uncorrected or undercorrected refractive error was responsible for blindness (presenting distance visual acuity <20/200 in the better eye) in 3 million persons and moderate visual impairment (presenting distance visual acuity <20/60 to 20/200 in the better eye) in another 37 million persons. In developing countries, the reasons for this high rate of visual impairment due to refractive error include a low rate of seeking refractive error correction, limited access to eye-care providers, and inability to afford spectacles. The reasons for visual impairment due to refractive error in the developed countries may be more complex. For example, in Australia, the government provides for spectacles, and the ratio of eye-care providers to the population is quite reasonable; yet visual impairment due to refractive error continues to exist.

Clinical Research Currently Under Way

Various approaches to arrest the onset and progression of myopia are being studied, including the use of either topical atropine or bifocal lenses with a plus lens for near work to reduce accommodation. So far no clear evidence exists that these strategies reduce myopia. Research is also being done to understand the interplay of genetics and environmental factors in the occurrence of myopia. Operations research is being performed in some parts of the developing world to assess the feasibility of detecting refractive error in the community and facilitating distribution of glasses and assessing the impact this might have on reducing blindness and visual impairment due to refractive error. More of such health services research is needed to provide answers about the logistics needed to provide spectacles to those who need them most.

CHAPTER 14

Cataract

Background

Cataract is the most common cause of blindness in the world. The "clouding" of the crystalline lens was thought in ancient times to be the result of fluid movement in the eye—hence, the Greek word for waterfall, *cataract*, to describe this condition. Very early references to surgery for cataract describe "couching techniques," or dislocating the lens into the vitreous. Couching was still commonly practiced in parts of Asia and Africa during the 20th century, but it is being supplanted by modern techniques as they become more accessible and demanded by the populations in need.

Surgery to restore vision lost to cataract can be done effectively and efficiently with excellent visual outcomes. Despite this, access to surgery, cost, and utilization of services continue to be problematic. Cataract remains a common cause of visual loss in all populations, and no gender, racial, or ethnic group is immune from age-related opacification of the lens.

Although congenital cataract can occur, and children and young adults may develop cataract secondary to trauma, the vast majority of cataract is age-related. In the United States, the primary onset of visually disabling cataract is in the older ages, 60 and above; by age 80, approximately 23% or more of the white population has had bilateral cataract surgery (compared with 11% of the black population). In other countries, notably India, the onset of cataract occurs earlier in life, and progression to visual loss is more rapid. The reasons for this difference in presentation and progression are unknown, but the consequences in terms of visual loss are profound. Clearly, the burden of cataract falls disproportionately on the developing world, which can least afford to manage the problem.

West SK, Muñoz B, Schein OD, et al. Racial differences in lens opacities. The Salisbury Eye Evaluation (SEE) project. *Am J Epidemiol*. 1998;148:1033–1039.

The three main types of age-related cataract are distinct anatomically and etiologically. Population-based studies have confirmed that nuclear and cortical cataract are the most common types and posterior subcapsular cataract (PSC) the least common type, although the latter is quite visually disabling and will occur in a surgical series of cases in disproportionate numbers. Several systems are used in research for grading the presence and severity of the different types of opacities. The primary systems are the Wilmer Grading System, Wisconsin Cataract Grading System, Lens Opacities Classification System (LOCS) series, and the Oxford Clinical Cataract Classification and Grading System;

each has been used for studies of cataract in numerous countries. The Wilmer Grading System for nuclear and cortical cataract is shown in Figures 14-1A and 14-1B. These detailed grading schemes are meant to be used with photographs and trained graders and can be the basis for objective analyses of digital images. The World Health Organization has developed a simple assessment system for nuclear, cortical, and PSC cataract, which incorporates several features of the other grading systems. It is meant to be used clinically in field studies, particularly in less developed countries. These grading schemes have been instrumental in epidemiologic studies of environmental and genetic risk factors for cataract.

Impact of Cataract

Magnitude of the Problem

An estimated 17 million persons are blind from cataract worldwide, making it the leading cause of visual loss. In countries in the developed world, such as the United States and Great Britain, cataract is still a common cause of visual loss, especially among African Americans and the elderly. In the future, the proportion of the population of the world aged 60 and older will increase as mortality rates and birth rates decline. With this aging will come a shift in the burden of eye diseases to age-related causes, resulting in an even greater proportion of visual loss due to cataract. By the year 2020, it is estimated, 40 million worldwide will have blinding cataract. Unless a preventive approach can be found that will effectively protect against the onset of cataract or delay its progression, it will continue as a leading cause of blindness well into the future.

> Brian G, Taylor H. Cataract blindness—challenges for the 21st century. *Bull World Health Organ.* 2001;79:249–256.

Economic Impact

The economic impact in developing countries of vision loss from cataract is huge, including loss of jobs and increase in custodial care. It is estimated that 1500% of the cost of cataract surgery could be generated in 1 year through increased economic productivity. In fact, cataract surgery is ranked as one of the most cost-effective public health interventions for the developing world.

> Javitt JC. Cataract. In: Jamison DT, Mosley WH, Measham AR, et al, eds. *Disease Control Priorities in Developing Countries.* OUP/World Bank: New York; 1993:635–645.

The advantages of intraocular lens (IOL) surgery, relative to the costs, were an issue for developing countries a decade ago. However, the evidence for superior visual outcome, high patient satisfaction, and the decline in costs of the surgery and IOLs have led to general acceptance of pseudophakia as the standard of care. In the developed countries, there has been a significant rise in the number of cataract operations, concomitant with a shift to the use of IOL for visual rehabilitation. At present, the major public health issues surrounding cataract surgery for most countries are increasing the volume and affordability of surgery, while ensuring high quality.

Nuclear opacity grades:
0: (less than Std 1)
1: (Std 1, less than Std 2)
2: (Std 2, less than Std 3)
3: (Std 3, less than Std 4)
4: (Std 4 or greater)

Cortical opacity grade: Percent of area involved in cortical opacification, expressed in 16ths (shadows visualized on red reflex image)

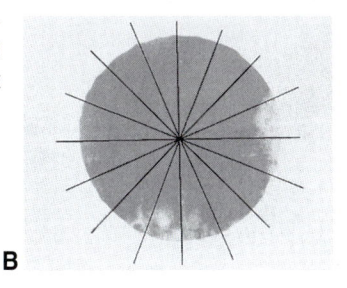

Figure 14-1 The Wilmer Grading System for cataract. **A,** For nuclear opacities and **B,** for cortical opacities. *(Photographs courtesy of Sheila West, PhD.)*

Utilization of cataract surgery is highly variable, even in developed countries where, presumably, high-quality surgery is accessible and affordable. In the United States in 1992, an estimated 1.2 million plus cataract surgeries were performed at a cost of over $3.4 billion. Nevertheless, there is evidence of underutilization of surgical services in the United States by minority populations, and barriers to access need to be addressed. For developing countries, surgical coverage of cataract blindness is estimated to be quite low. A survey across seven states in India revealed that half of those blind from cataract were not operated on, and of those who were, 92% received intracapsular cataract extraction. In China and Nepal, 46%–48% of those needing surgery had operations. In Africa, surgical coverage of cataract is even lower; in Malawi, one survey estimated that only 1 in 7 persons with bilateral cataract blindness has received surgery. The prevalence of prior cataract surgery in various populations is a function of both demand within the population and variation in coverage (Table 14-1). The highest prevalence rates of previous surgery are reported from India, which has a relatively low surgical coverage of cataract cases and a very high need and demand. The lowest rates are from Africa, where coverage (regardless of need or demand) is very low. Interestingly, in two studies where the annual rates of surgery were examined within one setting but among different ethnic groups, the rates of prior cataract surgery were highest in those of South Asian origin.

In developing countries, the cost of surgery depends on the type of surgery, the use of intraocular lenses, and the facility. In Nepal, the cost of cataract surgery with IOL is estimated at less than US$20. For many countries, the primary problem with access to surgery is the lack of trained surgical staff to deliver care. In parts of Africa, the ratio of surgeon to population is less than 1 to 1 million, with most of the surgeons in the urban centers; thus sufficient staff to even begin to address the problem of cataract surgery is simply not available.

Table 14-1 Prevalence Rates of Cataract Surgery in Population-based Studies Worldwide

Author	Country/Population	Age Group	Prevalence of Surgery
Leske et al[1]	Barbados/black	40–84	3% in one or both eyes
Murthy et al[2]	India	50+	13% in one or both eyes
Dandona et al[3]	India	50+	14.6% in one or both eyes
Li et al[4]	China	50+	1.6% in one or both eyes
He et al[5]	China	50+	2.0% in one or both eyes
Congdon et al[6]	Tanzania	40+	0.4% in one or both eyes
Rabiu et al[7]	Nigeria	40+	0.5% in one or both eyes
McCarty et al[8]	Australia	50+	4%
Mitchell et al[9]	Australia	49+	6% in one or both eyes
Deane et al[10]	England	55–74	2.0% in one or both eyes
Klein et al[11]	United States/white	43–84	3.6% in right eyes
West et al[12]	United States/white	65–84	12.2% bilateral surgery
	United States/black	65–84	4.8% bilateral surgery
Broman et al[13]	United States/Hispanic	40+	6.7% in one or both eyes
Sasaki et al[14]	Iceland	50+	4.7% bilateral surgery
Wong et al*[15]	Singapore/Indian	all ages	4/1000/year have surgery
	Singapore/Chinese	all ages	3.7/1000/year have surgery
	Singapore/Malayan	all ages	2.4/1000/year have surgery
Thompson et al*[16]	UK/Asians	65–69	12.8/1000/year have surgery
	UK/Caucasians	65–69	2.45/1000/year have surgery

* Rates for these two studies are not prevalence rates but estimates of annual surgical rates within the population; they are included to show potential ethnic differences.

[1] Leske MC, Connell AM, Wu SY, et al. Prevalence of lens opacities in the Barbados Eye Study. *Arch Ophthalmol*. 1997;115:101–111.
[2] Murthy GV, Gupta S, Ellwein LB, et al. A population-based eye survey of older adults in a rural district of Rajasthan: I. Central vision impairment, blindness, and cataract surgery. *Ophthalmology*. 2001;108:679–685.
[3] Dandona L, Dandona R, Naduvilath TJ, et al. Population-based assessment of the outcome of cataract surgery in an urban population in southern India. *Am J Ophthalmol*. 1999;127:650–658.
[4] Li S, Xu J, He M, et al. A survey of blindness and cataract surgery in Doumen County, China. *Ophthalmology*. 1999;106:1602–1608.
[5] He M, Xu J, Li S, et al. Visual acuity and quality of life in patients with cataract in Doumen County, China. *Ophthalmology*. 1999;106:1609–1615.
[6] Congdon N, West SK, Buhrmann RR, et al. Prevalence of the different types of age-related cataract in an African population. *Invest Ophthalmol Vis Sci*. 2001;42:2478–2482.
[7] Rabiu MM. Cataract blindness and barriers to uptake of cataract surgery in a rural community of northern Nigeria. *Br J Ophthalmol*. 2001;85:776–780.
[8] McCarty CA, Nanjan MB, Taylor HR. Operated and unoperated cataract in Australia. *Clin Experiment Ophthalmol*. 2000;28:77–82.
[9] Mitchell P, Cumming RG, Attebo K, et al. Prevalence of cataract in Australia: the Blue Mountains Eye Study. *Ophthalmology*. 1997;104:581–588.
[10] Deane JS, Hall AB, Thompson JR, et al. Prevalence of lenticular abnormalities in a population-based study: Oxford Clinical Cataract Grading in the Melton Eye Study. *Ophthalmic Epidemiol*. 1997;4:195–206.
[11] Klein BE, Klein R, Linton KL. Prevalence of age-related opacities in a population. The Beaver Dam Eye Study. *Ophthalmology*. 1992;99:546–552.
[12] West SK, Muñoz B, Schein OD, et al. Racial differences in lens opacities: the Salisbury Eye Evaluation (SEE) project. *Am J Epidemiol*. 1998;148:1033–1039.
[13] Broman A, Muñoz B, Rodriguez J, et al. Factors associated with accessing cataract surgery in a population-based study of Hispanics: Proyecto VER [ARVO abstract]. *Invest Ophthalmol Vis Sci*. 2001;42:S534. Abstract NR 2869.
[14] Sasaki H, Jonasson F, Kojima M, et al. The Reykjavik Eye Study—prevalence of lens opacification with reference to identical Japanese studies. *Ophthalmologica*. 2000;214:412–420.
[15] Wong TY. Cataract extraction rates among Chinese, Malays, and Indians in Singapore: a population-based analysis. *Arch Ophthalmol*. 2001;119:727–732.
[16] Thompson JR. The demand incidence of cataract in Asian immigrants to Britain and their descendants. *Br J Ophthalmol*. 198;73:950–954.

Foster A. Who will operate on Africa's 3 million curably blind people? *Lancet.* 1991;337: 1267–1269.

Quality of Cataract Surgery

The cost-effectiveness of quality cataract surgery has been demonstrated and shown to enhance visual function and quality of life. In the developed countries, severe complications of surgery were rare, as reported by the National Study of Cataract Outcomes, and achievement of 20/40 or better vision in the operated eye occurred in greater than 90%. In the developing countries, cataract surgery outcomes can also reflect low rates of severe complications and improvement in vision. Recently, however, some evaluations have suggested that desirable outcomes were not as large as expected, due to surgical complications, concurrent diseases, loss of aphakic spectacles, and development of posterior capsular opacification. Research from China and India suggests as many as one quarter to one third of eyes with cataract surgery have postoperative vision of <20/200. When the proportion of poor outcomes (visual acuity 20/400) is high, exceeding 10%, the causes need to be investigated to ensure maximum benefit in terms of visual recovery and satisfaction.

> Dandona L, Dandona R, Naduvilath TJ, et al. Population based assessment of the outcome of cataract surgery in an urban population in southern India. *Am J Ophthalmol.* 1999; 127:650–658.
> Limburg H, Foster A, Vaidyanathan K, et al. Monitoring the visual outcome of cataract surgery in India. *Bull World Health Organ.* 1999;77:455–460.
> Steinberg EP, Tielsch JM, Schein OD, et al. National study of cataract surgery outcomes. Variation in 4-month postoperative outcomes as reflected in multiple outcome measures. *Ophthalmology.* 1994;101:1131–1140.

Quality of Life

Cataract surgeons are well aware of reports before surgery by patients with cataract of the increasing difficulty they have in performing visually intensive tasks, interacting with others in social settings, and maintaining independent functioning. In addition, cataract, even in the early stages, appears to affect mobility, including the ability to drive. Cataract patients will avoid difficult driving circumstances, such as night driving or driving in bad weather conditions, because of their visual difficulties. All of these complaints fall into the domain of "quality of life" for these patients. Research has documented the improvement in performance of tasks involving vision and improvement in psychological well-being following cataract surgery. Some data indicate that the improvement in depressive symptoms following cataract surgery may be a major pathway for the improvement in quality of life in other domains.

> Owsley C, McGwin G Jr. Vision impairment and driving. *Surv Ophthalmol.* 1999;43:535–550.

In less developed countries where the quality of the surgery is high and patient visual outcomes are good, the improvement in patient-reported quality of life following cataract surgery is also marked. In populations of post–cataract surgery patients where gains in acuity were not high, changes in scores of self-reported function were not as strong.

Caution is required in using quality-of-life instruments in a culture other than the one in which they were developed. Quality-of-life concepts and questions with meaning for one culture—particularly in the realms of mental health, social functioning, and depressive symptoms—may have little to no applicability for another.

Clearly, opacification of the lens and subsequent visual loss does influence the quality of life for patients. High-quality, affordable, and accessible cataract surgery is one of the main goals of the VISION 2020 initiative of the World Health Organization Prevention of Blindness program and the prevention of blindness community. Ultimately, however, the prevention of cataract, or delay in the progression of cataract, will offer the most sustainable strategy for control of blinding cataract. The next sections provide an overview of the epidemiology and risk factors associated with cataract and the future of research needed to move the field toward cataract prevention.

> West S, Sommer A. Prevention of blindness and priorities for the future. *Bull World Health Organ.* 2001;79:244–248.

Epidemiology

Prevalence

Research on the prevalence of the different cataract types in various countries has been hampered by the absence of a uniform grading system for lens opacities and their visually disabling endpoint, cataract. Table 14-2 shows the prevalence rate of the three types of lens opacities in different populations and age groups (using the cataract grading scheme indicated). Because cataract onset is so age dependent, even 5 to 10 years' difference in the age categories, or differences in the age structure, of the populations may explain discrepancies. With these caveats, some differences do emerge. The highest rates of PSC opacities appear to be in people of Chinese origin. The prevalence of cortical opacity is higher in African Americans (and African Caribbeans) than in Caucasians, and the rates of nuclear and PSC opacities may be lower. The excess of cortical opacities in African Americans is not entirely explained by differences in risk factors, suggesting that exploration of racial and ethnic differences in risk may be a fruitful area for further research.

Risk Factors

Important advances have been made in the understanding of risk factors for the different types of cataract. (See Table 14-3.) Personal factors such as age, gender, ethnic group, and as-yet-unknown genetic factors are well-accepted risk factors for cataracts. It is likely that continued exploration into candidate genes and gene–environment interactions will yield the most fruitful research into preventive strategies for cataract.

> West SK, Valmadrid CT. Epidemiology of risk factors for age-related cataract. *Surv Ophthalmol.* 1995;39:323–334.

Environmental factors have been extensively studied for their role in cataractogenesis. Those factors that are relatively common in the population, such as smoking, exposure to light, or diabetes, are of greatest public health interest because preventive strategies

Table 14-2 Prevalence Rate of Different Types of Lens Opacities Within Different Study Populations

Author	Population	Age Group	Cataract Grading System	Prevalence of Nuclear Opacity	Prevalence of Cortical Opacity	Prevalence of PSC Opacity
Klein et al[1]	US/white	43–80	Wisconsin	17.3%	16.3%	6.0%
West et al[2]	US/white	65–84	Wilmer	46.3%	23.9%	5.4%
	US/black	65–84	Wilmer	31.0%	54.5%	2.6%
Leske et al[3]	Barbados/black	40–84	LOCS	19%	34%	4%
Congdon et al[4]	Tanzania/black	40+	WHO	15.6%	8.8%	1.9%
McCarty et al[5]	Australia/white	40+	Wilmer	11.6%	11.3%	4.1%
Mitchell et al[6]	Australia/white	49+	Wisconsin	51.7%	23.8%	6.3%
Sasaki et al[7]	Iceland/white	50+	JCCESGS*	15.7%	12.2%	2.4%
Deane et al[8]	UK/white	55–74	Oxford	100%†	36%	11%
Cheng et al[9]	Taiwan	50+	?	35.2%	7.8%	15.3%
Xu et al[10]	China	45+	LOCS	28.6%	30.3%	8.7%

* The classification system used was Japanese Cooperative Cataract Epidemiology Study Group System.
† Any white scatter was considered nuclear opacity.
[1] Klein BE, Klein R, Linton KL. Prevalence of age-related opacities in a population. The Beaver Dam Eye Study. *Ophthalmology*. 1992;99:546–552.
[2] West SK, Muñoz B, Schein OD, et al. Racial differences in lens opacities: the Salisbury Eye Evaluation (SEE) project. *Am J Epidemiol*. 1998;148:1033–1039.
[3] Leske MC, Connell AM, Wu SY, et al. Prevalence of lens opacities in the Barbados Eye Study. *Arch Ophthalmol* 1997;115:101–111.
[4] Congdon N, West SK, Buhrmann RR, et al. Prevalence of the different types of age-related cataract in an African population. *Invest Ophthalmol Vis Sci*. 2001;42:2478–2482.
[5] McCarty CA, Mukesh BN, Fu CL, et al. The epidemiology of cataract in Australia. *Am J Ophthalmol*. 1999;128:446–465.
[6] Mitchell P, Cumming RG, Attebo K, et al. Prevalence of cataract in Australia: the Blue Mountains Eye Study. *Ophthalmology*. 1997;104:581–588.
[7] Sasaki H, Jonasson F, Kojima M, et al. The Reykjavik Eye Study—prevalence of lens opacification with reference to identical Japanese studies. *Ophthalmologica*. 2000;214:412–420.
[8] Deane JS, Hall AB, Thompson JR, et al. Prevalence of lenticular abnormalities in a population-based study: Oxford Clinical Cataract Grading in the Melton Eye Study. *Ophthalmic Epidemiol*. 1997;4:195–206.
[9] Cheng CY, Liu JH, Chen SJ, et al. Population-based study on prevalence and risk factors of age-related cataracts in Peitou, Taiwan. *Zhonghua Yi Xue Zu Zhi* (Taipei). 2000;63:641–648.
[10] Xu J, Yu Q, Zhu S, et al. A population-based study of lens opacities. *Yan Ke Xue Bao*. 1996;12:115–117.

could be targeted to large, relevant groups. Cigarette smoking has now been linked to an increased risk of nuclear cataract in numerous studies, with a dose–response relationship and evidence that current smoking drives progression. Posterior subcapsular cataract may also be linked to smoking although the data are less well established. In 1995, it was estimated that 25% of the United States population were smokers, suggesting that as much as 20% of the cataract cases were attributable to smoking. Smoking rates are even higher in other countries, such as China, where 60% of men are smokers and every year

Table 14-3 Summary Table of Risk Factors for Different Cataract Types

Risk Factor	Cataract Type	Quality of Evidence
Personal Factors		
Age	nuclear, cortical, PSC	Conclusive for nuclear and cortical; PSC is less strongly age related
Female	cortical, nuclear	Robust for slight increased risk of cortical; data are weaker for nuclear
Ethnicity: black vs white Chinese vs white	cortical. less nuclear PSC	Robust for increased risk of cortical in blacks; some evidence for higher risk of nuclear and PSC in whites; limited evidence for excess PSC in Chinese
Genetic factors	cortical and nuclear	Robust evidence for genetic component to both cataract types in white populations; could be the source of racial variation
Environmental Factors		
Cigarette smoking	nuclear and PSC	Robust evidence with dose–response relationship for nuclear; some evidence for PSC
Ultraviolet B	cortical	Robust evidence with dose–response relationship for cortical
Nutrition/supplements	cortical, nuclear, PSC	Conflicting studies (protection, no association, risk reported); no consistent data
Low socioeconomic status/education/income	cortical, nuclear, PSC	Strong evidence linking markers of low socioeconomic status with all types of cataract
Alcohol use	PSC, nuclear	Conflicting; strongest evidence for heavy drinking and PSC, with protective effect of light intake; less clear for nuclear
Diabetes	cortical, PSC	Robust; risk related to duration of diabetes and level of control; associated with cataract surgery at an earlier age
Diarrhea/dehydration	"cataract"	Conflicting data reporting risk and no association; no type specified
Blood pressure/hypertension	nuclear, cortical, PSC	Limited; some evidence for risk of PSC with hypertension, possibly diastolic blood pressure elevation and cortical opacity in blacks
Steroid use	PSC	Robust; associated with high doses and prolonged use; inhaled steroids also likely a risk factor
Body mass index (BMI)	nuclear, cortical, PSC	Conflicting data on direction of risk with nuclear; limited data on higher BMI associated with greater risk of cortical, PSC
Gout/gout medications	mixed, nuclear, cortical	Limited, conflicting data on disease versus treatment, and cataract type
Protective Factors		
Aspirin	cataract	Unproven; clinical trial data do not support a protective effect
Hormone replacement therapy (women)	nuclear	Limited; evidence from prospective studies suggests no effect

there are 3 million new smokers. The projected increase in all smoking-related diseases, including cataract, in these countries is high.

Cortical cataract has been solidly linked to chronic ocular exposure to ultraviolet B radiation in sunlight. Even with the low levels of exposure typically encountered in the general population, a modest increased risk can be demonstrated.

People with diabetes are at increased risk for cataract, particularly cortical and likely PSC cataract. Research has shown an association of cataract with duration of diabetes and level of glycemic control. Incidence and progression of cortical opacities is greater in those with diabetes, and poorer level of control may further increase the risk. The incidence of cataract surgery, especially in the younger age groups, appears to be higher in patients with diabetes compared to those without. With a projected rise in the prevalence of diabetes in developing countries by 170%, this risk factor for cataract will take on an important dimension for control efforts in the future.

> King H, Aubert RE, Herman WH. Global burden of diabetes, 1995–2025: prevalence, numerical estimates, and projections. *Diabetes Care.* 1998;21:1414–1431.
>
> Klein BE, Klein R, Lee KE. Diabetes, cardiovascular disease, selected cardiovascular disease risk factors, and the 5-year incidence of age-related cataract and progression of lens opacities: the Beaver Dam Eye Study. *Am J Ophthalmol.* 1998;126:782–790.

In theory, antioxidant defense of lens proteins and membranes from oxidative stress should protect against cataractogenesis. However, studies on the role of diet or supplement use or serum levels of various antioxidants have provided conflicting data and do not strongly support any one micronutrient, supplement, or food source as particularly anticataractogenic. Results from clinical trials have found no evidence of a protective effect. At present, the promotion of any vitamin or mineral supplement to retard the onset or progression of cataract is unjustified.

The search for protective agents against the onset or progression of cataract has been disappointing to date. Initial hopes that aspirin could provide a protective effect were not confirmed in longitudinal studies and clinical trials. Interesting cross-sectional data suggested a role for hormone replacement therapy as protective for nuclear cataract in women, and estrogen receptor alpha has been demonstrated in lens epithelium. However, prospective studies have failed to confirm the association. At present, no pharmacologic agent is known to be safe and effective against the onset of age-related cataract.

Cataract and Mortality

Nuclear cataract, particularly nuclear cataract mixed with other types, appears to be an independent predictor of early mortality. The association is present in Caucasians, African Americans, and African Caribbeans. Other predictors of mortality, such as frailty, smoking, diabetes, and other chronic conditions, do not explain this association. Thus, the lens may provide an interesting window into the aging process, and there is considerable research interest in finding a common pathway between lens opacification and premortal events at the cellular or subcellular level.

> Hennis A, Wu SY, Li X, et al and the Barbados Eye Study Group. Lens opacities and mortality: the Barbados Eye Studies. *Ophthalmology.* 2001;108:498–504.

West SK, Muñoz B, Istre J, et al. Mixed lens opacities and subsequent mortality. *Arch Ophthalmol.* 2000;118:393–397.

Clinical Research Currently Under Way

Cataract will remain a significant problem, both in economic and social terms, for the foreseeable future. Research in this field can make major contributions. The most active clinical research is concentrated in the following areas:

- Risk factors for cataractogenesis: The most promising lines of research are the investigations into the genetic risk factors for cataract. It is likely that the interaction of genetic factors and environmental risk factors will explain a significant component of cataract. Researchers are actively investigating candidate genes, although most of their activity is focused on congenital or juvenile genetic cataract.
- Anticataract agents: Development of specific anticataract drugs is a high priority, but no new compounds are yet ready for extensive clinical testing. As compounds are created, the issue of appropriate clinical trials must be addressed. Cataract takes a relatively long time to progress and may result from insults that are lifelong or cumulative, thus raising the issue of when to start treatment and the time course for sustaining treatment. The likelihood of a pharmacologic agent that would be affordable or practical for use in developing countries is remote.
- Evaluations of cataract programs: The National Cataract Outcomes Study based in the United States provided critical information on the expected outcomes of cataract surgery and may serve as a benchmark on expected outcomes for the evaluation of other surgical programs. The finding of less satisfactory outcomes in other countries can stimulate inquiry into causes and possible remedies. Moreover, the role of health services research in determining optimal delivery of services, including using alternative staff and health care delivery approaches appropriate for less-developed country settings, is crucial for developing strategies to tackle blindness from cataract worldwide in a cost-effective manner.

CHAPTER 15

Ethnic Differences in Primary Open-Angle Glaucoma

Background

By the year 2020, an estimated 54 million persons aged 60 years and older will be blind worldwide. Glaucoma will be responsible for approximately 14% of these cases, following cataract and trachoma. Most glaucoma blindness in black and white populations is due to primary open-angle glaucoma (POAG). Due to the magnitude and public health impact of POAG, it is important to know its frequency and distribution in various populations, which may provide some clues to its etiology. This chapter summarizes epidemiologic data on primary POAG and its risk factors, as they relate to ethnic patterns of the disease.

Thylefors B, Négrel AD. The global impact of glaucoma. *Bull World Health Organ.* 1994;72: 323–326.

Prevalence and Incidence

Several large population-based epidemiologic studies have investigated POAG prevalence, with the majority being conducted in predominantly white populations. As seen in Table 15-1, the prevalence of primary POAG is generally low in these populations, ranging from 1% to 3%. Studies of Asian populations found comparable rates, with most POAG being classified as the "low tension" type. Clinical impressions, as well as data from blindness registries, have long suggested that POAG and POAG-related blindness are more frequent in black than white individuals. The presence of racial differences in POAG is supported by prevalence studies in populations of African origin, where rates are generally much higher, especially in African Caribbeans. After a small study conducted in Jamaica, West Indies, data from several large studies in Barbados, West Indies ($n = 4498$); Tanzania, Africa ($n = 3268$); Baltimore, Maryland ($n = 2395$); and St. Lucia, West Indies ($n = 1679$) also demonstrated the increased frequency of POAG in black populations, ranging from 3% to 9% (see Table 15-1).

Furthermore, POAG is a major cause of visual impairment and accounts for a higher percentage of blindness in black than white participants in these studies. In Baltimore, POAG was responsible for 19% ($n = 14$) of all blindness among African Americans and 6% ($n = 3$) among whites. After age adjustment, the blindness rate was 6 times higher

Table 15-1 Summary of Population-based Studies of Primary Open-Angle Glaucoma

Study	Year	Race*	Age Range (Years)	No. of Participants	POAG Criteria†	No. of Cases	Prevalence (%)
Ferndale, Wales[1]	1966	W	40–74	4231	GD, VF	20	<1
Framingham Eye Study[2] Framingham, Massachusetts, United States	1977	W	52–85	2433	VF	28	1.4
Dalby, Sweden[3]	1981	W	55–70	1511	GD, VF	13	<1
Beaver Dam Eye Study[4] Beaver Dam, Wisconsin, United States	1992	W	43–75+	4926	GD, VF, IOP	104	2.1
Roscommon, Ireland[5]	1993	W	50–80+	2186	GD, VF, IOP	41	1.9
Rotterdam Eye Study[6] Rotterdam, Netherlands	1994	W	55–85+	3062	GD, VF	34	1.1
Blue Mountains Eye Study[7] Sydney, Australia	1996	W	49–97	3654	GD, VF	108	3.0
Ponza, Italy[8]	1997	W	40–80+	1034	GD, VF, IOP	26	2.5

* W = white
† GD = glaucomatous disc, VF = visual field defects, IOP = elevated intraocular pressure
[1] Hollows FC, Graham PA. Intraocular pressure, glaucoma and glaucoma suspects in a defined population. *Br J ophthalmol.* 1966;50:570–586.
[2] Kahn HA, Leibowitz HM, Ganley JP, et al. The Framingham Eye Study. I. Outline and major prevalence findings. *Am J Epidemiol.* 1977;106:17–32.
[3] Bengtsson B. The prevalence of glaucoma. *Br J Ophthalmol.* 1981;65:46–49.
[4] Klein BE, Klein R, Sponsel WE, et al. Prevalence of glaucoma. The Beaver Dam Eye Study. *Ophthalmology.* 1992;99:1499–1504.
[5] Coffey M, Reidy A, Wormald R, et al. Prevalence of glaucoma in the west of Ireland. *Br J Ophthalmol.* 1993;77:17–21.
[6] Dielemans I, Vingerling JR, Wolfs RC, et al. The prevalence of primary open-angle glaucoma in a population-based study in The Netherlands. The Rotterdam Study. *Ophthalmology.* 1994;101:1851–1855.
[7] Mitchell P, Smith W, Attebo K, et al. Prevalence of open-angle glaucoma in Australia: The Blue Mountains Eye Study. *Ophthalmology.* 1996;103:1661–1669.
[8] Cedrone C, Culasso F, Cesareo M, et al. Prevalence of glaucoma in Ponza, Italy: a comparison with other studies. *Ophthalmic Epidemiol.* 1997;4:59–72.

(Continues)

Table 15-1 Summary of Population-Based Studies of Primary Open-Angle Glaucoma (Continued)

Study	Year	Race*	Age Range (Years)	No. of Participants	POAG Criteria[†]	No. of Cases	Prevalence (%)
Melbourne Visual Impairment Study[9] Melbourne, Australia	1998	W	40–90+	3271	GD, VF, IOP, Gl Hx	56	1.7
Nationwide Glaucoma Survey[10] Japan	1991	A	40–90+	8126	GD, VF	213	2.6
St. Lucia Eye Study[11] St. Lucia, West Indies	1989	B	30–70+	1679	VF	147	8.8
Baltimore Eye Survey[12] Baltimore, Maryland, United States	1991	B W	40–80+	2395 2913	GD, VF GD, VF	100 32	4.2 1.1
Barbados Eye Study[13] Barbados, West Indies	1994	B M	40–80+	4314 184	GD, VF GD, VF	302 6	7.0 3.3
Tanzania, East Africa[14]	2000	B	40–80+	3268	GD, VF	99	3.1

* W = white, B = black, A = Asian, M = mixed (black and white)
[†] GD = glaucomatous disc, VF = visual field defects, IOP = elevated intraocular pressure, Gl Hx = history of glaucoma
[9] Wensor MD, McCarty CA, Stanislavsky YL, et al. The prevalence of glaucoma in the Melbourne Visual Impairment Project. *Ophthalmology.* 1998;105:733–739.
[10] Shiose Y, Kitazawa Y, Tsukahara S, et al. Epidemiology of glaucoma in Japan—a nationwide glaucoma survey. *Jpn J Ophthalmol.* 1991;35:133–155.
[11] Mason RP, Kosoko O, Wilson MR, et al. National survey of the prevalence and risk factors of glaucoma in St. Lucia, West Indies. Part I. Prevalence findings. *Ophthalmology.* 1989;96:1363–1368.
[12] Tielsch JM, Sommer A, Katz J, et al. Racial variations in the prevalence of primary open-angle glaucoma. The Baltimore Eye Survey. *JAMA.* 1991;266:369–374.
[13] Leske MC, Connell AM, Schachat A, et al. The Barbados Eye Study. Prevalence of open-angle glaucoma. *Arch Ophthalmol.* 1994;112:821–829.
[14] Buhrmann RR, Quigley HA, Barron Y, et al. Prevalence of glaucoma in a rural East African population. *Invest Ophthalmol Vis Sci.* 2000;41:40–48.

among black than among white participants, and POAG prevalence was 4 times higher. In Barbados, POAG accounted for 28% ($n = 42$) of bilateral blindness and was the leading cause of visual loss. Further follow-up of the Barbados cohort has provided a measurement of incidence, which supports the high risk of developing POAG in this population, with a 4-year incidence rate of 2.2%.

> Leske MC, Connell AM, Wu SY, et al. Incidence of open-angle glaucoma: the Barbados Eye Studies. *Arch Ophthalmol.* 2001;119:89–95.

In sum, the results of these studies indicate large differences in prevalence and blindness rates between white and black populations in the United States and the Caribbean; they also suggest some variations in POAG occurrence among different black populations (see Table 15-1).

Comparisons Among Studies

Interpretation of the variability in POAG prevalence among studies must consider the differences in populations, diagnostic criteria, and participation rates. In addition, the small number of cases identified in some studies leads to wide confidence intervals in their rates. As a result, caution is needed when comparing results. The lack of a standardized classification scheme to define POAG is a major problem for valid interpretation. Generally, some degree of optic disc damage and/or visual field defect must be present for the definition. Although most current POAG criteria rely only on visual field and/or disc damage, others also include intraocular pressure (IOP) levels in their definitions, thus complicating comparability. In a study conducted in Dalby, Sweden, the criteria for POAG included repeatable visual field defects consistent with glaucoma and glaucomatous cupping of the optic disc. Based on this definition, less than 1% ($n = 13$) of the participants 55–70 years of age were found to have POAG. This finding was consistent with the prevalence rates reported in studies conducted in Wales (<1%); Framingham, Massachusetts (1.4%); Baltimore, Maryland (1.1%); and Rotterdam, The Netherlands (1.1%). Population-based studies in Melbourne, Australia; Roscommon, Ireland; Beaver Dam, Wisconsin; and Ponza, Italy, included high IOP levels among the POAG criteria and reported slightly higher prevalence rates (1.7%, 1.9%, 2.1%, and 2.5%, respectively). Although we cannot discount the possibility of other factors, it seems likely that the increased prevalence in these studies may be due, at least in part, to the inclusion of IOP in the POAG criteria. Another population-based study in Australia—the Blue Mountains Eye Study—reported a 3% prevalence of POAG, as defined by glaucomatous visual field loss combined with disc pathology. Although the overall rate is higher than reported in other studies of whites, black populations have higher age-specific rates.

The Barbados Eye Study

The largest investigation of eye diseases in people of African origin is the Barbados Eye Study (BES). It was designed to investigate the prevalence and risk factors for POAG and other ocular diseases in a predominantly black population, with the aim to prevent or control visual loss. The study included 4709 participants (84% of those eligible), randomly selected from among Barbadian-born citizens 40–84 years of age. Participants received an extensive standardized examination, including automated refraction, best-corrected visual acuity, Humphrey perimetry (suprathreshold screening test: C64 program; full-threshold tests: C24-2 and C30-2 programs), applanation tonometry, lens gradings, stereo fundus photography, blood pressure and anthropometric measurements, venipuncture for glycosylated hemoglobin, and an interview to ascertain potential risk factors, demographic information, and ocular and medical history. A 10% sample of all participants, as well as those with positive findings, such as abnormal perimetry, were referred for a comprehensive ophthalmologic examination. A high degree of data completeness was achieved, with 95% of the Barbados study participants completing perimetry, 97% having photographic or clinical gradings, and 93% of those referred having an ophthalmologic examination. Of those 40 years of age and older, 7% ($n = 302$) of black, 3% ($n = 6$) of mixed black and white ancestry, and less than 1% ($n = 1$) of white participants had POAG. The 309 participants with POAG represent the largest number of cases identified in any population-based study (see Table 15-1), thus allowing extensive risk factor analyses for black participants, with high statistical power.

Of note, the POAG prevalence in the study's mixed-race participants (3.3%; 95% CI (1.2, 7.0)) was similar to that reported for African Americans in Baltimore (4.2%; (3.4, 5.0)) and for Africans in Tanzania (3.1%; (2.5, 3.8)), but prevalence in black participants in the Barbados study was higher (7.0%; (6.3, 7.8)). The prevalence among the Barbados study's black participants was more comparable to the rate reported for participants in the St. Lucia study (8.8%; (7.5, 10.2)), thus supporting the existence of a high POAG prevalence in African Caribbeans.

To interpret the results of these four studies, it is useful to compare their definitions and protocols. In the Barbados study, the definition of POAG required the presence of visual field *and* optic disc criteria, with an ophthalmologic assessment to exclude other possible causes. This strict definition does not consider IOP. Visual field and optic disc criteria were used to define glaucoma in Baltimore and Tanzania as well, whereas the St. Lucia study based its definition on visual field abnormalities. Concerning protocols, the Barbados and Baltimore studies screened the visual field with Humphrey suprathreshold tests (using the C64 and full-field 120 programs, respectively), whereas the Tanzania study used a threshold-related, suprathreshold screening program (Dicon 1), and the St. Lucia study screened every third participant with the Humphrey full-field 120 program.

Subsequent testing for those with potential field loss involved full-threshold Humphrey tests in Barbados (C24 and C30) and St. Lucia, as compared with Goldmann perimetry in Baltimore and repeat Dicon testing in Tanzania. Optic disc classification was based on disc photographs and clinical gradings in Barbados and Baltimore and mainly on clinical evaluation in Tanzania and St. Lucia. Because visual field and disc findings were an integral part of the POAG definition in these studies, these protocol differences undoubtedly affected their respective prevalence estimates, thus contributing to the apparent variation in rates. Regardless of the specific estimate, the high rates in the Barbados study, which is the largest of these studies and conservatively required both visual field and optic disc damage to define POAG, clearly indicate the severity and extent of the glaucoma problem in populations of African origin. Hence, although differences in definitions, protocols, and data completeness may partly account for the differences in the reported prevalence of POAG, results indicate an increased prevalence in the very few black populations studied. As more research is conducted in diverse regions of Africa and in other areas of the world with populations of African origin, it is possible that different POAG rates will be found, given the expected genetic and environmental variability among black populations. To enhance comparability, future studies should use standard definitions and protocols.

Risk Factors

Few studies have evaluated risk factors for POAG in black populations. In addition to race, the Barbados study found that increasing age, male gender, higher IOP, a family history of POAG, myopia, and a history of cataract were all risk factors for POAG.

> Leske MC, Connell AM, Wu SY, et al. Risk factors for open-angle glaucoma. The Barbados Eye Study. *Arch Ophthalmol.* 1995;113:918–924.

The Barbados study also found that lean body mass was associated with POAG in this population, a finding not previously reported; indeed, few studies have evaluated the role of body size (or patterns of adiposity) in POAG. Although diabetes and hypertension were very frequent in Barbados study black participants, thus allowing extensive evaluations, they were unrelated to POAG. However, both were associated with elevated IOP.

> Wu SY, Leske MC. Associations with intraocular pressure in the Barbados Eye Study. *Arch Ophthalmol.* 1997;115:1572–1576.

Many studies have also shown that hypertension and diabetes are related to high IOP, but their independent relationship to POAG has not been proven conclusively. However, low blood pressure–IOP ratios and low diastolic blood pressure–IOP differences (an indicator of perfusion pressure) were related to POAG in the Barbados study; low blood pressure–IOP differences were also found in the Baltimore study. These findings may reflect the role of vascular factors in POAG or may simply reflect its strong association with IOP. In the Barbados study, mean IOP was significantly higher in black than white participants (18.0 mm Hg vs 16.7 mm Hg), which is consistent with mean IOP levels (17.7 mm Hg) among African Caribbeans in St. Lucia. In contrast, the Baltimore and Tanzania studies found that average IOP levels in their black participants were similar to those of whites (approximately 16 mm Hg). The increased POAG prevalence in African-origin populations is thus not explained solely by an elevated IOP.

Conclusions

Although it is difficult to compare studies due to inconsistency of methods, definitions, populations, and other factors, it is evident that marked ethnic and racial differences exist in the prevalence of POAG. To date, there is no clear explanation for this variability. Hypertension and diabetes, which are common in black populations, do not seem to be the reason; in addition, the racial differences cannot be attributed to IOP alone. Gene–environment interactions, yet to be elucidated, are likely to play a role. Research is ongoing to understand why ethnic differences are present, with the ultimate aim of developing strategies to prevent blindness.

CHAPTER 16

Primary Angle-Closure Glaucoma

Background

History

The main emphasis of modern glaucoma research has been on the variant of the disease most commonly found in the populations of Europe and North America: primary open-angle glaucoma (POAG). It has recently been recognized that, on a worldwide scale, primary angle-closure glaucoma (PACG) may affect more people than POAG because of its higher prevalence in the densely populated nations of East and Southeast Asia.

Seminal descriptions of PACG have originated in Europe and North America and may not accurately depict the entity as it exists worldwide. Because of its low prevalence and incidence in the West, population-based studies of PACG are difficult. Furthermore, it is not certain that the condition has the same natural history in Asians as in Europeans. The latter factor especially has hindered efforts to tackle the problem of PACG blindness effectively on a global scale.

Although the classification of POAG has enjoyed progressive and logical revision, textbook descriptions of PACG have lagged behind.

Context

Traditionally, PACG has been classified according to symptoms into four categories:

- *Suspects* with a narrow drainage angle
- *Intermittent* or *subacute* PACG with a narrow drainage angle and remitting symptoms of anterior segment congestion
- *Acute* PACG with symptoms that are not self-aborting
- *Chronic* PACG in people with an occludable drainage angle and either raised IOP *or* glaucomatous optic neuropathy

Recent population-based research in Asia and Africa has shown repeatedly that glaucomatous visual loss in PACG is usually an asymptomatic condition. The florid presentation with pain, redness, reduced visual acuity, and an unreactive, mid-dilated pupil familiar to those reading Western textbooks of ophthalmology is less common. As the majority of people worldwide afflicted with PACG suffer asymptomatic loss of sight, the traditional classification is being reconsidered.

Foster PJ, Buhrmann R, Quigley HA, et al. The definition and classification of glaucoma in prevalence surveys. *Br J Ophthal.* 2002;86:238–242.

The most important feature of the disease, from both the individual's perspective and the community's (in terms of loss of livelihood, dependence on family, and use of health service resources), is loss of sight due to glaucomatous optic neuropathy. Anterior segment damage, such as lens opacities and iris sphincter dysfunction, and nonglaucomatous optic atrophy are less common causes of visual loss.

The diagnosis of POAG now requires evidence of "end-organ damage." Such emphasis in the diagnosis of PACG would aid the epidemiologic description of visual morbidity in the community and the design of public health policy aimed at reducing this. It would also set the study of PACG on a more scientific footing and assist development of logical management algorithms.

Primary angle closure (PAC) is characterized by contact between the iris and the trabecular meshwork associated with anatomic or physiologic features not found in the normal population. The presence of PAC confers an increased (but as yet unquantified) risk of developing glaucomatous optic neuropathy in exactly the same way as raised intraocular pressure (IOP) does. Making a distinction between these two causes may seem pedantic to the clinical ophthalmologist, as both PAC and glaucomatous optic neuropathy require treatment. However, the distinction is important when considering public health initiatives aimed at reducing blindness from PACG because the skills and infrastructure required will differ. To prevent PACG, the goal would almost certainly be to alter the configuration of the iridotrabecular angle on the assumption that this would significantly reduce the risk of developing glaucomatous optic neuropathy. Once PACG is established, the goal of all treatment is to reduce the IOP.

The following concepts are suggested for pursuing epidemiologic and public health research into PACG:

- *Primary angle-closure suspect:* A narrow, crowded anterior chamber angle in which appositional contact between the peripheral iris and posterior trabecular meshwork is considered possible but without signs of optic neuropathy
- *Primary angle closure*
    - *Nonischemic, chronic:* An occludable or partly closed drainage angle and features suggesting trabecular dysfunction, such as peripheral anterior synechiae, elevated IOP, or iris pigment deposition on the trabecular surface. The optic disc and visual field are normal.
    - *Ischemic, congestive:* The acute phase of anterior segment ischemia may be due to a sudden angle closure or a gradual closure, with IOP reaching a stage that causes ischemia. Typically, no optic neuropathy or visual field defect is demonstrable up to 3 months after the event. The presence of iris whorling, stromal atrophy, or glaukomflecken signify previous "acute" PAC. However, as these are areas of ischemic necrosis, "ischemic PAC" is likely the correct description. Differentiating between nonischemic and ischemic PAC is supported by experimental evidence that the iris and ciliary body are the ocular tissues most sensitive to pressure-induced ischemia. Damage to the optic nerve occurs only at higher pressures, and, therefore, anterior segment ischemic sequelae indicate that ischemic optic neuropathy may have occurred, but they do not confirm it.

- *Primary angle-closure glaucoma:* Glaucomatous optic atrophy with a characteristic visual field defect in the presence of an occludable drainage angle or signs of PAC

Anderson DR, Davis EB. Sensitivities of ocular tissues to acute pressure-induced ischemia. *Arch Ophthalmol.* 1975;93:267–274.

Pathogenesis

The evolution of PAC and associated glaucoma is conceptually divided into three phases:
- An anatomic predisposition to iridotrabecular contact
- Actual closure of the iridotrabecular recess
- Glaucomatous optic neuropathy in some individuals

Establishing the mechanism of closure is fundamental to managing the condition effectively and preventing visual loss. In PAC, at least two mechanisms cause closure of the angle.

Pupillary Block

Pupillary block can occur only when the plane of the pupil is anterior to the iris root. In such a situation, there may be a relative resistance to aqueous flow from the posterior to anterior chamber, resulting in a pressure gradient across the iris. Depending on the flexibility of the iris and on the pressure gradient, the iris may become bowed anteriorly. This bowing may cause part or all of the trabecular meshwork to be occluded by peripheral iris.

Non–Pupillary Block

Non–pupillary block has two subdivisions:

- *Plateau iris mechanism:* Anterior angulation of the peripheral iris caused by anterior rotation of the ciliary processes
- *Peripheral iris crowding and prominent last iris roll:* Mass effect of a thick iris being thrown into peripheral, circumferential folds with dilation

It has been stated previously that plateau iris configuration is common in East Asians. However, in population-based studies of gonioscopic anatomy in Mongolia and Singapore, a plateau iris configuration was found in only 8% of people in each population. A study in Mongolia of prophylaxis of PAC in eyes with occludable drainage angles found that 98% of angles were no longer occludable after laser iridotomy. This suggests that PAC in East Asian people, at least in the early stages, has a large component of pupillary block mechanism.

Epidemiology

Incidence

Incidence is the rate at which new cases of disease occur in a population. Figure 16-1 depicts the incidence of acute symptomatic PAC in Chinese Singaporean individuals 30

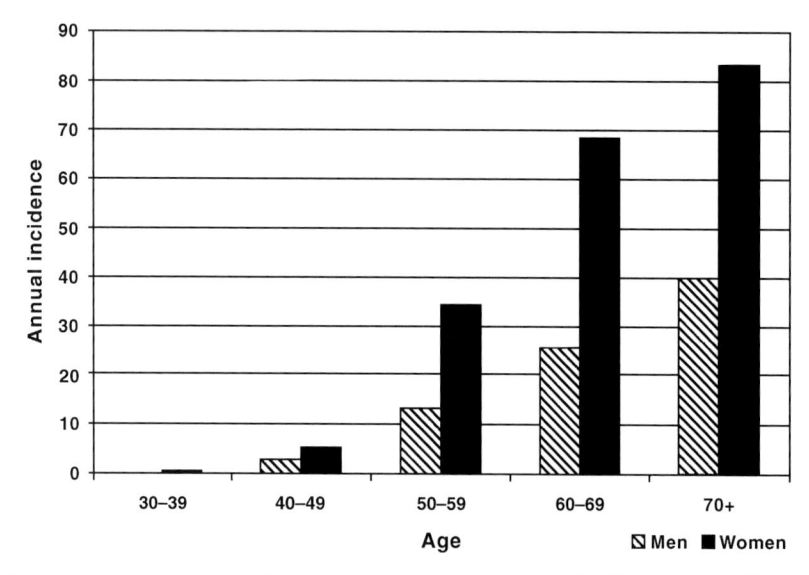

Figure 16-1 Age- and sex-specific incidence of symptomatic PAC (per 100,000 per year) in Chinese Singaporeans. Figures relate to the population aged 30 years and older. *(Data used with permission from Seah SK, Foster PJ, Chew PT, et al. Incidence of acute primary angle-closure glaucoma in Singapore: an island-wide survey. Arch Ophthalmol. 1997;115:1436–1440. Copyrighted 1997, American Medical Association.)*

years and older. The age and gender standardized incidence rate rises with age and is higher in women than men.

Data on incidence of symptomatic PAC ("acute" PACG) from five other countries give some insight into the role of ethnicity in angle closure. Finland had the lowest incidence of 4.7 per 100,000 per year in the population aged 30 years and older. The incidence is higher in Thailand (7.0), Israel (10.7), and Japan (11.4). The highest recorded incidence is found in the multiethnic population of Singapore (12.2). Among the Chinese population of Singapore, the incidence is 15.5. It is surprising that the incidence of symptomatic PAC is lower in the Southeast Asian population of Thailand than in Israel. There are several possible explanations for this:

- The Thai study may have failed to identify all eligible cases.
- One group of the multiethnic population of Israel may have a disproportionately high rate of angle closure and therefore may have skewed the figures.
- The population in Southeast Asia may, indeed, have a lower rate of PAC than other ethnic groups, especially the Chinese population of Singapore.

The data cited do not have the power to address this question. However, in a subsequent study of hospital discharge data for cases of PAC in Singapore, annual rates of 12.2 in Chinese, 6.0 in Malay, and 6.3 in people of Indian origin were found (all cited per 100,000 in the population aged 30 years and older). If one assumes that most hospital admissions for PACG are made on the grounds of symptomatic disease, these figures suggest that the Malay and Indian populations of Singapore do indeed have incidence rates of symptomatic PAC about half that of the Chinese population.

Seah SK, Foster PJ, Chew PT, et al. Incidence of acute primary angle-closure glaucoma in Singapore: an island-wide survey. *Arch Ophthalmol.* 1997;115:1436–1440.

Wong TY, Foster PJ, Seah SK, et al. Rates of hospital admissions for primary angle closure glaucoma among Chinese, Malays, and Indians in Singapore. *Br J Ophthalmol.* 2000;84: 990–992.

Prevalence

Prevalence of disease is the rate of existing cases in a population. The data on prevalence of PACG have recently been expanded to cover many different regions and ethnic groups. All figures reported here use the traditional classification and do not signify the rate of glaucomatous optic neuropathy; therefore, they represent rates of PAC with or without optic neuropathy. Figures cited apply to the population aged 40 years and older. Among people of European origin, prevalence of PACG ranges between 0.1% and 0.6%. The populations of Asia suffer higher rates, ranging from 0.4% in Japan to 1.4% in both Beijing, China, and Hövsgöl, northern Mongolia. The highest prevalence of PACG is reported among the Inuit living in arctic regions of Alaska, Canada, and Greenland, in whom the prevalence ranges from 2.6% to 3.5%.

Africa has not been adequately studied to allow a comprehensive statement about PACG prevalence to be made. Generalization is inappropriate because of the degree of genetic variation in the continent. One study in South Africa in a population of mixed African, European, and Southeast Asian heritage ("Cape-Malay" people) found a PACG prevalence of 2.3%. In a rural population in Tanzania (East Africa), the prevalence of the disease was 0.6%. Extrapolation to the rest of Africa is not appropriate.

Buhrmann RR, Quigley HA, Barron Y, et al. Prevalence of glaucoma in a rural East African population. *Invest Ophthalmol Vis Sci.* 2000;41:40–48.

Salmon JF, Mermoud A, Ivey A, et al. The prevalence of primary angle-closure glaucoma and open angle glaucoma in Mamre, western Cape, South Africa. *Arch Ophthalmol.* 1993;111: 1263–1269.

Reliable data for the Indian subcontinent are similarly lacking. The rate of PACG in the southern Indian state of Andhra Pradesh has been reported as 1.1%. In contrast, in nearby Tamil Nadu, the prevalence of the disease was reported as 4.3%. This striking difference in prevalence of disease in neighboring regions is probably due to differing diagnostic criteria.

Dandona L, Dandona R, Mandal P, et al. Angle-closure glaucoma in an urban population in southern India. The Andhra Pradesh Eye Disease Study. *Ophthalmology.* 2000;107: 1710–1716.

Jacob A, Thomas R, Koshi SP, et al. Prevalence of primary glaucoma in an urban south Indian population. *Indian J Ophthalmol.* 1998;46:81–86.

Risk Factors

The risk factors for PAC have been well established in Europeans and in Greenland Inuits. A crowded anterior segment is generally held to be the major predisposing factor. This is characterized by both axial and limbal shallowing of the anterior chamber, a smaller corneal diameter, and a tendency toward hypermetropic refraction with a short axial length. None of these factors is an absolute requirement, however, and one may find myopic subjects with a relatively long axial length who have PAC.

The tendency toward PAC may be familial. A study of patients with PAC and their first-degree relatives (siblings and children) compared ocular dimension in affected individuals and relatives with that of normal subjects closely matched for age, sex, and refractive error. The anterior chamber depth (ACD), lens thickness, and corneal diameter all differed significantly between normal people and the affected individuals and their families. The authors concluded that the anatomic tendency toward angle closure was a heritable trait. Alsbirk carried out a detailed study of the inheritance patterns of ACD in Inuits and Danes. Cautious extrapolation suggested that around 70% of age- and sex-independent variation in ACD was attributable to additive polygenic inheritance.

> Alsbirk PH. Primary angle-closure glaucoma. Oculometry, epidemiology, and genetics in a high risk population. *Acta Ophthalmol Suppl.* 1976;5–31.
>
> Tomlinson A, Leighton DA. Ocular dimensions in the heredity of angle-closure glaucoma. *Br J Ophthalmol.* 1973;57:475–486.

The anatomic predisposition toward PAC seems quite clear. However, the exact sequence of events triggering the condition is not well understood. Onset of symptomatic PAC has been associated with numerous drugs that affect the autonomic nervous system, including nebulized bronchodilators, tricyclic antidepressants, anti-Parkinsonian drugs, and even nasal decongestants. As many of these compounds are derived from naturally occurring substances (eg, belladonna alkaloids), it is possible that traditional herbal remedies may also play a role in triggering closure of the drainage angle. There have been several reports of an association between the climate and symptomatic PAC. The common trend is that attacks tend to be more frequent at times of temperature extremes (either high or low) and during times of prolonged darkness.

The major determinants in the development of optic neuropathy and visual field loss remain the degree of elevation of IOP and its duration.

Clinical Presentation and Findings

In most countries without a well-developed vision screening service, PACG often occurs as painless visual loss in one eye, found to have end-stage field loss. The other eye usually has some degree of glaucomatous neuropathy. These eyes are typically white, with clear corneas and reactive pupils. The limbal ACD is very shallow, being less than 10%–15% of corneal thickness. Screening IOP may be within normal limits or may be grossly elevated (even with a clear cornea). Glaucomatous optic neuropathy and associated visual field loss closely resemble that seen in POAG. The less prevalent clinical pattern, with which most hospital-based ophthalmologists are familiar, is that of the "acute" symptomatic presentation—a painful red eye with corneal edema and an unreactive pupil. The appearance of the optic disc may range from classically cupped to a pale, atrophic flat disc suggestive of anterior ischemic optic neuropathy.

Gonioscopy is the definitive examination in detecting PAC. Signs of prolonged iridotrabecular contact include geographic blotches of iris pigment on the surface of the trabecular meshwork or a broad band of pigment along Schwalbe's line. Peripheral anterior synechiae vary in width and height. At the earliest stage, they extend onto the scleral spur with a narrow sawtooth profile. These must be distinguished from iris processes by noticing that they distort the iris stroma. See BCSC Section 10, *Glaucoma*.

There is often a delay of several days before help is sought. In Singapore, the median time from onset of symptoms to presentation was 3 days (range 1 to 99 days). A delay in presentation of more than 24 hours is associated with an increased risk of 2.8 times of developing glaucoma after symptomatic PAC.

>   Wong JS, Chew PT, Alsagoff Z, et al. Clinical course and outcome of primary acute angle-closure glaucoma in Singapore. *Singapore Med J.* 1997;38:16–18.

Prevention

The number of people affected by PACG demands that methods of prevention be explored. The developing economies of East and Southeast Asia are home to the majority of sufferers. This means that reliance on detection in general optometric and ophthalmic practice is unlikely to have a significant impact on the problem. Inadequate access to eye care is a major problem in parts of the world, and avoidable blindness may occur. Therefore, large-scale, structured screening programs are needed. The decision to implement these initiatives, which would undoubtedly require significant staff, equipment, and administrative resources, would almost certainly have to be politically motivated and based on calculation of cost–benefit ratio.

Screening

A successful structured screening program for PACG would probably use demographic data to narrow the target population. Overall, women are more than twice as likely to be affected as men. The risk of glaucomatous loss is greatest in the 60- to 69-year-old age group, suggesting that preventive efforts should be focused on those 1 to 2 decades younger. Screening should aim at detecting evidence of an early, asymptomatic form of PACG (ie, PAC) for which simple, effective therapy could be administered. Three techniques can be used to detect early PAC. The first technique, and most promising of these, is measurement of axial anterior chamber depth.

Figure 16-2 shows the distribution of ACD in Mongolians, highlighting those with PAC. It can be seen that people with PAC typically have an ACD in a shallower range than that found in the population as a whole.

>   Congdon NG, Quigley HA, Hung PT, et al. Screening techniques for angle-closure glaucoma in rural Taiwan. *Acta Ophthalmol Scand.* 1996;74:113–119.
>   Devereux JG, Foster PJ, Baasanhu J, et al. Anterior chamber depth measurement as a screening tool for primary angle-closure glaucoma in an East Asian population. *Arch Ophthalmol.* 2000;118:257–263.

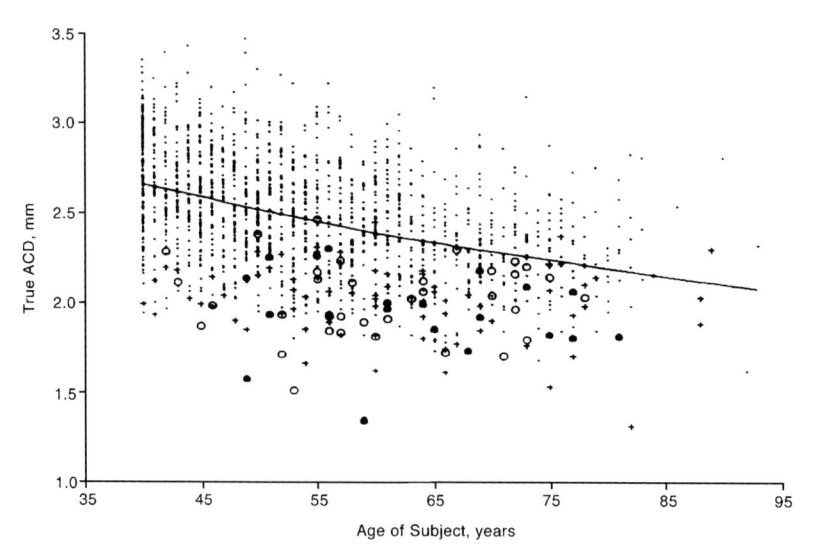

Figure 16-2 Anterior chamber depth against age in Mongolians, highlighting those with occludable drainage angles *(crosses)*, PAC *(open circles)*, and PACG *(filled circles)*. The trend in ACD with age is summarized by a LOWESS line. *(Reproduced with permission from Devereux JG, Foster PJ, Baasanhu J, et al. Anterior chamber depth measurement as a screening tool for primary angle-closure glaucoma in an East Asian population. Arch Ophthalmol. 2000;118:257–263. Copyrighted 2000, American Medical Association.)*

The performance of screening tests may also be evaluated graphically. Receiver operating characteristic (ROC) plots compare false-positive error rate (1 − specificity) on the *x*-axis with sensitivity on the *y*-axis. The area under the curve is a global index of test performance. The curve representing a test that has a performance no better than chance runs as a straight line from the bottom left to the top right corner. As a general rule, the closer the curve approaches the top left corner, the better the test performs.

Figure 16-3 is a ROC curve illustrating the efficacy of three methods of ACD measurement in detecting PAC. It shows that optical pachymetric measurements and ultrasound measures made with the probe mounted on a tonometer both perform well. However, measurements made using handheld ultrasound perform less well.

The second technique, estimating limbal chamber depth (the "van Herick" test), is a rapid testing tool that performs well in identifying PAC. In this test, a slit beam is shone onto the temporal limbus, perpendicular to the ocular surface. The observer judges the peripheral ACD and expresses this as a fraction of corneal thickness. A limbal chamber depth of less than a quarter of corneal thickness is indicative of a narrow drainage angle and deserves gonioscopic examination (it should be noted that this test is not intended as a substitute for detailed gonioscopic examination in clinical practice). Figure 16-4 is a ROC plot for limbal chamber depth as a screening tool for detection of PAC.

Both measurement of axial ACD and estimation of limbal chamber depth currently rely on relatively sophisticated equipment. The third technique is a simpler approach: assessing central ACD with a penlight held at the lateral canthus. This test is effective in skilled hands, but it does require experience to reach optimal performance.

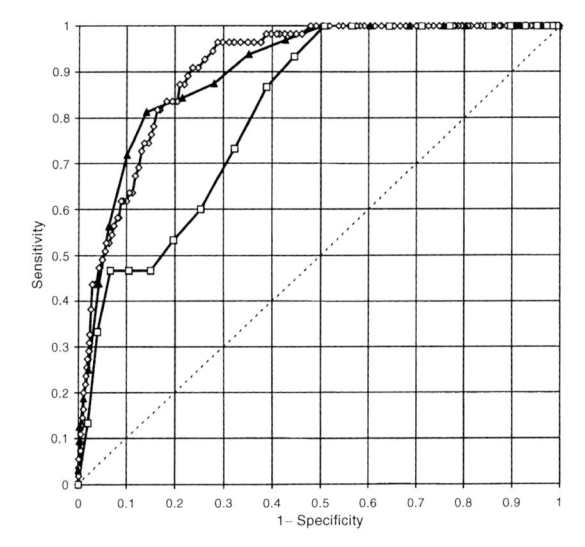

Figure 16-3 A receiver operating characteristic (ROC) curve showing the performance of ACD measurement as a screening tool for PAC. The diamonds represent the performance of optical pachymetry; triangles, a tonometer-mounted ultrasound probe; and squares, data for handheld ultrasound measurement. An ideal test would have a ROC curve passing through the top left corner of the plot. *(Redrawn with permission from Devereux JG, Foster PJ, Baasanhu J, et al. Anterior chamber depth measurement as a screening tool for primary angle-closure glaucoma in an East Asian population. Arch Ophthalmol. 2000;118:257–263. Copyrighted 2000, American Medical Association.)*

Treatment

Once detected, effective treatment of PAC must be delivered. In developing countries with a sizeable rural population, this means surgery. Surgical iridectomy is undoubtedly an effective method of managing the condition. However, it does carry with it the risks of intraocular surgery. Nd:YAG laser iridotomy is a highly attractive alternative. Laser units are portable and effective. Current opinion holds that any degree of iridotrabecular apposition justifies iridotomy or iridectomy although the scientific validity of this assertion remains to be proven in clinical trials. Recent follow-up studies of patients treated in Mongolia suggest that Nd:YAG laser iridotomy is effective in controlling IOP and preventing further closure of the angle in 98% of cases with PAC. Once glaucomatous optic neuropathy has developed, a peripheral iridotomy will be successful in controlling pressure and synechial closure in only 47%. These data are potentially confounded by "lead time bias," which is induced by detection and treatment at an early stage of disease taking longer to progress to "end stage."

> Nolan WP, Foster PJ, Devereux JG, et al. YAG laser iridotomy treatment for primary angle-closure in east Asian eyes. *Br J Ophthalmol.* 2000;84:1255–1259.
> Wilensky JT, Ritch R, Kolker AE. Should patients with anatomically narrow angles have prophylactic iridectomy? *Surv Ophthalmol.* 1996;41:31–36.

The optimal management of PAC that is not satisfactorily controlled by iridotomy with or without medication has not been fully elucidated. Trabeculectomy is not an appropriate management for symptomatic PAC where the IOP cannot be controlled. A study in Singapore (mean follow-up of 22 months) found that if satisfactory IOP control was not achieved preoperatively, only 66% of people undergoing trabeculectomy were likely to achieve pressures less than 21 mm Hg with or without medication.

> Aung T, Tow SL, Yap EY, et al. Trabeculectomy for acute primary angle closure. *Ophthalmology.* 2000;107:1298–1302.

Figure 16-4 A receiver operating characteristic (ROC) curve showing the performance of limbal chamber depth estimation in the detection of PAC. The solid line indicates the performance of the augmented grading scheme. The broken line indicates the performance of the traditional grading scheme. An ideal test would have an ROC curve passing through the top left corner of the plot. *(Redrawn with permission from the BMJ Publishing Group. From Foster PJ, Devereux JG, Alsbirk PH, et al. Detection of gonioscopically occludable angles and primary angle closure glaucoma by estimation of limbal chamber depth in Asians: modified grading scheme.* Br J Ophthalmol. *2000;84:186–192.)*

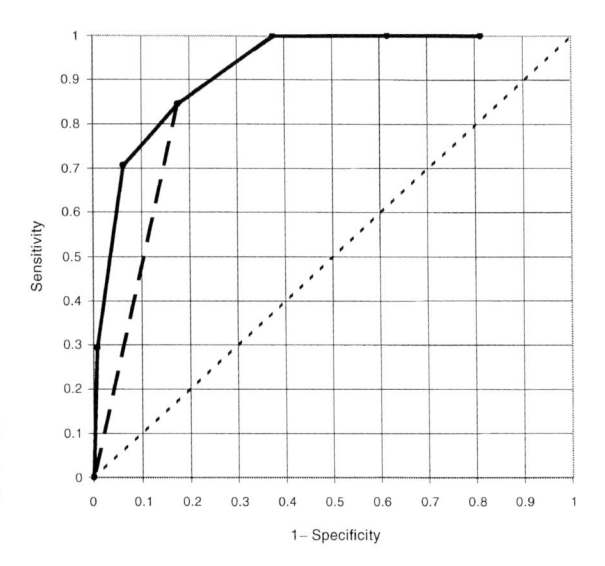

Cataract extraction and posterior chamber lens implantation has been proposed as a method of managing PAC. Combination phacoemulsification and goniosynechialysis has also been proposed. Although these recommendations are based on uncontrolled case series, removal of the lens is a logical therapeutic maneuver, as PAC is associated with a thick, anteriorly positioned lens. Furthermore, in developing countries, ophthalmic surgical services are invariably centered around provision of cataract surgery. Trabeculectomy often requires intensive postoperative follow-up and intervention to achieve optimal results. The more straightforward postoperative care of cataract patients is a strong advantage of this technique. The efficacy of iridectomy, trabeculectomy, and cataract surgery in the management of PAC(G) requires further evaluation in randomized, controlled clinical trials.

The Asymptomatic Narrow Angle and the "Fellow Eye"

In a multicenter prospective study of asymptomatic patients in the United States with ACD less than 2 mm or drainage angles that were potentially occludable, only 6% developed signs or symptoms consistent with PAC over a mean period of 2.7 years. A population-based study of Greenland Inuits, who have a high prevalence of PAC, found that fewer than 10% of untreated people with high-risk characteristics had developed PAC over a 10-year period (less than 1% annual risk of significant angle closure). It would therefore appear that an individual's risk of developing visually threatening sequelae is low on a year-to-year basis. However, it is now accepted practice to perform a laser iridotomy on patients with early gonioscopic evidence of angle closure, reflecting the perceived (although unproven) high benefit–risk ratio for this procedure. This view is probably justified when the potential for late-presentation diagnosis or misdiagnosis under nonophthalmologic care and the low incidence of sight-threatening complications of laser iridotomy are considered.

The management of an eye whose fellow has suffered an episode of symptomatic PAC is subject to little debate. Two European studies give overwhelming evidence in favor of prophylactic iridotomy. One describes 113 such "fellow" eyes, 58 of which developed symptomatic PAC (half within a 5-year period). Twenty-six of these 58 were using topical pilocarpine. A second study of 250 patients with PAC found that 72 did not have prophylactic peripheral iridectomy. Forty-three developed PAC (33 symptomatic, 10 asymptomatic or unknown), 33 of them within 6 years. There are no published studies of a similar nature dealing with Asian or African populations, but it would probably be unethical to carry out such a trial.

Lowe RF. Acute angle-closure glaucoma. The second eye: an analysis of 200 cases. *Br J Ophthalmol.* 1962;46:641–650.

Snow JT. Value of prophylactic peripheral iridectomy on the second eye in angle-closure glaucoma. *Trans Ophthalmol Soc UK.* 1977;97:189–191.

Wilensky JT, Kaufman PL, Frohlichstein D, et al. Follow-up of angle-closure glaucoma suspects. *Am J Ophthalmol.* 1993;115:338–346.

Research Currently Under Way

The field of PACG research has enjoyed renewed interest in the last decade. The basic epidemiology is now much better understood, and there now exist sufficient data to design trials for screening for and preventing the disease. Such trials should be assessed according to their impact on the visual function of the population. Several important questions remain to be addressed. An "occludable angle" remains a poorly characterized entity; further study is needed to determine when a narrow drainage angle becomes potentially occludable and how this affects the risk of glaucomatous visual loss. The natural history of both treated and untreated PAC and PACG need to be studied in much greater detail to decide the optimal timing and nature of medical intervention. However, public health efforts to prevent blindness from PACG offer much greater hope of success than has been the case with POAG.

CHAPTER 17

Application of Findings in Diabetic Retinopathy Studies: The Iceland Experience

Background

The Diabetic Retinopathy Study (DRS) was the first multicenter, prospective, randomized clinical trial in ophthalmology. The study was initiated because of the prevalence of blindness due to diabetic retinopathy, which is the leading cause of blindness in the United States and the United Kingdom among people aged 20–74 years. In Denmark, legal blindness in insulin-treated patients with type 1 diabetes was estimated to be 50 to 80 times greater than that in similar-aged patients without diabetes.

> The diabetic retinopathy study [editorial]. *Arch Ophthalmol.* 1973;90:347–348.
> Sjølie AK, Green A. Blindness in insulin-treated diabetic patients with age at onset less than 30 years. *J Chron Dis.* 1987;40:215–220.

The outcomes of the DRS showed the benefit of panretinal photocoagulation in the clinical management of advanced nonproliferative diabetic retinopathy (NPDR) and proliferative diabetic retinopathy (PDR), confirming a treatment strategy that reduced blindness as compared with the natural clinical course without panretinal photocoagulation treatment. See BCSC Section 12, *Retina and Vitreous*.

> Flynn HW Jr, Smiddy WE. *Diabetes and Ocular Disease. Past, Present, and Future Therapies.* Ophthalmology Monograph 14. San Francisco: American Academy of Ophthalmology; 2002.

In follow-up to the DRS, the Early Treatment Diabetic Retinopathy Study (ETDRS) addressed three issues:

- The timing of panretinal photocoagulation: Is earlier photocoagulation helpful?
- The value of acetylsalicylic acid in the prevention of progression of diabetic retinopathy
- The benefit of laser treatment for diabetic macular edema

The ETDRS results of early scatter photocoagulation showed a small reduction in risk of severe visual loss with severe NPDR and early PDR. This benefit appeared to be especially evident in patients with type 1 diabetes. The ETDRS showed reduced risk of visual acuity loss with focal/grid photocoagulation for diabetic macular edema.

The Diabetes Control and Complication Trial (DCCT) compared intensive versus conventional insulin treatment of type 1 diabetes mellitus. In 9 years, a 76% reduction of diabetic retinopathy progression was found in the intensive group compared with the conventional treatment group. In eyes with mild or moderate retinopathy at baseline, the intensive treatment group had a 61% reduction in progression to preproliferative or proliferative retinopathy and a 59% reduction in photocoagulation for macular edema when compared with the conventional treatment group.

The Wisconsin Epidemiologic Study of Diabetic Retinopathy (WESDR) provided data on the prevalence, incidence, and progression of diabetic retinopathy. It reported that, in addition to duration of disease, progression of diabetic retinopathy is associated with higher levels of blood glucose and elevated baseline glycosylated hemoglobin (HbA_{1c}) levels.

> Klein R, Klein BE, Moss SE. Relation of glycemic control to diabetic microvascular complications in diabetes mellitus. *Ann Intern Med.* 1996;124(1 pt 2):90–96.

The United Kingdom Prospective Diabetes Study (UKPDS) showed that intensive glycemic control from treatment with either a sulfonylurea or insulin is associated with a reduced risk of development of diabetic retinopathy and reduced progression of diabetic retinopathy in type 2 diabetes mellitus. In addition, a 29% reduction in retinal photocoagulation was found in the intensive group compared to the conventional group.

> Intensive blood-glucose control with sulphonylureas or insulin compared with conventional treatment and the risk of complications in patients with type 2 diabetes (UKPDS 33). United Kingdom Prospective Diabetes Study Group. *Lancet.* 1998;352:837–853.

These data suggest that prevention of diabetic retinopathy is attainable once the diagnosis of diabetes mellitus is made and intensive treatment instituted. However, the Visual Impairment Project in Melbourne, Australia, reveals that fewer than 50% of the people with diabetes are receiving timely and appropriate eye examinations. In a Hong Kong study using oral glucose tolerance testing, only 38% of workers with diabetes in an industrial company had been previously diagnosed. An alarming number of people have undiagnosed or latent type 2 diabetes mellitus, which perhaps is due to the insidious onset of this disease.

> Cockram CS, Woo J, Lau E, et al. The prevalence of diabetes mellitus and impaired glucose tolerance among Hong Kong Chinese adults of working age. *Diabetes Res Clin Pract.* 1993;21:67–73.

Pathogenesis

Refer to BCSC Section 1, *Update on General Medicine,* and BCSC Section 12, *Retina and Vitreous.*

Epidemiology

The incidence and prevalence of diabetes mellitus varies in different populations. The age-adjusted mean annual incidence of type 1 diabetes mellitus per 100,000 for the 20-year period 1970–1989 in Iceland was 9.4 (95% confidence interval [CI], 7.8–11.3). The incidence in Icelandic children under 15 years of age is low, especially in type 1, in comparison with Norway, Denmark, Sweden, and Finland, whose incidence per 100,000 person-years was 22, 23, 24, and 36, respectively.

The age-standardized prevalence of type 2 diabetes mellitus in Icelandic males aged 34–79 years is 2.9% (95% CI, 2.5–3.2) and 2.1% (1.8–2.5) for females.

> Helgason T, Danielsen R, Thorsson AV. Incidence and prevalence of type I (insulin-dependent) diabetes mellitus in Icelandic children 1970–1989. *Diabetologia.* 1992;35:880–883.
>
> Vilbergsson S, Sigurdsson G, Sigvaldason H, et al. Prevalence and incidence of NIDDM in Iceland: evidence for stable incidence among males and females 1967–1991—the Reykjavik Study. *Diabet Med.* 1997;14:491–498.
>
> WHO Study Group. *Prevention of Diabetes Mellitus.* Technical Report Series No. 844. Geneva: WHO; 1994:4.

Populations with some of the highest published prevalence of type 2 diabetes mellitus include the Pima Indians of Arizona, 50%; Fiji Asian Indians, 22%; Micronesians of Nauru, 17%; and the Mauritian Chinese, 13%. In these populations, glucose concentrations and obesity were the best predictors of type 2 diabetes mellitus risk.

> Dowse GK. Incidence of NIDDM and the natural history of IGT in Pacific and Indian Ocean populations. *Diabetes Res Clin Pract.* 1996;(suppl 34):S45–S50.

Prevalence of Diabetic Retinopathy

In Iceland, the crude prevalence of diabetic retinopathy detected with fundus photography in 205 patients with type 1 diabetes was 52%. The prevalence of diabetic retinopathy is related to the duration of diabetes (Fig 17-1).

> Kristinsson JK. Diabetic retinopathy. Screening and prevention of blindness. A doctoral thesis. *Acta Ophthalmol Scand Suppl.* 1997;(suppl 223):1–76.

In the population-based Rotterdam Study, the prevalence of diabetic retinopathy was 4.8% (296 of the 6191 participants 55 years of age or older).

> Stolk RP, Vingerling JR, Paulus TVM, et al. Retinopathy, glucose and insulin in an elderly population: the Rotterdam study. *Diabetes.* 1995;44:11–15.

The prevalence of clinically significant diabetic macular edema also is observed to increase with duration of diabetes and, after 25 years or more with diabetes, about 25% have developed diabetic macular edema (Fig 17-2).

After 20 years of diabetes, between 30%–40% of patients with type 1 have PDR (Fig 17-3).

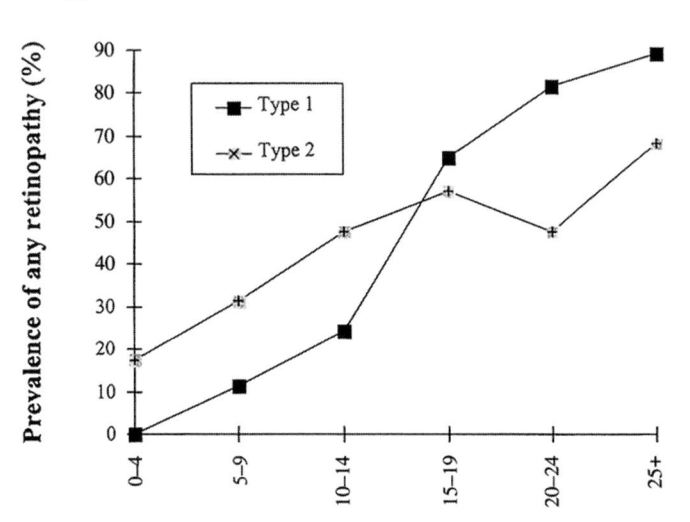

Figure 17-1 Prevalence of diabetic retinopathy as a function of duration of diabetes in the Icelandic population. *(Reproduced with permission from Blackwell Publishing. From Stefánsson E, Bek T, Porta M, et al. Screening and prevention of diabetic blindness. Acta Ophthalmol Scand. 2000;78:374–385.)*

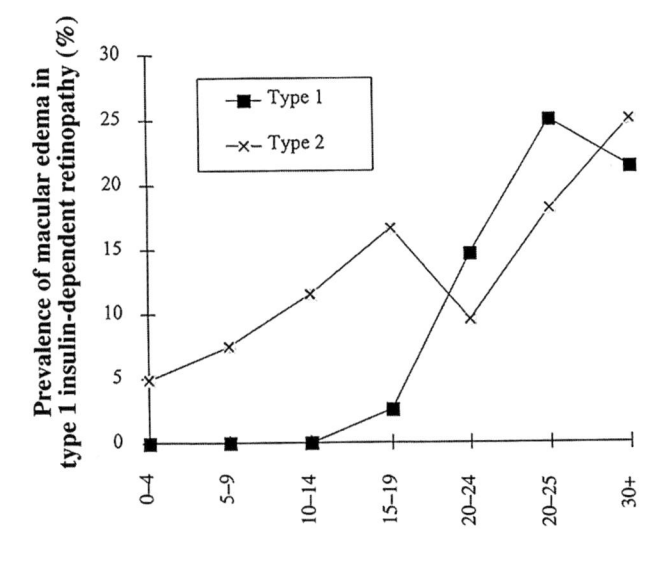

Figure 17-2 Prevalence of diabetic macular edema as a function of duration of diabetes in the Icelandic population. *(Reproduced with permission from Blackwell Publishing. From Stefánsson E, Bek T, Porta M, et al. Screening and prevention of diabetic blindness. Acta Ophthalmol Scand. 2000;78:374–385.)*

Incidence of Diabetic Retinopathy

The incidence of any diabetic retinopathy, proliferative diabetic retinopathy, and clinically significant diabetic macular edema was somewhat less in Iceland when compared with that observed by WESDR. Although we cannot be certain of the explanation, the mean HgA_{1c} was 7.5% in the Iceland sample and 12.5% in the WESDR study (Fig 17-4).

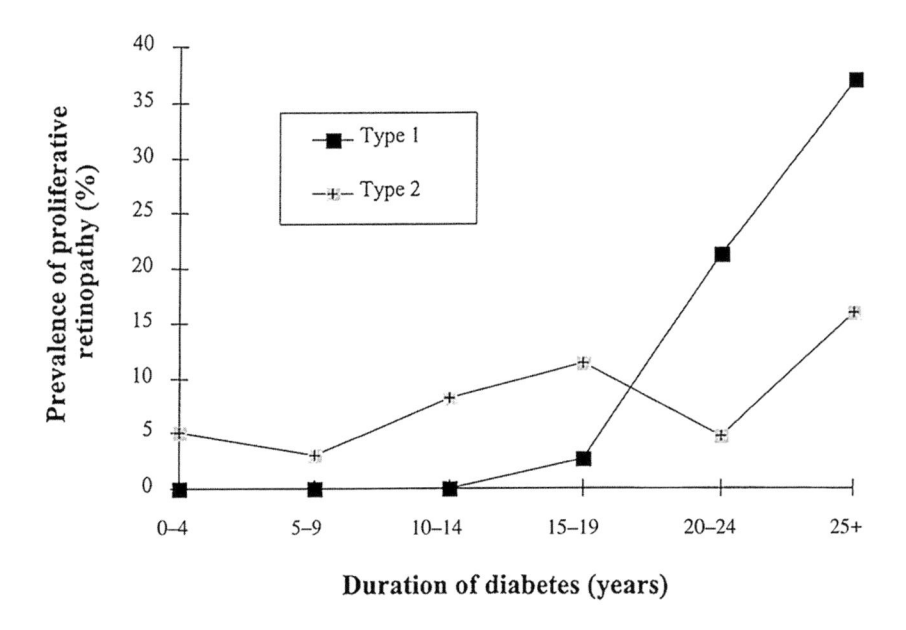

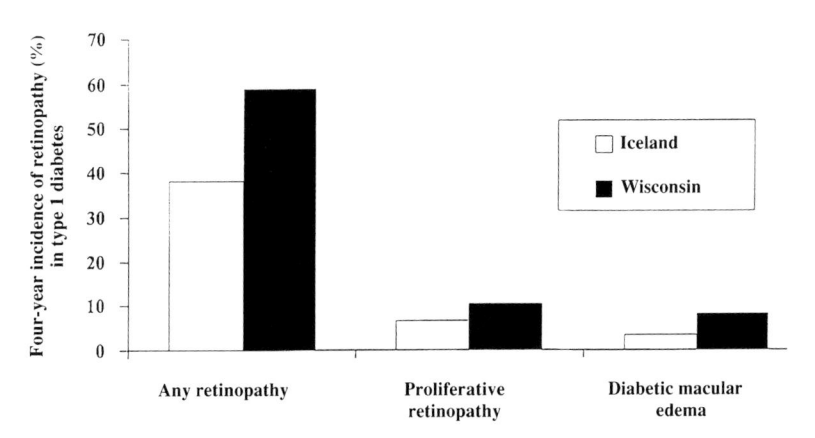

CHAPTER 17: Application of Findings in Diabetic Retinopathy Studies • 193

Figure 17-4 Incidence of diabetic retinopathy in Iceland and Wisconsin over 4 years. *(Reproduced with permission from Blackwell Publishing. From Stefánsson E, Bek T, Porta M, et al. Screening and prevention of diabetic blindness.* Acta Ophthalmol Scand. *2000;78:374–385.)*

Screening for Diabetes Mellitus

A general screening program for diabetes mellitus must be medically effective and economically sound and cost-effective. (See BCSC Section 1, *Update on General Medicine.*) An ideal screening test should be both highly sensitive and specific; however, because these parameters are inversely related, a compromise is required. A highly sensitive screening test will correctly identify subjects with the disease. A highly specific screening test will correctly identify normal subjects. A screening test can be misleading if the test result indicates positive but the disease is absent (false positive) or negative when the disease is present (false negative).

Risk Factors

In the United Kingdom, the British Diabetic Association recommends that screening be restricted to subjects between 40 and 75 years of age and be repeated only every 5 years. If a risk factor such as obesity, family history of diabetes, older age, being a member of certain ethnic groups, or women with a history of gestational diabetes or high-birthweight children is present, the screening should be repeated every 3 years if the screening test is normal.

> Paterson KR. Population screening for diabetes mellitus. Professional Advisory Committee of the British Diabetic Association. *Diabet Med.* 1993;10:777–781.

Screening selected members of a population with high-risk factors for diabetes is most cost-effective. The choice of a particular method could be based on cost, convenience, and availability.

Treatment

The DCCT reported the value of intensive insulin therapy in lowering the incidence of severe retinopathy and reducing the risk of severe nonproliferative and proliferative retinopathy in type 1 diabetes mellitus when compared with conventional insulin therapy. The Stockholm Diabetes Intervention Study and a meta-analysis of six similar prospective randomized clinical trials showed that the risk of diabetic retinopathy progression and the risk of requiring photocoagulation for proliferative diabetic retinopathy was significantly reduced in patients with type 1 diabetes who received intensive therapy treatment compared with those in the conventional treatment group. The UKPDS demonstrated conclusively that intensive glycemic control showed a reduction in diabetic complications in type 2 diabetes mellitus. In Japan, the Kumamoto University Study compared an intensive insulin treatment group of nonobese patients with type 2 diabetes with a conventional insulin treatment group over a 6-year period. Data showed a mean HbA_{1c} of 7.1% and a mean fasting blood sugar (FBS) of 157 mg/dL in the intensive treatment group, compared with a HbA_{1c} of 9.4% and FBS of 221 mg/dL in the conventional group. Progression of diabetic retinopathy and the need for retinal photocoagulation was reduced in the intensive insulin treatment group.

> Ohkubo Y, Kishikawa H, Araki E, et al. Intensive insulin therapy prevents the progression of diabetic microvascular complications in Japanese patients with non–insulin-dependent diabetes mellitus: a randomized prospective 6-year study. *Diabetes Res Clin Pract.* 1995;28: 103–117.
>
> Wang PH, Lau J, Chalmers TC. Meta-analysis of effects of intensive blood-glucose control on late complications of type I diabetes. *Lancet.* 1993;341:1306–1309.

The Iceland Experience

In Iceland, an effective diagnostic and therapeutic program for diabetes mellitus has been established in a centralized University Hospital clinic in Reykjavik. This clinic serves more than 95% of known patients with diabetes in Iceland and offers educational support to those patients. It has been an established practice at the clinic to strive for near-normal blood glucose levels in patients with the disease. In 1988 and 1990, the mean HbA_{1c} in clinic patients with type 1 diabetes mellitus was 7.0 ± 1.3% and 7.4 ± 1.4%, compared with WESDR patients, who had a baseline mean HbA_{1c} of 12.5 ± 2.6%. This difference reflects tighter control of the Icelandic patients with type 1 diabetes mellitus.

> Hreidarsson AB. *Diabetes Mellitus in Iceland: Prevalence, Incidence, Organization of Services, Treatment and Long-term Complications.* Reykjavik, Iceland: Ministry of Health and Social Security; 1995:9–17. (56 pages.)

Hypertension in patients with diabetes is also a risk factor for vision impairment. An important part of the UKPDS was the Hypertension in Diabetes Study. This multicenter randomized controlled clinical trial of 1148 patients compared tight blood pressure control (<150/85 mm Hg) with control that was not as tight (<180/105 mm Hg). Over the study period (median follow-up of 8.4 years), the mean blood pressure was 144/82 mm Hg in the tight group compared with 154/87 mm Hg in the less-tight group ($P < 0.0001$). After 7.5 years, the tight control group showed a 34% reduction in the risk of progression of retinopathy and a 47% reduction in the risk of loss of three lines of ETDRS visual acuity.

> Tight blood pressure control and risk of macrovascular and microvascular complications in type 2 diabetes: UKPDS 38. UK Prospective Diabetes Study Group. *BMJ.* 1998;317:703–713.

Patient education and compliance is an essential part of good glycemic and blood pressure control in diabetes mellitus. Inability to attend health visits without assistance and failure to attend appointments, however, increase the risk of complications.

Screening for Diabetic Retinopathy

A screening program for diabetic eye disease was established in Iceland in 1980. The number of patients with diabetes seen regularly has increased considerably since then, with 70%–80% of patients in the country with type 1 participating in the program in 1990, increasing to over 90% in 1994. About a fifth of those with type 2 diabetes mellitus in Iceland participated in the program in 1990; it is not possible to make a direct comparison of diabetic retinopathy screening between Iceland and the United States. The 1987 National Health Interview Survey showed that 51% of participants with diabetes in the United States had not received a dilated eye examination in the preceding year.

> Brechner RJ, Cowie CC, Howie LJ, et al. Ophthalmic examination among adults with diagnosed diabetes mellitus. *JAMA.* 1993;270:1714–1718.

The prevalence of legal blindness due to all diabetic retinopathy in Iceland in 1980 and 1994 is compared in Figure 17-5.

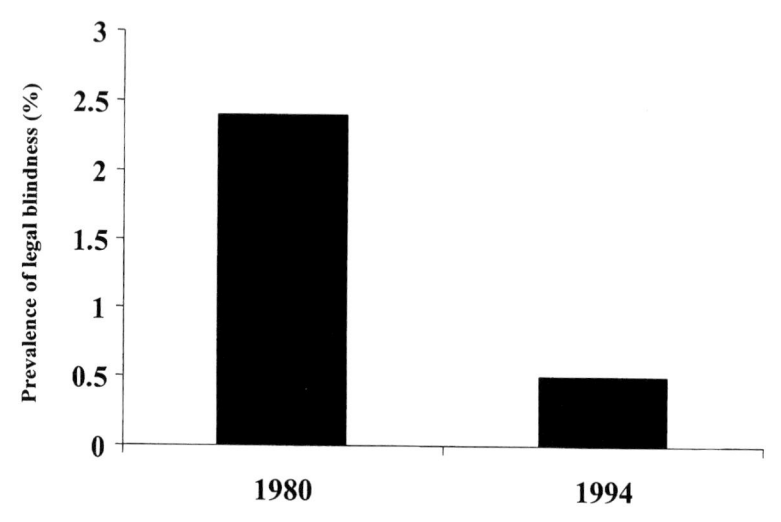

Figure 17-5 Prevalence of legal blindness in patients with diabetes in Iceland in 1980, at the beginning of the screening program, and 14 years later, in 1994. *(Reproduced with permission from Blackwell Publishing. From Stefánsson E, Bek T, Porta M, et al. Screening and prevention of diabetic blindness.* Acta Ophthalmol Scand. *2000;78:374–385.)*

In Iceland, an attempt has been made to make the screening program more efficient by identifying subgroups at low risk of developing diabetic ocular complications that require treatment and therefore need less frequent screening. The results in Iceland indicate that children with diabetes under the age of 12 years do not need regular screening for eye disease. Biannual examinations, including annual eye examinations and fundus photography, seem to suffice in type 1 and type 2 diabetes mellitus without retinopathy. Laser treatment is actively administered for proliferative retinopathy and diabetic macular edema according to the DRS and ETDRS criteria.

An analysis of the medical and economic implications of alternative screening strategies for detecting retinopathy in a diabetic population indicated that an annual examination of all patients with diabetes and a semiannual examination of those with retinopathy may be more effective than an annual examination with fundus photography. This screening strategy is consistent with the Preferred Practice Pattern for diabetic retinopathy of the American Academy of Ophthalmology.

Diabetic Retinopathy. Preferred Practice Patterns. San Francisco: American Academy of Ophthalmology; 2003.

Javitt JC, Canner JK, Frank RG, et al. Detecting and treating retinopathy in patients with type I diabetes mellitus. A health policy model. *Ophthalmology.* 1990;97:483–494.

Other screening options include community-wide fundus photography for early detection of diabetic retinopathy by mobile teams. Photography through dilated pupils is offered free of charge at 80 primary health care centers in Stockholm. This method of early diagnosis is feasible, acceptable, and offers twice the utilization as the usual referral-based system of care. It is now planned to extend this service to cover the whole of Sweden.

Backlund LB, Algvere PV, Rosenqvist U. Early detection of diabetic retinopathy by a mobile retinal photography service working in partnership with primary health care teams. *Diabet Med.* 1998;15 (suppl 3):S32 –S37.

Cost-effectiveness

Although intensively treating hyperglycemia may double the cost, this increase in cost is offset by reductions in the expense of managing complications, the increased productivity of a healthier person, and the value of an improved quality of life for the patient. Incorporating data from population-based epidemiologic studies and multicenter clinical trials using computer models, screening and treatment of eye disease in patients with diabetes mellitus costs US$3190 per quality-adjusted life-year (QALY) saved. This average cost is a weighted average (based on disease prevalence) of the cost-effectiveness of detecting and treating diabetic eye disease in those with type 1 diabetes mellitus (US$1996 per QALY), those with type 2 who use insulin for glycemic control (US$2933 per QALY), and those with type 2 who do not use insulin for glycemic control (US$3530 per QALY). This analysis indicates that in the United States, prevention programs aimed at improving eye care for persons with diabetes result in substantial federal budgetary savings and are highly cost-effective health investments for society. Diabetes screening is more cost-effective than many routinely provided health interventions. In remote areas, where access to providers is limited, the cost-effectiveness of 7-field fundus photographic screening improves access, and this mobile screening method offers some distinct advantages.

Javitt JC, Aiello LP. Cost-effectiveness of detecting and treating diabetic retinopathy. *Ann Intern Med.* 1996;124(1 Pt 2):164–169.

Martin JD, Yidegiligne HM. The cost-effectiveness of a retinal photography screening program for preventing diabetic retinopathy in the First Nations diabetic population in British Columbia, Canada. *Int J Circumpolar Health.* 1998;57(suppl 1):379–382.

Outcomes

In 1990, 10 years after the establishment of the Iceland diabetic retinopathy screening program, the prevalence of visual acuity ≤6/60 due to diabetic retinopathy in type 1 and type 2 diabetes mellitus was reported at 1.0% and 1.6%, respectively. In 1994, 174 patients (85%) completed the four annual screening examinations. Visual acuity remained quite stable and no one became legally blind—that is, ≤6/60. The 4-year incidence of any retinopathy was observed in 38% (32 patients out of 84). The 4-year incidence of proliferative diabetic retinopathy was 6.6% (10 patients out of 152). The 4-year incidence of macular edema was 3.4% (5 patients out of 149). All patients with proliferative diabetic retinopathy had had panretinal photocoagulation.

Kristinsson JK, Hauksdóttir H, Stefánsson E, et al. Active prevention in diabetic eye disease: a 4-year follow-up. *Acta Ophthalmol Scand.* 1997;75:249–254.

The utilization of diabetes services may have been better in Iceland than in Wisconsin during the late 1970s and 1980s. In the WESDR at baseline, 33% of participants with diabetes had not seen an ophthalmologist in the previous 2 years. Also at baseline, 41% of the younger-onset group and 70% of the older-onset group with DRS high-risk characteristics had not been treated with photocoagulation. Surprisingly, 4 years later, more than half of these groups still had not been treated with photocoagulation.

> Klein R, Moss SE, Klein BE, et al. The Wisconsin Epidemiologic Study of Diabetic Retinopathy: VIII. The incidence of retinal photocoagulation. *J Diabet Complications.* 1988;2:79–87.

In the WESDR, the group of patients with young-onset (<30 years) diabetes had a 4-year incidence of blindness of 1.5%. This difference is not statistically significant because of the small numbers in the Iceland sample. However, the WESDR 4-year incidence results for patients with type 1 diabetes mellitus were higher than those observed in Iceland: for any retinopathy in type 1 diabetes mellitus, 59% (160 patients out of 271); for proliferative retinopathy, 10.5% (75 patients out of 713); and for macular edema, 8.2% (50 patients out of 610).

> Klein R, Klein BE, Moss SE, et al. The Wisconsin Epidemiologic Study of Diabetic Retinopathy. IX. Four-year incidence and progression of diabetic retinopathy when age at diagnosis is less than 30 years. *Arch Ophthalmol.* 1989;107:237–243.

Utilization of Eye-Care Services

Iceland has few barriers to eye-care services. Access is good because of a good physician–patient ratio, adequate medical equipment infrastructure, and efficient clinical services. Other important issues influencing utilization elsewhere, such as regional poverty, poor education, cultural beliefs, and ethnic barriers, are not major barriers in Iceland. In Iceland, however, as in most places, distance, work, dependence, mobility, and weather may influence utilization of services by patients.

Study Strengths and Weaknesses

The standardized and centralized medical management of the diabetic population in Reykjavik is a strength of the Iceland experience. This is reflected in the high attendance at follow-up visits, near-normal fasting blood glucose levels, and mean glycosylated hemoglobin levels near 7%. The WESDR reported that over 70% of participants with diabetes after 10 years in the study reported not having a dilated eye examination because "they had no problems with their eyes." In addition, nearly 1 in 3 participants in the WESDR reported that they were not told that they needed an eye examination.

> Moss SE, Klein R, Klein BE. Factors associated with having eye examinations in persons with diabetes. *Arch Fam Med.* 1995;4:529–534.

Active diabetic retinopathy screening and the application of the DRS and ETDRS laser treatment guidelines are also strengths of the Iceland practice.

The most obvious weakness of the Iceland data is the small numbers in the sample populations. In addition, the lower prevalence of diabetes in the population and the homogeneous ethnic composition of the Icelandic population raise concern about the transferability of the findings to other populations.

Although only 14% were lost to follow-up in the Iceland study, this is an important group when the sample is small.

Conclusion

The Iceland studies provide important data on screening for diabetes mellitus and diabetic retinopathy and for managing the disease. By applying the findings from the DRS, ETDRS, DCCT, and the UKPDS, and through early detection of high-risk patients with diabetes, we can greatly reduce the incidence of blindness from diabetic retinopathy.

The success of the Iceland program may be credited to the dedicated effort of one man. Thorir Helgason was born in Reykjavik in 1932 and received his medical degree from the University of Iceland in 1959. He did postgraduate training in internal medicine and endocrinology in the United Kingdom. He returned to his native Iceland in the early 1970s and immediately took the lead in diabetology in Iceland. He was instrumental in the establishment of The Icelandic Diabetic Association in 1971, and in 1974 he became the first chief physician of a newly established ambulatory care facility for people with diabetes in The University Hospital in Reykjavik. He ran the diabetes clinic with unparalleled enthusiasm and vigor. From the beginning, he axiomatically determined that keeping blood glucose levels close to the physiologic levels was the main goal of treatment, and he provided his patients with the drugs, diet, and discipline necessary to achieve this goal.

The campaign against diabetic complications in Iceland has also had good results. Diabetic nephropathy has become uncommon; the perinatal death rate in diabetic pregnancies has decreased from 10% in the 1960s to 2.3% in the 1980s; and, from 1983 to 1999, no mother with diabetes lost a child in pregnancy or delivery.

Thorir Helgason was decades ahead of his time in his insight into the pathophysiology of diabetic complications. The value of striving for euglycemia was not widely recognized in the 1970s, and it was only in the 1990s that this approach was validated in the DCCT.

Dr Helgason assembled a team of endocrinologists, residents, nurses, dietitians, and podiatrists for the diabetes clinic. It was never a large team, but it was very dedicated; it managed to care for almost all patients with type 1 diabetes and for a large number of those with type 2 diabetes in a facility comprising a few rooms in the hospital outpatient clinic. This is a prime example of what a small group of health care workers with limited resources can accomplish and at the same time shows the value of leadership and insight.

A physician's career is relatively short. It is gratifying to know that in this time a physician can approach a problem, even a nationwide problem of public health; analyze the problem; create the instruments to deal with it; and live to see the benefits.

PART IV

Preventable Infectious Causes of Vision Impairment

Introduction

Infectious diseases have always had a prominent place in the history of ophthalmology, as they are often prevalent, easily recognizable, and treatable. Here, we cover a spectrum of ocular infections important in the developing world, some of which are now so rare in the United States and Western Europe that they seem Historical and some whose full importance internationally may not yet be recognized.

Credé prophylaxis for ophthalmia neonatorum (discussed in Part II of this volume) was one of the major public health achievements of the 19th century. The enrollment in blindness schools in Europe dropped considerably in the first few decades after its introduction—there are estimates that a quarter of vision impairment at the time was due to gonorrhea. Some have worried, however, that we have grown complacent with coverage and that many are not benefiting from this simple, remarkably effective public health measure.

Trachoma is one of the oldest diseases known to man; its presence is recorded in an early medical papyrus from Egypt. Indigenous active trachoma has not been seen in Western Europe and the United States for decades, but it is still prevalent in poor, dry areas of Africa, Australia, the Middle East, and Southeast Asia. Trachoma prevention is interesting epidemiologically, in part because prevention can be primary (hygiene to prevent infection), secondary (antibiotics to clear infection), or tertiary (surgery for entropion/trichiasis). Although trachoma is an infectious disease in its own right, caused by recurrent episodes of chlamydial conjunctivitis, most vision impairment is probably caused by secondary infections resulting in bacterial or fungal corneal ulcers. Some may argue that we should also concentrate on prophylaxis and treatment of the corneal ulcers due to end-stage trachoma *(quaternary prevention?).*

Corneal ulcers resulting from microbial keratitis are a major, perhaps underappreciated, cause of vision impairment worldwide, even if we don't include those due to trachoma. They are particularly common in agricultural areas. Often individuals don't seek medical attention until it is too late or unless the second eye is involved. As most treatment is empirical, it is important to know the common etiologies—they are remarkably different in different areas. Corneal ulcers may not be an inevitable occurrence in poor areas; prophylaxis of all abrasions with inexpensive antibiotics has recently been shown to reduce the incidence of ulcers at the population level.

In HIV, as with trachoma, it is not the original infection that causes vision impairment but rather a secondary infection, most commonly from cytomegalovirus (CMV) retinitis. The distribution of CMV retinitis cases is not always similar to that of HIV. CMV retinitis was a major cause of vision impairment with AIDS in the 1980s in the developed world; its incidence has recently decreased remarkably with highly active antiretroviral therapy (HAART). However, even with the huge burden of HIV and the scarcity of treatment in sub-Saharan Africa and Southeast Asia, CMV retinitis has never been an important cause of vision impairment in these areas, perhaps because the average lifespan with AIDS is so much shorter. As treatment improves for other AIDS-related diseases and lifespans are extended, it will be important to monitor the incidence of CMV retinitis cases in the developing world.

Onchocerciasis is found in a relatively small geographical area. In these areas, however, its effects are devastating. The two-pronged approach to its elimination—eliminating the vector and eliminating the infection itself—has proven remarkably successful. The donation of antibiotics by a pharmaceutical company has been the model for other diseases, including trachoma. Although the long life cycle of *Onchocerca volvulus* will delay elimination, the disease is apparently now well on its way to disappearing.

The infectious causes of vision impairment discussed in this section have placed different burdens on the developing world than on the developed world. The current state of these diseases ranges from nearly eliminated to not yet fully appreciated—but with all of them, relatively simple public health measures may yield great benefits.

Thomas M. Lietman, MD

CHAPTER 18

Trachoma

Background

History

Trachoma was first described in Egypt in the 16th-century BC Ebers Papyrus. The infectious potential of *Chlamydia trachomatis* was demonstrated by experimental transmission of the agent from an Indonesian case of trachoma to an orangutan in 1907 and was first grown in culture by T'ang in Beijing in 1957. Several of Europe's largest eye hospitals were founded in the 19th century to care for trachoma cases. Trachoma had disappeared from Europe in the early 1900s and from the last areas in the United States (Appalachia and the Southwest) by the 1960s. However, it is still present in much of the developing world and, after cataract, is one of the leading causes of vision impairment worldwide. In addition, only relatively recently has *C trachomatis* been identified as an important cause of sexually transmitted disease.

Context

Trachoma is essentially two diseases. *Active trachoma* is caused by infection with *C trachomatis* and is found more frequently in children (Fig 18-1). *Cicatricial trachoma* is the result of multiple episodes of active trachoma and is seen most often in adults (Fig 18-2).

Economic Impact

Cost of treatment

Because reinfection is so common, it is not productive simply to treat individual cases of active trachoma. Rather, treatment efforts have to be directed toward a community and include the costs of identifying high-risk communities, educating these communities concerning the importance of hygiene, purchasing and distributing antibiotics, identifying trichiasis cases, and performing corrective surgery. Efforts are under way to reduce the costs of tetracycline ointment and systemic azithromycin for trachoma control programs. Azithromycin is considerably more expensive than topical tetracycline; it has been donated by the government in Australia and by Pfizer Inc in countries chosen by the International Trachoma Initiative.

Corrective surgery for trichiasis can be performed in about 15 minutes for approximately US$10–$20.

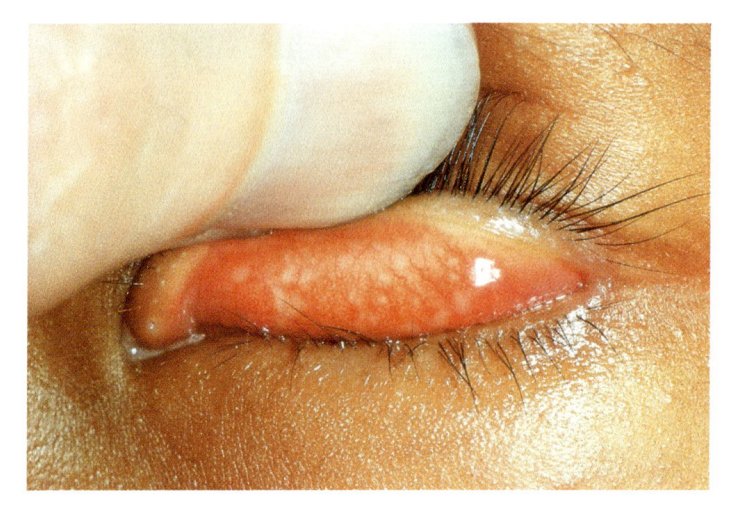

Figure 18-1 Follicular trachoma (TF): five follicles, each greater than 0.5 mm, in the upper tarsal conjunctiva. Both TF and TI (Fig 18-5) are considered to be *active trachoma*. *(Photograph courtesy of Thomas M. Lietman, MD.)*

Cost of lost productivity

Although vision impairment from trichiasis is rare in those under 30 years old and much more common in the elderly, it can still be particularly costly to families and communities, as younger, productive members of the community have to care for the blind.

Pathogenesis

C trachomatis ocular infections (serovars A, B, and C) are transmitted by hand-to-eye contact (and perhaps to some extent by face flies) and cause a follicular conjunctivitis (active trachoma) (see Fig 18-1). Chronic inflammation from recurrent infections leads to conjunctival scarring (cicatricial trachoma; Fig 18-2) by late childhood or early adulthood. Progressive scarring and contraction of existing scars can distort the upper tarsus, leading to cicatricial entropion and trichiasis (Fig 18-3). Trichiasis predisposes individuals to bacterial and fungal corneal ulcers. In addition, decreased mucin and tear production from the scarred conjunctiva and lacrimal glands are a risk factor for corneal ulcers. Although pannus alone occasionally leads to decreased vision, central corneal ulcers are the most frequent cause of visual loss in trachoma.

Epidemiology

Surveys to Determine Prevalence/Incidence

Trachoma has been estimated by the World Health Organization (WHO) to cause 15% of world blindness. It is a leading cause of preventable eye disease. Approximately 150 million people are infected with ocular chlamydia, 10 million have trachomatous trichi-

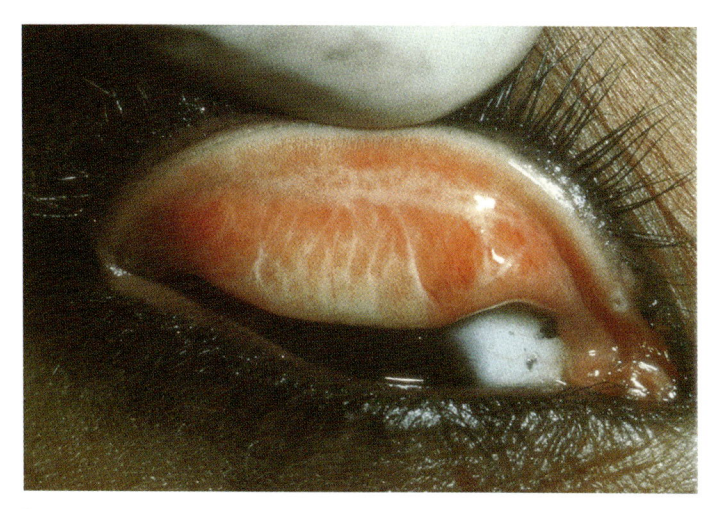

Figure 18-2 Cicatricial trachoma (TS): presence of scarring in the upper tarsal conjunctiva. *(Photograph courtesy of Thomas M. Lietman, MD.)*

asis, and 6 million are blind (<20/400) from trachoma. Hyperendemic trachoma, with more than 30% active trachoma in children, has been found in many countries, including Egypt, Tanzania, The Gambia, Morocco, Mali, and Nepal (Fig 18-4). In some communities, up to 60% of children have active trachoma, and essentially all adults have some degree of conjunctival scarring. Trachoma programs are often focused in areas where the prevalence of active trachoma is greater than 10% in children aged 10 years and under because lower prevalences may be due to background (causes of conjunctivitis other than *C trachomatis*) and because less frequent infection may be less likely to lead to cicatricial disease and vision impairment.

Risk Factors

Geographic
Trachoma is found in poor communities with no access to water. It is most prevalent in sub-Saharan Africa and along the Nile River but is also found in central Australia; northeastern Brazil; areas of the Indian subcontinent, such as Nepal; and areas of Southeast Asia, such as Vietnam (see Fig 18-4).

Environmental
Although flies are not necessary for the transmission of trachoma, recent studies suggest that fly control may reduce active trachoma. Hyperendemic trachoma is found only in extremely arid areas. A lack of access to potable water has been shown to be a risk factor for active trachoma. In many areas, active trachoma is markedly increased at certain times of the year—for example, immediately before the rainy season.

Social
Within a community, age is by far the largest risk factor in acquiring active trachoma. The prevalence of active trachoma peaks at 3–6 years old and then decreases monotonically to

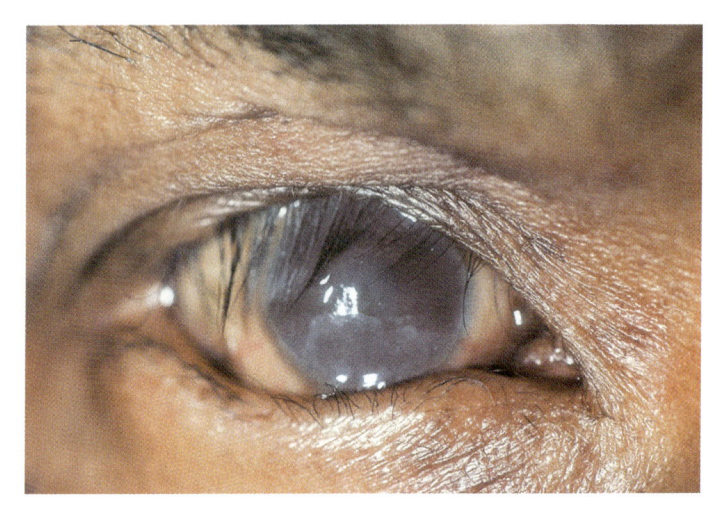

Figure 18-3 Trachomatous trichiasis (TT): at least one eyelash touching the globe. *(Photograph courtesy of Thomas M. Lietman, MD.)*

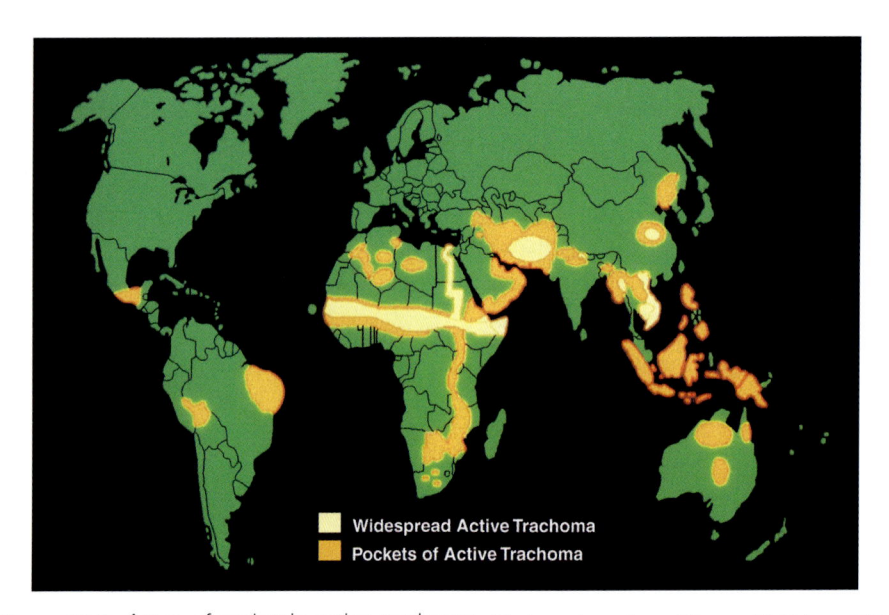

Figure 18-4 Areas of endemic active trachoma. *(Photograph courtesy of Thomas M. Lietman, MD.)*

very low levels in adulthood (presumably from a combination of acquired immunity and behavioral changes).

Children with clean faces are significantly less likely to have active trachoma, although it has been difficult to demonstrate a large immediate effect with face-cleanliness campaigns alone.

As with many infectious diseases, transmission is felt to occur frequently within the household. It has been shown that the risk of a child having active trachoma doubles if a sibling has active trachoma. In some areas, both active and cicatricial trachoma are more common in females, presumably because older sisters and mothers more frequently care for the younger children, who are most prone to transmitting infection.

Ethnic differences

Although trachoma is clearly more prevalent in certain ethnic groups (for example, among the Tharu people in Nepal), it may well be that this has more to do with socioeconomic differences than genetic or even cultural differences. Although several groups have tried to demonstrate a tendency for cicatricial scarring with certain HLA types, the relationship between host genetic factors and trachoma is not at all clear.

Clinical Presentation and Findings

After infection with *Chlamydia*, a 1–2 week latent period is followed by a period of active trachoma, in which there is characteristically a follicular conjunctivitis (see Fig 18-1) that may have a marked papillary reaction (Fig 18-5). The follicular reaction is apparent in both the upper and lower palpebral conjunctiva and may persist for 4–6 weeks, even after *Chlamydia* can no longer be isolated by even the most sensitive laboratory tests. After repeated infections, a network of scars can be seen, most easily in the upper tarsal conjunctiva (see Fig 18-2). Less frequently, a band of scarring in the watershed area between the marginal and peripheral conjunctival vascular arcades forms and is called an *Arlt's line* (Fig 18-6). The remnants of limbal follicles within a pannus can cause oval depressions in the peripheral cornea and are known as *Herbert's pits* (Fig 18-7). These are most commonly seen superiorly but can be seen at any location. Although Arlt's line and Herbert's pits are the most common signs associated with trachoma, they have limited epidemiologic significance. Conjunctival scarring can distort the tarsus and lead to

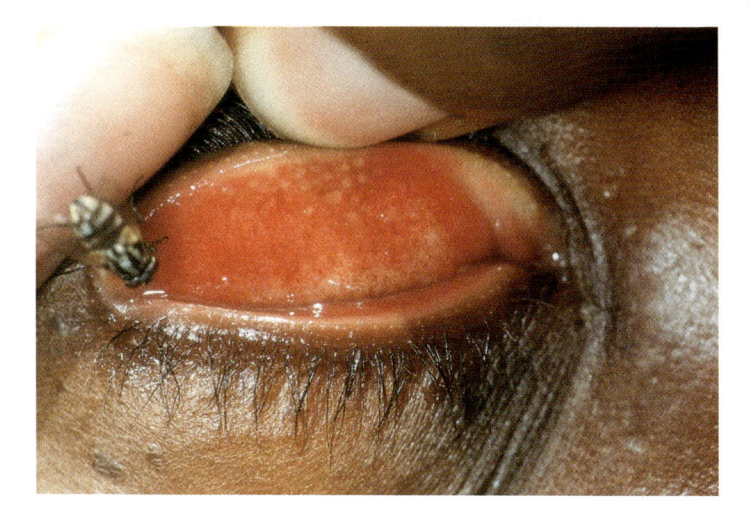

Figure 18-5 Intense trachoma (TI): inflammatory thickening (papillary hypertrophy) obscuring more than one half of the underlying conjunctival vasculature. Flies, in particular *Musca sorbens*, are thought by some to play a role in the transmission of trachoma. *(Photograph courtesy of Thomas M. Lietman, MD.)*

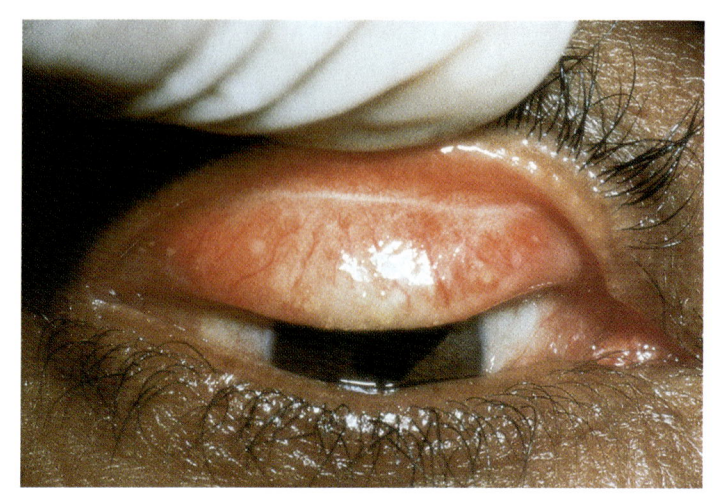

Figure 18-6 Arlt's line: a horizontal linear scar found in the watershed area between the marginal and peripheral conjunctival vasculature. *(Photograph courtesy of Thomas M. Lietman, MD.)*

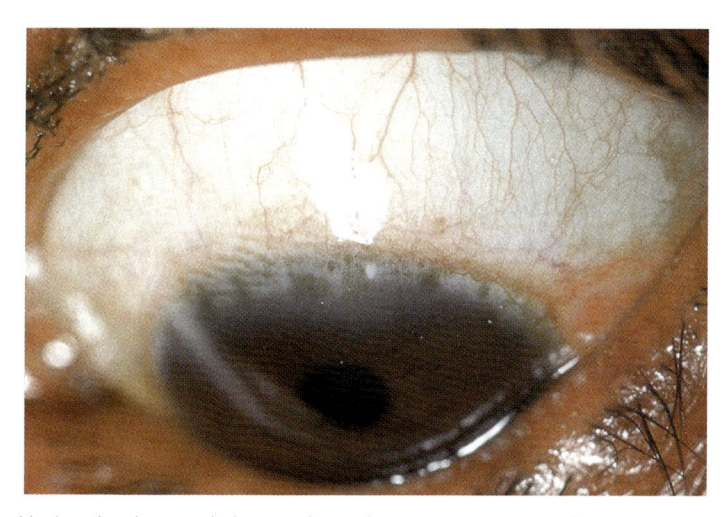

Figure 18-7 Herbert's pits: oval depressions that are remnants of limbal follicles. *(Photograph courtesy of Thomas M. Lietman, MD.)*

a cicatricial entropion with trichiasis (see Fig 18-3). Trichiasis, along with mechanical abrasion, loss of mucin production from a scarred conjunctiva, and loss of tears due to scarred lacrimal ductules, predisposes individuals to both bacterial and fungal corneal ulcers. These ulcers are the major cause of a loss of vision.

Prevention

Trachoma programs are based on prevention of scarring by eliminating active disease and on prevention of corneal ulcers by correcting trichiasis. Active trachoma can be eliminated from an individual with a 42-day course of twice-daily tetracycline ointment. Unfortunately, compliance is very low. A single dose of oral systemic azithromycin (Zithromax, 20 mg/kg for children, 1 g for adults) has been found to be extremely effective and compliance is not an issue. However, reinfection is the rule, so all those at risk in the community must be treated. Proposed distribution strategies for azithromycin now include:

- Treatment of all members of the community, once per year
- Treatment of all children aged 10 and under, once per year
- Identification and treatment of children with active trachoma, along with treatment of members of their household, with the identification and treatment repeated annually

Current Treatment Programs

Screening

Active trachoma

Although new DNA amplification techniques that use the polymerase chain reaction (PCR) or the ligase chain reaction (LCR) are becoming the gold standard for diagnosing ocular *C trachomatis* infection, these tests are relatively expensive to perform, do not give immediate results, and are not readily available in areas of the world where trachoma is prevalent. Thus, active trachoma is most commonly diagnosed by clinical examination. Currently, most control programs use the WHO simplified grading system (Table 18-1). Conjunctival examination with loupes (1.8–2.5× magnification at 10–14 inches) can be used to identify the typical pattern of follicles and the degree of papillary inflammation on the upper palpebral conjunctiva. The presence of five or more follicles greater than 0.5 mm in size on the lower portion (upper portion after the lid is everted) of the upper conjunctival tarsal plate constitutes *follicular trachoma* (TF; see Fig 18-1). A papillary reaction in the upper palpebral conjunctiva that obscures more than half of the underlying conjunctival vasculature is designated as *intense trachoma* (TI; see Fig 18-5). In

Table 18-1 World Health Organization Simplified Trachoma Grading System

Abbreviation	Sign	Definition
TF	Trachoma follicular (see Fig 18-1)	The presence of 5 or more follicles in the upper tarsal conjunctiva
TI	Trachoma intense (see Fig 18-5)	Pronounced inflammatory thickening of the upper tarsal conjunctiva that obscures more than half the normal deep tarsal vessels
TS	Trachomatous scarring (see Fig 18-2)	The presence of scarring in the tarsal conjunctiva
TT	Trachomatous trichiasis (see Fig 18-3)	At least one eyelash rubbing on the eyeball
CO	Corneal opacity (see Fig 18-8)	Easily visible corneal opacity over the pupil

hyperendemic areas, a clinical examination consistent with TF or TI is 77%–79% sensitive and 65%–89% specific in identifying chlamydial infection (as determined by DNA amplification tests), with a positive predictive value of 65%–75%. Unfortunately, the positive predictive value of the clinical examination decreases as the prevalence of disease decreases—TF and TI seem to be less indicative of infection in areas of low prevalence.

Cicatricial trachoma

Scars on the upper tarsus of individuals who live in communities with endemic trachoma are recognized as cicatricial trachoma and designated TS (see Fig 18-2). The presence of eyelashes touching the globe is considered trichiasis and is designated as TT (see Fig 18-3), and the presence of a central corneal opacity overlying any part of the pupil is designated as CO (Fig 18-8).

Strengths, Weaknesses, and Results of Treatment Programs

The World Health Organization has instituted a prevention and treatment program entitled the *S.A.F.E. strategy* (*s*urgery, *a*ntibiotics, *f*ace cleanliness, and *e*nvironmental improvements). Bilamellar tarsal rotation has been found to be the most effective corrective surgery, preventing recurrence of trichiasis in up to 80% of people at 2 years; recurrence is possible, and a repeat procedure is often necessary.

Tetracycline is effective at eliminating *Chlamydia*, but few can comply with the 42-day treatment course. Azithromycin has been found to be effective in eliminating *Chlamydia* from individuals and, with mass drug administration, from a community. However, azithromycin is expensive, and if nothing else in a community is changed, then the disease can be expected to return eventually to its previous levels. Although *Chlamydia* has so far remained sensitive to macrolides and azalides, including azithromycin, other bacteria may develop resistance, and there is some concern that large-scale trachoma

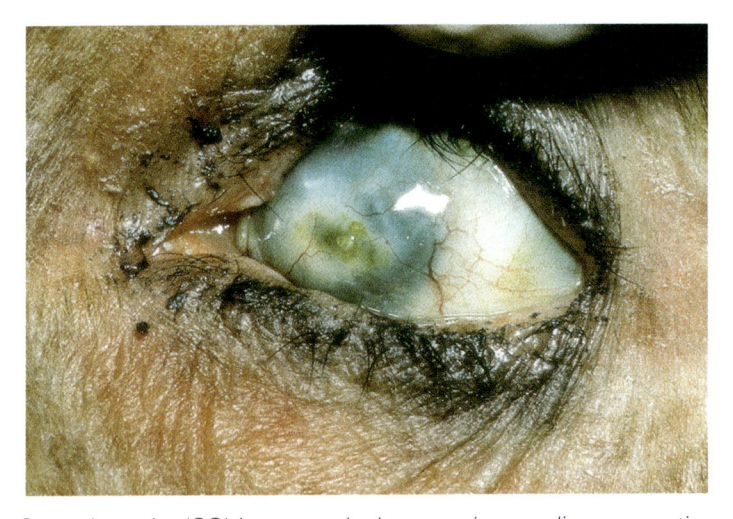

Figure 18-8 Corneal opacity (CO) is reported when scarring overlies any portion of the pupil. The black kohl has been added to the lids for cosmetic reasons. *(Photograph courtesy of Thomas M. Lietman, MD.)*

programs may interfere with bacterial flora. Resistance of *C trachomatis, Streptococcus pneumoniae,* and *Streptococcus pyogenes* will have to be carefully monitored during mass drug administrations.

Face-cleanliness campaigns, improved water availability, and fly control have been implemented with varying degrees of success. It is hoped that annual treatment with systemic azithromycin, in conjunction with the other measures, will permanently reduce the burden of active trachoma. Even if this program is successful, however, the current generation of trichiasis patients will need to have corrective surgery and be followed.

Clinical Research Currently Under Way

Research is currently being conducted in Nepal, Tanzania, The Gambia, Morocco, and many other countries to answer the following questions:

- What are the optimal strategies for antibiotic distribution (who in a community should be treated)?
- Can multiple mass drug administrations eliminate *Chlamydia* from a community?
- Is fly reduction a viable and effective control measure?
- What is the long-term efficacy of trichiasis surgery?

Bailey RL, Arullendran P, Whittle HC, et al. Randomised controlled trial of single-dose azithromycin in treatment of trachoma. *Lancet.* 1993;342:453–456.

Emerson PM, Lindsay SW, Walraven GE, et al. Effect of fly control on trachoma and diarrhoea. *Lancet.* 1999;353:1401–1403.

Lietman TM, Porco T, Dawson C, et al. Global elimination of trachoma: how frequently should we administer mass chemotherapy? *Nat Med.* 1999;5:572–576.

Mabey D, Fraser-Hurt N. Trachoma. *BMJ.* 2001:323;218–221.

Muñoz B, West S. Trachoma: the forgotten cause of blindness. *Epidemiol Rev.* 1997;19: 205–217.

Schachter J, West SK, Mabey D, et al. Azithromycin in control of trachoma. *Lancet.* 1999; 354:630–635.

Taylor HR, Rapoza PA, West S, et al. The epidemiology of infection in trachoma. *Invest Ophthalmol Vis Sci.* 1989;30:1823–1833.

Thylefors B, Dawson CR, Jones BR, et al. A simple system for the assessment of trachoma and its complications. *Bull World Health Organ.* 1987;65:477–483.

West S, Muñoz B, Lynch M, et al. Impact of face-washing on trachoma in Kongwa, Tanzania. *Lancet.* 1995;345:155–158.

CHAPTER 19

Microbial Keratitis

Background

History

Although corneal blindness in the developing world has traditionally been attributed to trachoma, xerophthalmia, measles, neonatal ophthalmia, and leprosy, the importance of superficial corneal trauma in agricultural work, which frequently leads to rapidly progressing corneal ulceration and visual loss, has been overlooked as a worldwide cause of monocular vision impairment. It has been estimated that up to 5% of all blinding conditions are directly related to ocular trauma. Children may be at even greater risk than adults. A recent study in Uganda indicates that corneal ulceration is second only to cataract as the main cause of vision impairment in the younger age group. Examination of 1135 children with subnormal vision revealed that 30.7% had visual impairment secondary to cataracts or poor surgical outcome, whereas 22.0% had visual loss following corneal ulceration.

>   Thylefors B. Epidemiological patterns of ocular trauma. *Aust N Z J Ophthalmol.* 1992;20: 95–98.
>   Waddell K. Childhood blindness and low vision in Uganda. *Eye.* 1998;12:184–192.

Context

The social and economic impact of corneal ulceration is insidious because the disease only infrequently causes bilateral vision impairment. The individuals most commonly affected are farmers or laborers; males are slightly more at risk than females; and the ulcers occur predominantly in middle-aged individuals who are in their most productive years. Because microbial keratitis most often affects the working poor in the developing world, it is underreported and often neglected. By conservative estimates, there are at least 1.5 million new cases of unilateral vision impairment worldwide every year due to microbial keratitis. These individuals are truly victims of a silent epidemic.

Economic Impact

Cost of treatment

The medical costs of treating microbial keratitis are prohibitively expensive in many circumstances, especially in the case of fungal ulceration, where medications are expensive and the visual outcome is usually disappointing. Approximately one half of eyes with fungal ulceration that receive appropriate treatment still develop blinding sequelae secondary to perforation, phthisis, and severe scarring. Those with bacterial ulcers fare somewhat better, but central corneal scarring effectively means that the individual is unilaterally vision impaired for life because of the prohibitive cost of corneal transplant surgery in most developing countries, the lack of facilities and trained surgeons, and the scarcity of donor tissue.

Cost of lost productivity

The true economic costs of unilateral vision impairment secondary to corneal ulceration are not known. The individual is undoubtedly at greater risk for injury to the other eye and more prone to accidents in general. In the case of bilateral vision impairment in children, the social and economic impact over a lifetime is incalculable.

Pathogenesis

The majority of corneal ulcers in the developing world occur after relatively minor corneal trauma. Microbial pathogens are introduced into the corneal stroma by contamination of the object producing the abrasion or by the presence of these pathogens in the environment or on the patient's conjunctiva and lids. Immediately after the corneal abrasion occurs, a window of opportunity opens, during which the microbial invasion can be treated before a keratitis develops. If an infection becomes established in the corneal stroma, the rapid growth of the microbial pathogens and the resulting tissue necrosis make it more difficult to reverse the process with medical treatment. The inflammatory mechanisms called into play by the body invariably produce rapid necrosis of the corneal stroma, which then heals slowly, with severe scarring developing over weeks to months.

Epidemiology

Surveys to Determine Prevalence/Incidence

Surveys in the developing world that investigate the prevalence of corneal ulceration are rare. The spectrum of microbial pathogens producing ulceration varies from population to population (Table 19-1), but large studies in Asia have demonstrated that the most common bacterial pathogen causing microbial keratitis is *Streptococcus pneumoniae*. In a large study from southern India, half of all ulcers were shown to be caused by fungal pathogens, with *Fusarium* spp the most commonly isolated organisms. Only one population-based retrospective incidence survey has been reported from a developing country. Gonzales et al found that the incidence of corneal ulceration in Madurai District, southern India, was 113 per 100,000, or ten times the incidence in the United States. Generalizing these findings to all of India, an estimated 840,000 people a year in that country develop a corneal ulcer.

Table 19-1 **Central Corneal Ulcers in the Developing World (Geographic Comparison)**

	South Africa[1]	South Africa[2]	Nepal[3]	Bangladesh[4]	West Africa[5]	South India[6]
Date of study	1985	1987	1991	1994	1995	1997
Number of ulcers	91	131	405	142	199	434
Culture positive (%)	68	65	80	82	57	68
Organisms cultured						
Bacteria (%)	90	96	79	66	49	47
Most frequent pathogens*						
Streptococcus pneumoniae	40	16	31	32	13	44
Staphylococcus spp	13	61	22	3	29	16
Pseudomonas spp	17	6	11	48	25	14
Other bacteria	30	17	36	17	33	26
Fungi (%)	10	4	21	34	51	53

* Each species as a percent of the total number of bacteria cultured

[1] Carmichael TR, Wolpert M, Koornhof HJ. Corneal ulceration at an urban African hospital. *Br J Ophthalmol.* 1985;69:920–926.
[2] Ormerod LD. Causation and management of microbial keratitis in subtropical Africa. *Ophthalmology.* 1987;94:1662-1668.
[3] Upadhyay MP, Karmacharya PC, Koirala S, et al. Epidemiologic characteristics, predisposing factors, and etiologic diagnosis of corneal ulceration in Nepal. *Am J Ophthalmol.* 1991;111:92–99.
[4] Dunlop AA, Wright ED, Howlader SA, et al. Suppurative corneal ulceration in Bangladesh: a study of 142 cases examining the microbiological diagnosis, clinical and epidemiological features of bacterial and fungal keratitis. *Aust NZ J Ophthalmol.* 1994;22:105–110.
[5] Hagan M, Wright E, Newman M, et al. Causes of suppurative keratitis in Ghana. *Br J Ophthalmol.* 1995;79:1024–1028.
[6] Srinivasan M, Gonzales CA, George C, et al. Epidemiology and aetiological diagnosis of corneal ulceration in Madurai, south India. *Br J Ophthalmol.* 1997;81:965–971.

Risk Factors

A number of risk factors may predispose an individual in a developing country to develop microbial keratitis. Geographic, environmental, social, and ethnic differences are usually of great importance. Undoubtedly, however, the most important risk factor is a history of corneal trauma. Unlike in the industrialized world, where contact lens wear is the main risk factor for corneal ulcers, in the developing world, contact lenses are worn by a relatively small portion of the population. In contrast, the majority of the population is involved in agricultural labor, and the opportunities for repeated incidences of corneal trauma are numerous.

Geographic areas that are consistently warm and humid, such as southern India, tend to have a greater number of fungal ulcers. Regions with more temperate climates, such as the mountainous areas of Nepal, have a preponderance of bacterial ulcers. Farmers, day laborers, and brick or stone workers tend to be especially prone to frequent corneal abrasions. Often, ethnic groups at the bottom of the socioeconomic order are at higher risk for microbial keratitis because of their occupational exposure and their lack of ready access to the health care system.

Clinical Presentation and Findings

Microbial keratitis, by definition, is a suppurative infection of the corneal stroma with an associated epithelial defect and signs of inflammation. The pathogens responsible are usually bacterial, fungal, or parasitic. The herpesviruses and other viral pathogens are generally excluded from this group. Despite a lack of good epidemiologic evidence, herpes simplex is rarely thought to be a cause of corneal vision loss in developing countries. Patients present with a history of redness, pain, and sensitivity to light, along with an associated decrease in vision. Even though the distinction between central corneal ulcers and peripheral ulcers is somewhat arbitrary, microbial keratitis does not have to occupy the visual axis to be included in the corneal ulceration category.

There is always a white or yellowish stromal infiltrate or infiltrates with an associated epithelial defect. The eye exhibits signs of inflammation: injection, an anterior chamber reaction, and possibly a hypopyon. The patient is in pain and usually presents as an acute emergency. If treatment is delayed, as was seen frequently in the study in Nepal, where patients sometimes had to walk for weeks to reach the hospital, there may be total corneal necrosis on presentation, with corneal perforation and endophthalmitis.

Because of the delay in diagnosis and treatment, microbial keratitis in developing countries is often much more severe on initial presentation. Both bacterial and fungal ulcers may show large areas of central necrosis and significant hypopyons. Satellite lesions and soft feathery edges may still be prominent in fungal ulceration (Fig 19-1), but, in general, the ulcers are much more aggressive than those seen in industrialized countries and perforate quickly. Likewise, bacterial ulcers progress rapidly to involve the entire cornea (Fig 19-2). Medical treatment then becomes problematic because even if the ulcer is sterilized, the necrosis has become so advanced that surgical intervention may be necessary to maintain the integrity of the eye.

Even if culture facilities are not available, corneal scrapings can be very helpful in making a tentative etiologic diagnosis. A smear from a bacterial ulcer can be stained with

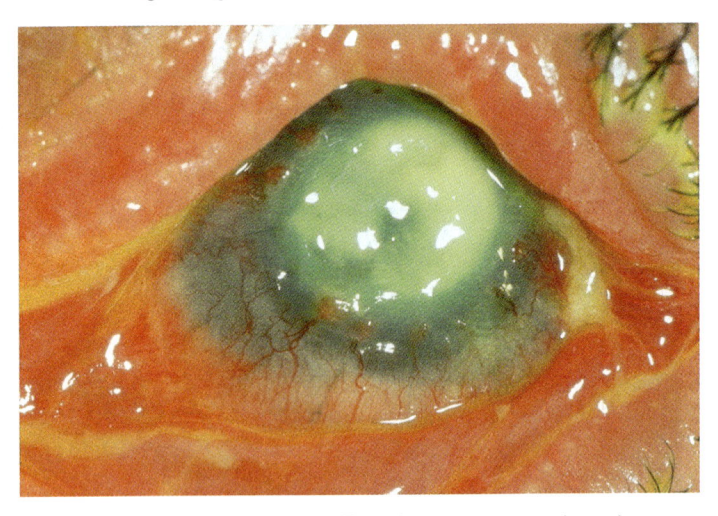

Figure 19-1 Fungal corneal ulcer from which *Fusarium* spp were cultured. *(Photo courtesy of Aravind Eye Hospital, Madurai, India.)*

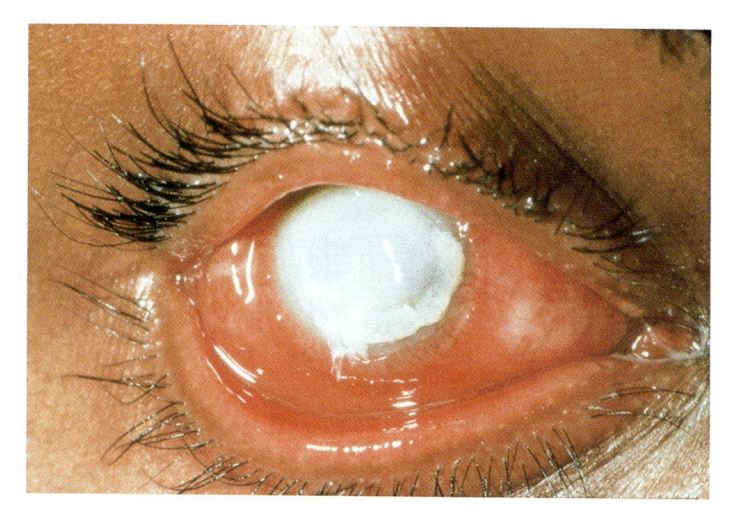

Figure 19-2 Central bacterial corneal ulcer in a patient with severe conjunctival and corneal scarring from trachoma. *Streptococcus pneumoniae* was cultured. *(Photo courtesy of Proctor Foundation, San Francisco.)*

Gram or Giemsa stains with minimal equipment. Examining corneal scrapings from fungal ulcers is greatly facilitated by using a KOH wet mount. Fortunately, *Acanthamoeba* is a rare cause of corneal ulceration in the developing world, but if the organisms are present, they can be identified from direct corneal scrapings stained with Giemsa.

Prevention

Because of the often prohibitive cost of treating microbial keratitis in a developing country and the invariable corneal scarring that the disease causes, prevention would be the ideal approach for reducing the epidemic numbers of corneal ulceration now occurring. Theoretically, the majority of ulcers could be prevented if a combination antibiotic-antifungal ointment were instilled into the eye immediately after an individual suffers a corneal abrasion. A large-scale program could be implemented through the existing village health care systems in many countries, and public awareness of ulcer prevention could be increased using the eye health education programs already in place. Unfortunately, a commercially available antibiotic-antifungal eye ointment does not exist at the present time, and no study has been done to prove that the incidence of corneal ulceration could be significantly reduced. However, the application of chloramphenicol ointment in eyes after corneal abrasion in a defined urban population has been observed to reduce the numbers of both bacterial and fungal ulcers.

Current Treatment Programs

Screening

The problem of microbial keratitis in the developing world should be handled at the grassroots level. Many of the ulcers in southern India are treated by village healers and nonophthalmologists who have little knowledge of Western medicine. Remedies used by traditional healers often enhance the development of microbial keratitis after corneal abrasion by introducing bacterial or fungal pathogens in contaminated solutions or organic materials. With simple training, most health care workers could learn how to administer prophylactic ointment after corneal abrasions and how to recognize early corneal ulcers just as they are beginning to develop. In most cases, personnel are already in place, but they need better training and specific instructions for referring suspected cases of microbial keratitis.

Strengths, Weaknesses, and Results of Treatment Programs

In general, physicians and health care workers in developing countries are incredibly dedicated. However, they often lack skills and even simple resources. Equipment and instruments are frequently antiquated or in need of repair, and medications are limited and prohibitively expensive. Successful treatment of microbial keratitis is problematic under the best of circumstances. In the setting of a developing country, where everything is in short supply, the odds are stacked against successful therapy.

Because laboratory facilities are often inadequate or unavailable, the treatment of corneal ulcers is frequently empirical. The choice of antibiotics for the treatment of bacterial ulcers must cover *S pneumoniae* because this is the most common corneal pathogen in many parts of the world. However, because of the severity of ulceration they produce, the gram-negative pathogens, such as *Pseudomonas*, cannot be overlooked. Any empirical therapy for a bacterial ulcer should include cefazolin or the equivalent to cover gram-positive organisms and a fluoroquinolone or an aminoglycoside to cover gram-negative pathogens. Antifungal medications are more problematic because they are frequently unavailable. Pimaricin in a 5% solution may sometimes be in stock, and amphotericin B drops can be made up in a 0.15% topical medication. The two are frequently used together for filamentous fungi. Yeasts respond best to amphotericin.

Clinical Research Currently Under Way

Until recently, the enormity of the problem of microbial keratitis in the developing world was not appreciated. Population-based studies sponsored by the World Health Organization are now under way in several countries in Southeast Asia to define the true incidence of corneal ulceration, to examine the importance of risk factors, and to determine the most common pathogens responsible for ulceration in each geographic area. As the epidemiology of microbial keratitis in the developing world becomes better understood, prevention and treatment programs that are evidence-based can be implemented. By that time, it is hoped, new antifungal-antibiotic medications will be available for large-scale prevention programs, and more effective antimicrobial agents will be available at an affordable cost for treating those ulcers that elude prevention.

Gonzales CA, Srinivasan M, Whitcher J, et al. Incidence of corneal ulceration in Madurai district, south India. *Ophthal Epidemiol*. 1996;3:159–166.

Srinivasan M, Gonzales CA, George C, et al. Epidemiology and aetiological diagnosis of corneal ulceration in Madurai, south India. *Br J Ophthalmol.* 1997;81:965–971.

Upadhyay MP, Karmacharya PC, Koirala S, et al. The Bhaktapur eye study: ocular trauma and antibiotic prophylaxis for the prevention of corneal ulceration in Nepal. *Br J Ophthalmol.* 2001;85:388–392.

Upadhyay MP, Karmacharya PC, Koirala S, et al. Epidemiologic characteristics, predisposing factors, and etiologic diagnosis of corneal ulceration in Nepal. *Am J Ophthalmol.* 1991;111:92–99.

Whitcher JP, Srinivasan M. Corneal ulceration in the developing world—a silent epidemic. *Br J Ophthalmol.* 1997;81:622–623.

CHAPTER 20

HIV/AIDS and Global Blindness

Background

History

The human immunodeficiency virus (HIV) appears to have been transmitted from chimpanzees to humans in Central Africa. Human infections were probably sporadic until the 1970s, when rapid urbanization of the African interior resulted in regional epidemics. Intercontinental travel, together with the widespread practices of unprotected sexual intercourse and intravenous drug use, led quickly to the globalization of HIV infection in the late 1970s and early 1980s. The acquired immune deficiency syndrome (AIDS), now recognized to represent advanced HIV infection, was first described in 1981. Dr Gary Holland and associates at UCLA provided the first description of the ocular complications in an HIV-positive cohort in 1982. HIV itself was independently isolated by researchers in France and the United States in 1983 and 1984, respectively.

Context

As of December 2001, the Joint United Nations Programme on HIV/AIDS (UNAIDS) and the World Health Organization (WHO) estimated that 40 million people were living with HIV worldwide (Fig 20-1). Approximately 95% of HIV-positive people live in the developing world, particularly in sub-Saharan Africa and South and Southeast Asia (see Fig 20-1; Table 20-1). Roughly half of all HIV-positive people living in North America and Europe, and more than 90% of infected people living in the developing world, are unaware of their HIV status.

Up to 75% of patients with HIV/AIDS eventually develop ocular complications related to their disease. Opportunistic infections, such as cytomegalovirus (CMV) retinitis and herpes zoster ophthalmicus (HZO), occur most often; but unusual neoplasms, including Kaposi sarcoma and intraocular lymphoma, and vascular abnormalities, such as HIV retinopathy and retinovascular occlusion, may also affect the eye and limit vision.

Economic Impact

Cost of treatment

Modern treatment of HIV/AIDS includes long-term use of three or more antiretroviral agents, an approach termed *combination* or *highly active antiretroviral therapy (HAART)*. The cost of such therapy currently exceeds $10,000 per year in the United States. Treatment

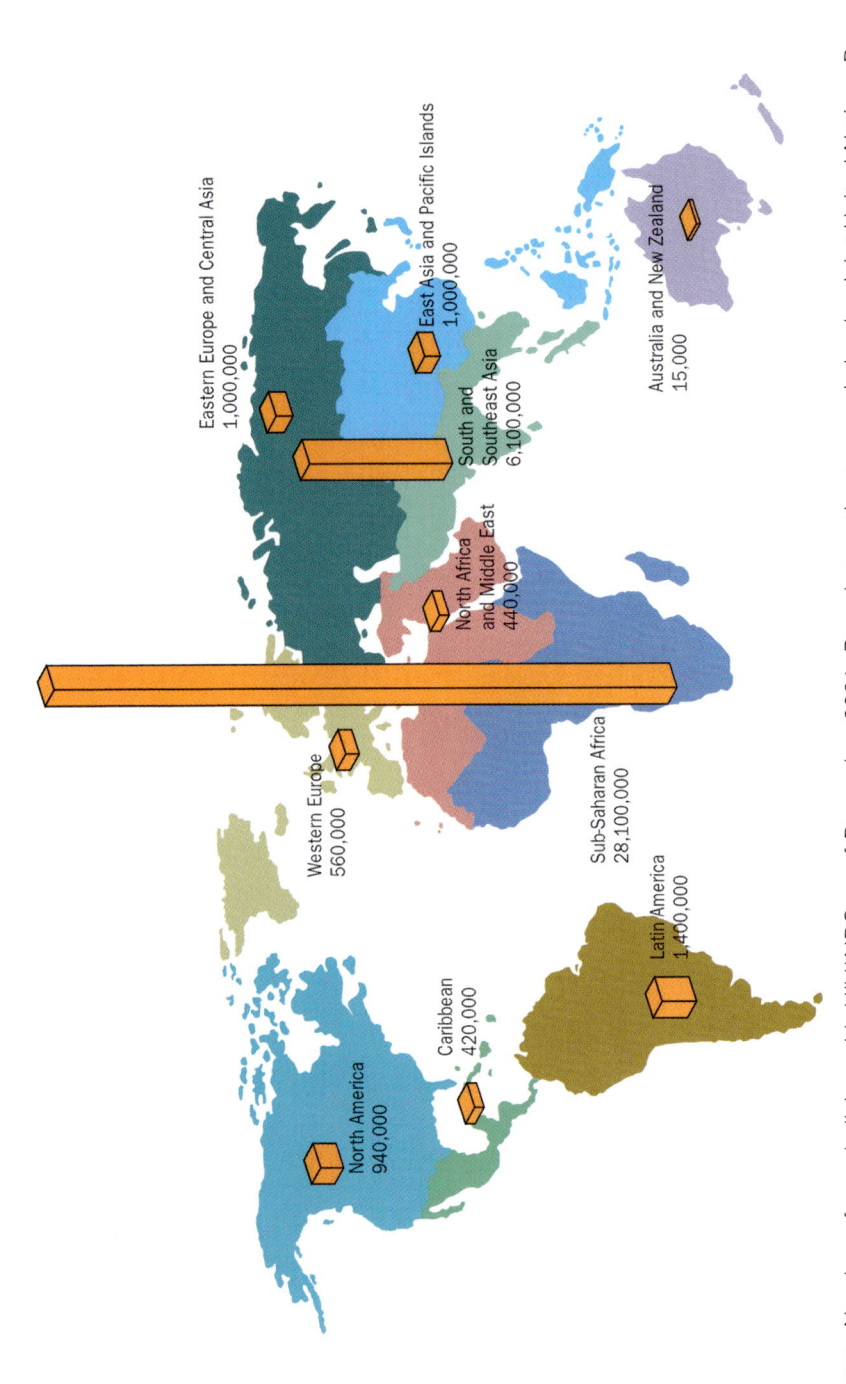

Figure 20-1 Number of people living with HIV/AIDS as of December 2001. Based on estimates made by the Joint United Nations Programme on HIV/AIDS and the World Health Organization. *(Modified with permission after Mann JM, Tarantola DJM. HIV 1998: the global picture. Sci Am. 1998;279:82–83. Data taken from Joint United Nations Programme on HIV/AIDS: AIDS Epidemic Update. Geneva: UNAIDS; December 2001).*

Table 20-1 UNAIDS Joint United Nations Programme on HIV/AIDS Regional Summary December 2001

Region	Epidemic Started	Adults and Children Living With HIV/AIDS in 2000	Adults and Children Infected With HIV During 2000	Adult Prevalence Rate*	Percentage of HIV-Positive Adults Who Are Women	Main Modes of Spread Among Adults
North America	Late 1970s Early 1980s	940,000	45,000	0.6%	20%	IDU, MSM, MSW
Western Europe	Late 1970s Early 1980s	560,000	30,000	0.3%	25%	IDU, MSM
Eastern Europe and Central Asia	Early 1990s	1 million	250,000	0.5%	20%	IDU
Latin America	Late 1970s Early 1980s	1.4 million	130,000	0.5%	30%	IDU, MSM, MSW
Australia and New Zealand	Late 1970s Early 1980s	15,000	500	0.1%	10%	MSM
East Asia and Pacific Islands	Late 1980s	1 million	270,000	0.1%	20%	IDU, MSM, MSW
Caribbean	Late 1970s Early 1980s	420,000	60,000	2.2%	50%	MSM, MSW
South and Southeast Asia	Late 1980s	6.1 million	800,000	0.6%	35%	IDU, MSW
North Africa and Middle East	Late 1980s	440,000	80,000	0.2%	40%	IDU, MSW
Sub-Saharan Africa	Late 1970s Early 1980s	28.1 million	3.4 million	8.4%	55%	MSW

* Proportion of adults (defined as 15–49 years of age) living with HIV/AIDS in 2001, using 2001 population numbers
IDU = intravenous drug use; MSM = men having sex with men; MSW = men having sex with women
(From Joint United Nations Programme on HIV/AIDS: *AIDS Epidemic Update*. Geneva: UNAIDS; December 2001.)

of opportunistic disorders, such as CMV retinitis, is similarly expensive. Such high costs have limited the availability of both HAART and other HIV-related therapies to those countries and regions where private or governmental health coverage is available to help meet the costs of therapy, most notably the United States, Western Europe, and selected countries in South America, such as Brazil and Argentina. The vast majority of patients with HIV/AIDS, who live in the developing world, go untreated. In fact, most patients with ocular complications of HIV infection are left to live the remainder of their lives with partial or complete loss of vision.

Cost of lost productivity

HIV/AIDS has had an enormous economic impact on the world. Roughly half of all HIV-positive patients become infected by their 25th birthday, adversely affecting both individual productivity and, in countries where infection is common, gross national productivity. Moreover, in some countries in sub-Saharan Africa, HIV infection is so common that overall life expectancy has dropped by more than 20 years over the past 2 decades, essentially reversing 50 years of social progress. In many of these countries, illness and death related to AIDS have become the most common reasons why employees leave a company, replacing both relocation and retirement as more traditional reasons for ending employment.

Infection of large numbers of relatively young adults with HIV also affects children and future generations, both because a significant number of children born to HIV-positive women will themselves be infected by the virus and because many children, whether infected or not, will ultimately lose their parents to HIV disease. Recent estimates suggest that there are over 1 million HIV-positive children and nearly 12 million HIV/AIDS orphans worldwide.

Pathogenesis

HIV preferentially resides and replicates in $CD4^+$ T lymphocytes. The risk of transmission, therefore, is greatest with exposure to contaminated blood or blood products. Transmission can also occur with exposure to semen, breast milk, saliva, or tears from HIV-infected patients, but this is less common. Among children born to HIV-positive women, 20%–50% will themselves become infected by the virus. Postexposure or perinatal treatment with antiretroviral agents significantly reduces the risk of infection.

The natural history of untreated HIV infection may be divided into three phases (Fig 20-2). The first phase represents primary infection and lasts weeks to months. The second phase is characterized by clinical latency and typically lasts years. The third phase, or AIDS, begins with the development of opportunistic illnesses and usually ends with death within a year if patients fail to receive antiretroviral therapy.

Primary HIV infection produces a burst of viral replication and widespread lysis of infected T lymphocytes. These events result in an intense viremia, a marked dip in circulating $CD4^+$ T lymphocytes, and, in most patients, a moderately severe flulike illness that occurs 2–4 weeks after infection. Common symptoms include fever, lymphadenopathy, rash, pharyngitis, headache, nausea, and diarrhea. An immune response directed against HIV occurs within 4–8 weeks and results in a decrease in circulating virus levels and partial restoration of peripheral $CD4^+$ T lymphocytes (see Fig 20-2).

Clinical latency follows primary infection. Latency lasts for at least 10 years in 25%–50% of untreated patients in the United States and Europe, but the time period can be considerably shorter for children and for HIV-infected patients in developing countries. During this time, viral replication continues in both reticuloendothelial tissue and peripheral lymphocytes even though the virus may be difficult to measure in plasma. If untreated, $CD4^+$ T-lymphocyte counts continue to decline, and virtually all patients eventually develop symptoms of impaired T-cell immunity, including generalized lymph-

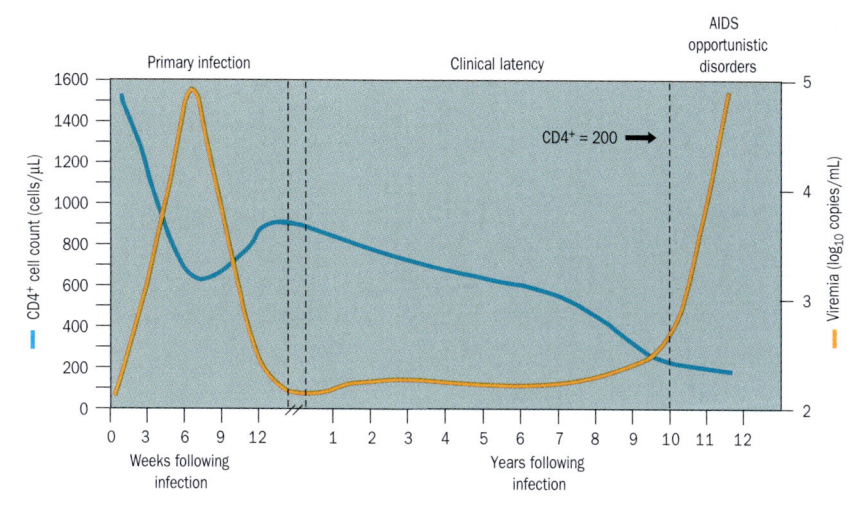

Figure 20-2 The natural history of untreated human immunodeficiency virus (HIV) infection. Clinical phases include primary infection, clinical latency, and the acquired immune deficiency syndrome (AIDS). The Centers for Disease Control and Prevention defines AIDS as the occurrence of an opportunistic infection or neoplasm, or a CD4+ T-lymphocyte count of less than 200 cells/mm³. *(Modified with permission of American College of Physicians–American Society of Internal Medicine from Fauci AS, Pantaleo G, Stanley S, et al: Immunopathogenic mechanisms of HIV infection.* Ann Intern Med. *1996;124:654–663.)*

adenopathy, recurrent fevers, night sweats, malaise, or an opportunistic infection or neoplasm. The best predictor for rapid progression to AIDS appears to be a persistently high viral load.

The end result of continued HIV replication is AIDS. Lymph node architecture is disrupted, CD4+ T lymphocytes approach near total depletion, and circulating virus levels climb as the patient's ability to combat the infection fails. Such a profound decline in immune function is accompanied by a greatly increased susceptibility to opportunistic illnesses, many of which can affect the eye, the ocular adnexa, or visual centers in the brain (Table 20-2).

The advent in 1996 of HAART has altered the natural history of HIV infection in two very important ways. First, patients have begun to live longer, with higher CD4+ T-lymphocyte counts and low, or even undetectable, viral loads. Second, many patients with preexisting CD4+ T-lymphocyte depletion have experienced immune reconstitution, characterized by significant and sustained elevations in circulating CD4+ cell counts and a regained immunologic ability to control opportunistic illnesses (Fig 20-3). Together, these two HAART-related effects have produced a 50%–80% decrease in the prevalence of ocular complications of HIV in those areas where combination therapy is available. The number of HIV-positive patients continues to grow, however, even in the developed world. Hence, although a lower proportion of HIV-infected patients in the United States and Europe will develop opportunistic disorders, the ever-increasing prevalence of HIV infection is bound to produce an overall increase in the number of HIV-related complications. That is, a 50% decline in any one patient's risk of developing CMV retinitis as a result of improved antiretroviral therapy eventually will be completely negated, at least

Table 20-2 Ophthalmic Manifestations of HIV Infection by CD4⁺T-Lymphocyte Count

CD4⁺ Cell Count	Complication
<500 cells/mm³	Herpes zoster, ophthalmicus Kaposi sarcoma Lymphoma
<200 cells/mm³	Coccidioidomycosis Cryptococcosis Histoplasmosis Pneumocystosis Toxoplasmosis Tuberculosis
<100 cells/mm³	Cytomegalovirus retinitis Microsporidiosis *Mycobacterium avium intracellulare* infection Progressive multifocal leukoencephalopathy Retinal/conjunctival microvasculopathy Varicella zoster virus retinitis

(Modified with permission from Bartlett JG: *The Johns Hopkins Hospital 1998–1999 Guide to Medical Care of Patients With HIV Infection*. 8th ed. Baltimore, MD: Williams & Wilkins; 1999; and modified with permission from Cunningham ET Jr, Margolis TP. Ocular manifestations of HIV infection. *New Engl J Med*. 1998;339:236–244. Copyright © 1998 Massachusetts Medical Society. All rights reserved.)

in terms of the absolute number of patients with CMV retinitis, by a doubling in the total number of HIV-positive patients.

Epidemiology

Surveys to Determine Prevalence

Cohort-based prevalence studies have suggested that up to 75% of HIV-positive patients eventually develop ocular complications of their disease. Most of these studies have been done in the United States and Europe, where the most common vision-threatening complication of HIV infection is CMV retinitis (Fig 20-4A). In the absence of HAART, CMV retinitis affects 30%–40% of patients, typically as CD4⁺ T-lymphocyte counts drop below 50 cells/mm³. Vision-threatening disorders encountered much less frequently in association with HIV infection but still seen in an appreciable number of HIV-positive patients include varicella zoster virus retinitis (Fig 20-4B), herpes simplex virus retinitis, toxoplasmic retinochoroiditis (Fig 20-4C), HZO (Fig 20-4D), Kaposi sarcoma of the eyelids (Fig 20-4E) or conjunctiva, herpetic keratitis or keratouveitis, fungal keratitis, and syphilitic uveitis. Conjunctival and retinal microvascular changes develop in more than 50% of patients with advanced HIV disease but seldom affect vision. The prevalence of each of these complications has decreased by 50%–80% since the introduction of HAART.

Fewer prevalence surveys are available from developing nations. Prospective, cohort-based studies from Africa, India, and Brazil have each suggested, however, that both CMV retinitis and HIV retinopathy affect roughly half the proportion of patients infected by

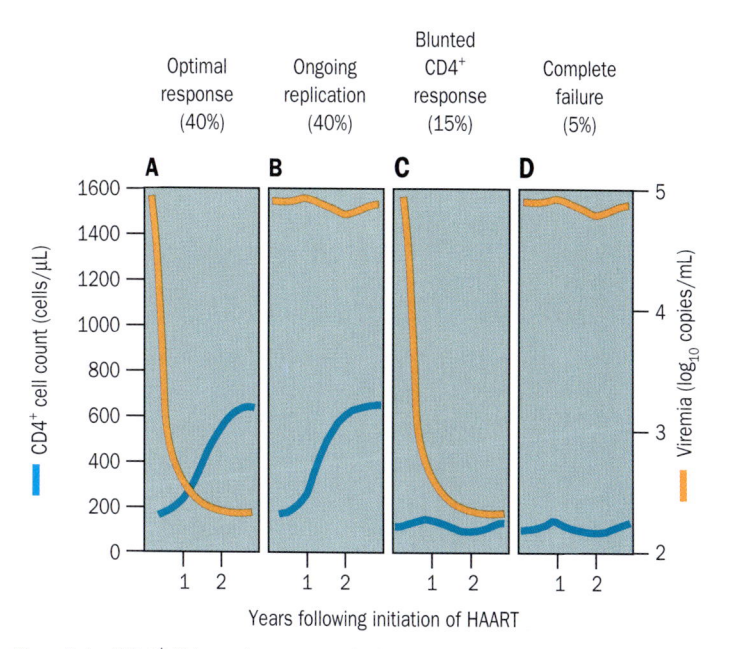

Figure 20-3 Possible CD4+ T-lymphocyte and viral load responses to HAART in patients with AIDS. **A,** Approximately 40% of patients experience optimal response, including increased CD4+ T-lymphocyte counts and marked viral suppression. **B,** Another 40% of patients experience increased CD4+ cell counts despite ongoing viral replication. **C,** Approximately 15% of patients experience a blunted CD4+ cell-count response despite viral control. **D,** Up to 5% of patients experience complete treatment failure. Predictors of treatment failure are incompletely understood but appear to include poor adherence to HAART, prior exposure to antiretroviral medications as single or dual therapy, sequential addition of drugs to a failing regimen, and adverse interactions among drugs used. *(Modified with permission from Perrin L, Telenti A. HIV treatment failure: testing HIV resistance in clinical practice.* Science. *1998;280:1871–1873. Copyright © 1998 American Association for the Advancement of Science.)*

HIV in these regions as compared to North America and Europe. Conversely, other opportunistic disorders, such as HZO, fungal keratitis, and papillomavirus-associated conjunctival squamous-cell tumors in Africa or toxoplasmic retinochoroiditis in Brazil, affect a higher proportion of patients with HIV disease. The reasons for these differences are complex but appear to be related most directly to differences in the prevalence of various opportunistic infections in different regions and to the fact that relatively few HIV-positive patients live long enough in developing countries to reach the profound levels of immunosuppression required to put themselves at risk for CMV retinitis and HIV retinopathy.

Risk Factors

Geographic

The prevalence of HIV infection and AIDS varies dramatically around the globe (see Fig 20-1, Table 20-1). More than 90% of HIV-positive patients live in sub-Saharan Africa and South and Southeast Asia. Large numbers of infected people also live in the Americas

230 • International Ophthalmology

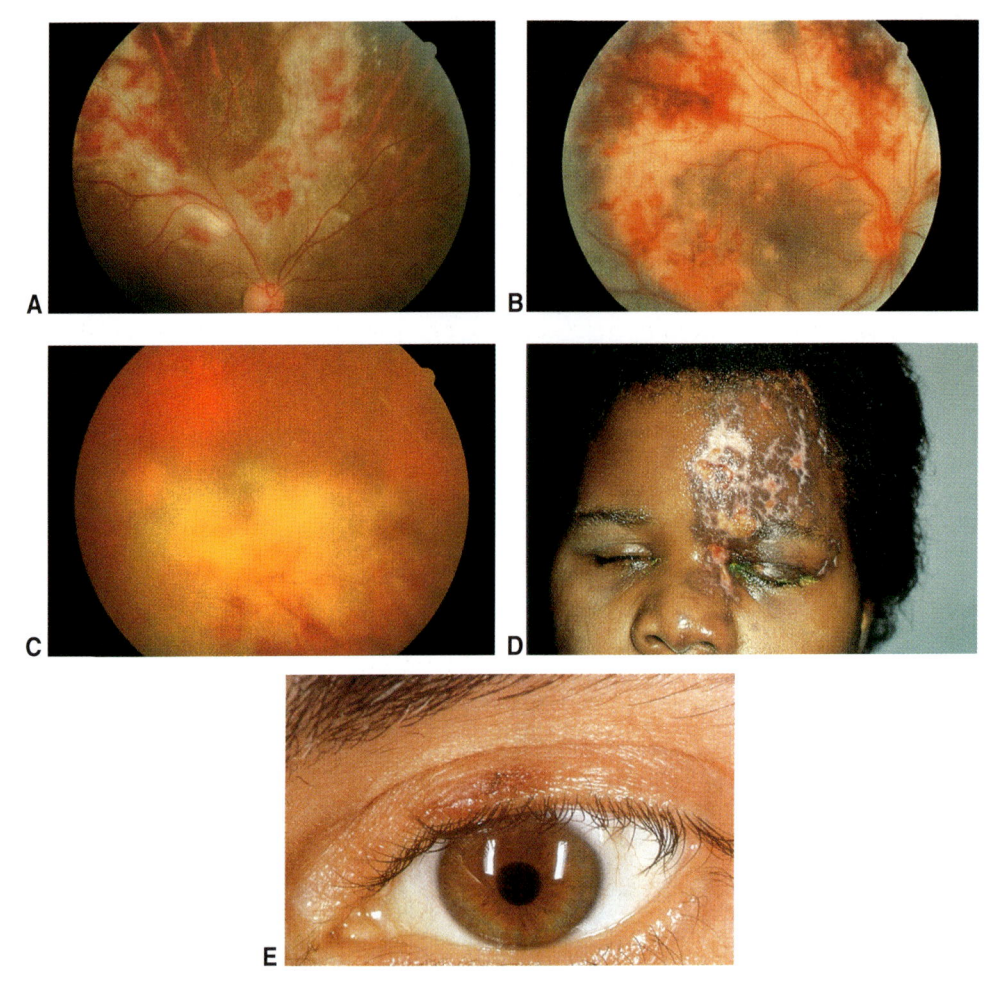

Figure 20-4 The most common forms of ocular disease observed in HIV-positive patients include the following. **A,** Cytomegalovirus (CMV) retinitis is characterized by retinal whitening and hemorrhage, often with satellite lesions at the advancing edge. **B,** Varicella zoster virus retinitis tends to produce large, confluent, and multiple areas of retinal whitening and hemorrhage that progress rapidly. **C,** Toxoplasmic retinochoroiditis usually results in a single area of retinal whitening with hemorrhage, often accompanied by moderate to severe vitreous inflammation. Although not present in this case, many patients with toxoplasmic retinochoroiditis will also have adjacent or nearby retinochoroidal scars. Both CMV retinitis and toxoplasmic retinochoroiditis tend to progress slowly, whereas varicella zoster virus and herpes simplex virus retinitis show rapid progression. **D,** Herpes zoster ophthalmicus (HZO) in an HIV-positive woman; HZO occurs worldwide but appears to be a particularly common presenting sign of HIV infection in certain parts of sub-Saharan Africa. **E,** Kaposi sarcoma of the upper eyelid in an HIV-positive man; periocular Kaposi sarcoma occurs in approximately 5% of HIV-infected patients in North America and Europe but is relatively uncommon in Africa, Asia, and South America. *(Photographs courtesy of Emmett T. Cunningham, MD.)*

and Europe. Asia, Eastern Europe, and South Africa are currently experiencing the most rapidly rising rates of infection.

Studies from developing countries suggest that CMV retinitis is less common in these countries than in North America and Europe, affecting 5%–25% of patients. This difference appears to be due to HIV-infected patients in developing countries often dying before their $CD4^+$ T-lymphocyte counts fall low enough to put them at risk for CMV reactivation. Kaposi sarcoma is also less common in Africa, Asia, and Brazil, due most probably to a lower prevalence of the causative agent, human herpesvirus 8, in these populations. Herpes zoster ophthalmicus, fungal keratitis, and papillomavirus-associated conjunctival squamous cell tumors, in contrast, are relatively more common in Africa. In fact, in Africa more than three fourths of patients who develop HZO, fungal keratitis, or squamous cell lesions of the conjunctiva are found to be HIV-positive when tested. Ocular complications of *Mycobacterium tuberculosis* and *Cryptococcus neoformans* infection are also more common in the developing world.

Social

Most HIV is transmitted sexually. In North America and Western Europe, the majority of HIV-positive patients are either gay or bisexual white men, although recent surveys have suggested rapidly growing HIV-positive heterosexual and minority populations. Risk factors include receptive anal intercourse; a high number of sexual partners; rectal trauma; or a history of an ulcerating anogenital infection, as might occur with gonorrhea, syphilis, or herpes simplex virus infection. Outside of North America and Western Europe, most HIV transmission occurs in the setting of heterosexual intercourse. Risk factors include multiple sex partners, unprotected intercourse with commercial sex workers, sex with intravenous drug users, or a history of prior sexually transmitted disease.

Injection drug use is a major risk factor for the transmission of HIV, particularly in major metropolitan areas in the Americas, Europe, South, and Southeast Asia. Needle sharing appears to be the primary mode of transmission, although this may be amplified by practices of unprotected sex and the occurrence of sexually transmitted diseases in these populations. Children born to women who practice intravenous drug use are also at increased risk of HIV infection.

Receipt of HIV-contaminated blood or blood products and of organs transplanted from HIV-positive patients is associated with a rate of seroconversion that approaches 100%. Fortunately, however, infection by these routes is now extremely low in most developed nations due, in large part, to self-deferral of potential donors who are known to be either infected or at high risk of infection, improved donor interviewing regarding high-risk behaviors, maintenance of regularly updated donor lists, and routine use of sensitive and specific HIV antibody screening tests. In countries where such practices are not employed, however, the risk of infection associated with receiving blood, blood products, or whole organs can be quite high.

Mother-to-child transmission of HIV accounts for over 90% of the more than 1 million children currently living with HIV/AIDS worldwide. Such vertical transmission may occur prepartum, intrapartum, or postpartum through breast feeding. Intrapartum transmission probably accounts for the greatest number of infections, although up to 15% of HIV-positive children are believed to have seroconverted following breast feeding.

Rates of mother-to-child transmission vary from approximately 15% in Europe, to 20%–30% in the United States, to as high as 50% in some African countries. The risk of transmission appears to be higher with advanced disease and lower $CD4^+$ T-lymphocyte counts in the mother. Use of perinatal antiretroviral agents dramatically decreases the risk of HIV transmission to the infant.

Biologic

Total $CD4^+$ T-lymphocyte count appears to be the best predictor of the risk of ocular complications in HIV/AIDS (Table 20-2). Moreover, the risk of opportunistic infections appears to decrease as counts of total $CD4^+$ cells climb in the setting of HAART and immune reconstitution.

Children are at relatively low risk for developing CMV retinitis, which affects only about 5% of HIV-infected children in North America and Europe. Children with HIV disease develop more bacterial infections than adults, however.

Contribution of HIV/AIDS to Global Blindness

It is difficult to assess with certainty the contribution of HIV/AIDS to global vision impairment. If one makes the conservative assumption that CMV retinitis affects, on average, 10% of all HIV-infected patients worldwide at some point during their illness and extrapolates that complication rate to the nearly 40 million people currently living with HIV/AIDS, then 4 million people in the world will develop CMV retinitis in at least one eye. Moreover, the Studies of Ocular Complications of AIDS (SOCA), which was done in the United States, found that CMV retinitis was bilateral in about 40% of affected patients at presentation. Given that CMV retinitis leads inexorably to blindness if untreated and that HIV infection and its complications tend to go untreated in most parts of the world, such prevalence estimates would suggest that perhaps 1 to 2 million people in the world are currently living with bilateral vision impairment as a result of CMV retinitis. These figures could easily double if other potentially blinding HIV-associated conditions are included.

Clinical Presentation and Findings

The clinical manifestations of the ocular complications of HIV/AIDS have been reviewed in detail elsewhere in this series (see BCSC Section 9, *Intraocular Inflammation and Uveitis*). Cytomegalovirus retinitis, the most common vision-threatening complication, almost always occurs at $CD4^+$ T-lymphocyte counts less than 100 cells/mm^3 and usually at counts of 50 cells/mm^3 or less. Patients with CMV retinitis tend to have a mild to moderate anterior chamber and vitreous inflammatory reaction and one or two foci of full-thickness retinitis, often associated with intraretinal hemorrhage. Small satellite lesions are usually seen at the advancing edge of retinitis; these can help distinguish CMV infection from other causes of retinal whitening (see Fig 20-4A). Diseases that can mimic CMV retinitis include varicella zoster virus (see Fig 20-4B) and herpes simplex virus retinitis, both of which progress rapidly; toxoplasmic retinochoroiditis (see Fig 20-4C), which is often seen in the setting of adjacent or nearby retinochoroidal scars and tends to produce a moderate to severe inflammatory reaction; syphilitic retinitis; tuberculous retinochoroiditis; and intraocular lymphoma. Herpes zoster ophthalmicus (see Fig 20-4D) is also common in HIV-positive patients and is characterized by the occurrence of a vesiculobullous dermatitis involving the ophthalmic distribution of the trigeminal nerve. Pain is typically severe. Concurrent or delayed keratitis, scleritis, uveitis, or retinitis can also occur and may significantly limit vision in more than 50% of patients. Unlike CMV retinitis, HZO may occur at any $CD4^+$ cell count and often develops while patients are still relatively healthy. Kaposi sarcoma (see Fig 20-4E) affects approximately 5% of HIV-positive patients in North America and Europe but is relatively uncommon in Africa, Asia, and Latin America.

Prevention

A number of strategies are available to help prevent the spread of HIV. Latex condoms are inexpensive and are an effective barrier against sexually transmitted HIV when used consistently and correctly. Transmission among intravenous drug users decreases when needle sharing is avoided. The rate of transmission from mother to child may be lowered by treating both the mother and the child with antiretroviral agents before, during, and after delivery. Health care providers should use latex gloves and practice handwashing before and after patient examinations and procedures. In addition, postexposure antiretroviral agents are generally advised for patients and physicians who have had high-risk exposures. Treatment guidelines change frequently as new antiretroviral agents and combination treatment regimens become available. Current recommendations may be obtained from the CDC (www.cdc.gov); from the HIV/AIDS National Clinicians Consultation Center, located at San Francisco General Hospital (1-888-448-4911); or from state or local infection control offices.

Current Treatment Programs

Screening

Although neither the efficacy nor the cost effectiveness of screening strategies has been demonstrated in a controlled fashion, most authorities recommend annual dilated screening examinations for those HIV-positive patients whose $CD4^+$ T-lymphocyte counts remain above 100 cells/mm³ and screenings every 3–4 months for those patients with T-cell counts falling below 100 cells/mm³. When $CD4^+$ T-lymphocyte counts rise in response to HAART, the scheduling of dilated fundus examinations may be extended to reflect the elevated T-cell count and immune reconstitution. Once eye involvement has occurred, the frequency of visits varies considerably, depending on the type and extent of disease.

Therapy

Treatment of HIV-related ocular disorders is complicated and depends largely on the type and extent of disease. Almost all patients should be encouraged to initiate combination therapy with HAART, however, because immune recovery significantly lowers the risk of opportunistic illnesses. Optimal management requires a close working relationship among the ophthalmologist, the patient, and the patient's primary care provider.

Belfort R Jr. The ophthalmologist and the global impact of the AIDS epidemic. LV Edward Jackson Memorial Lecture. *Am J Ophthalmol.* 2000;129:1–8.

The Centers for Disease Control and Prevention website on HIV/AIDS prevention (www.cdc.gov).

Cunningham ET Jr. Uveitis in HIV positive patients. *Br J Ophthalmol.* 2000;84:233–235.

Cunningham ET Jr, Belfort R Jr. *HIV/AIDS and the Eye: A Global Perspective.* Ophthalmology Monograph 15. San Francisco: American Academy of Ophthalmology; 2002.

Cunningham ET Jr, Margolis TP. Ocular manifestations of HIV infection. *N Engl J Med.* 1998;339:236–244.

Fauci AS. The AIDS epidemic—considerations for the 21st century. *N Engl J Med.* 1999; 341:1046–1050.

Fauci AS, Pantaleo G, Stanley S, et al. Immunopathogenic mechanisms of HIV infection. *Ann Intern Med.* 1996;124:654–663.

Gayle HD, Hill GL. Global impact of human immunodeficiency virus and AIDS. *Clin Microbiol Rev.* 2001;14:327–335.

The global HIV and AIDS epidemic, 2001. *MMWR.* 2001;50:434–439.

Joint United Nations Programme on HIV/AIDS website (www.unaids.org).

Kestelyn P. The epidemiology of CMV retinitis in Africa. *Ocul Immunol Inflamm.* 1999;7: 173–177.

Kestelyn PG, Cunningham ET Jr. HIV/AIDS and blindness. *Bull World Health Organ.* 2001; 79:208–213.

Lewallen S, Courtright P. HIV and AIDS and the eye in developing countries: a review. *Arch Ophthalmol.* 1997;115:1291–1295.

Perrin L, Telenti A. HIV treatment failure: testing HIV resistance in clinical practice. *Science.* 1998;280:1871–1872.

Piot P, Bartos M, Ghys PD, et al. The global impact of HIV/AIDS. *Nature.* 2001;410:968–973.

CHAPTER 21

Onchocerciasis

Background

Onchocerciasis is a parasitic infection caused by the filarial nematode *Onchocerca volvulus*. It is transmitted by the vector *Simulium* spp, or blackfly, which breeds in fast-flowing rivers and streams. Often called *river blindness*, it is a devastating disease that occurs in communities living along rivers, usually in remote, rural areas of tropical Africa, the Arabian Peninsula, and in foci in Latin America (Fig 21-1).

Various attempts have been made in the past to control onchocerciasis because of its public health importance but with little success. Then, in 1974, the Onchocerciasis Control Programme (OCP), which applies vector control as its main strategy, was begun in West Africa (see Fig 21-1). The program has been very successful and has eliminated onchocerciasis as a disease of public health importance in this West African subregion. The program uses helicopters and fixed-wing aircraft to spray the vector blackfly breeding sites in riverbeds with biodegradable larvicides. Although the program has been very cost-effective, it has not been possible to replicate the strategy elsewhere.

Two drugs have been available for treating onchocerciasis: diethylcarbamazine (DEC), a microfilaricide, and suramin, a macrofilaricide. However, both cause very serious adverse reactions and are, thus, unsuitable for mass treatment. The advent of ivermectin (Mectizan), a safe microfilaricide suitable for use in large-scale treatment, has proven an effective alternative. The drug has made it possible for public health personnel to pursue onchocerciasis control in African countries where the disease is endemic outside the West African program area, as well as in areas of Latin America and the Arabian Peninsula. As ivermectin is only microfilaricidal, population treatment needs to continue during the entire lifespan of the adult worm, which can be up to 14 years. The donation of ivermectin by its manufacturer, Merck & Co Inc, to onchocerciasis control programs for as long as necessary to eliminate the disease as a public health problem is unprecedented. It is a unique model that is being emulated by other public health programs.

Life Cycle of *O volvulus*

The human being is the definitive host of *O volvulus*. An individual is infected when he or she is bitten by a female blackfly in search of a blood meal. As the fly feeds, it ingests microfilariae (mf), or L_1 (the first larval stage), found in the skin (Fig 21-2). After passing from the gut to the flight muscles, the L_1 molts twice to the infective L_3 stage in 6–12 days (Fig 21-3). The L_3 larvae migrate back to the mouthparts, where they may be

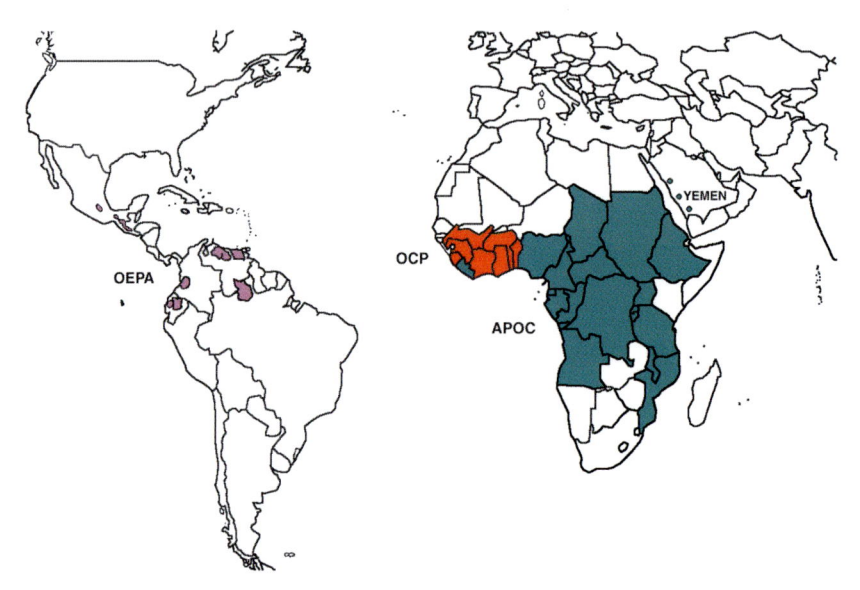

Figure 21-1 Two onchocerciasis control programs carry out onchocerciasis control in 30 endemic countries in Africa:

The *Onchocerciasis Control Programme (OCP)* operates in 11 West African endemic countries: Benin, Burkina Faso, Côte d'Ivoire, Ghana, Guinea-Bissau, Guinea-Conakry, Mali, Niger, Senegal, Sierra Leone, and Togo. Liberia and Nigeria, which are also in West Africa, are not included in the OCP.
The *African Programme for Onchocerciasis Control (APOC)* operates in the remaining 19 endemic countries outside the OCP: Angola, Burundi, Cameroon, Central African Republic, Chad, Congo Brazzaville, Democratic Republic of Congo, Ethiopia, Equatorial Guinea, Gabon, Kenya, Liberia, Malawi, Mozambique, Nigeria, Rwanda, Sudan, Tanzania, and Uganda.
In Latin America, the *Onchocerciasis Elimination Program for the Americas (OEPA)* covers 6 countries: Brazil, Ecuador, Colombia, Guatemala, Mexico, and Venezuela.
In Yemen, on the Arabian Peninsula, a national program controls onchocerciasis.

(Courtesy of Yankum Dadzie, MD.)

transmitted with the next blood meal. In the human, the L_3 larvae molt twice to become adult worms with lifespans of 9–14 years. The adult worms are significantly different in size; females are 30–80 cm long and 0.3 mm in diameter, whereas the males are 3–5 cm in length (see Fig 21-2). The coiled adults are found in fibrous nodules, which are often subcutaneous, visible, and palpable, called *onchocercomata*. The adult female *O volvulus* produces an estimated 700–1500 mf per day, which migrate from the nodules to the skin, eyes, and other organs.

History

The first scientific record of onchocerciasis appeared in 1875, when microfilariae were discovered in the skin of patients from Ghana, West Africa. Soon thereafter, filarial worms, named *Onchocerca volvulus*, were found in tumors removed from patients from the same country. Although the vector, *Simulium*, was described at the beginning of the last century, transmission of the disease was established only in 1926, also in West Africa.

CHAPTER 21: Onchocerciasis • 237

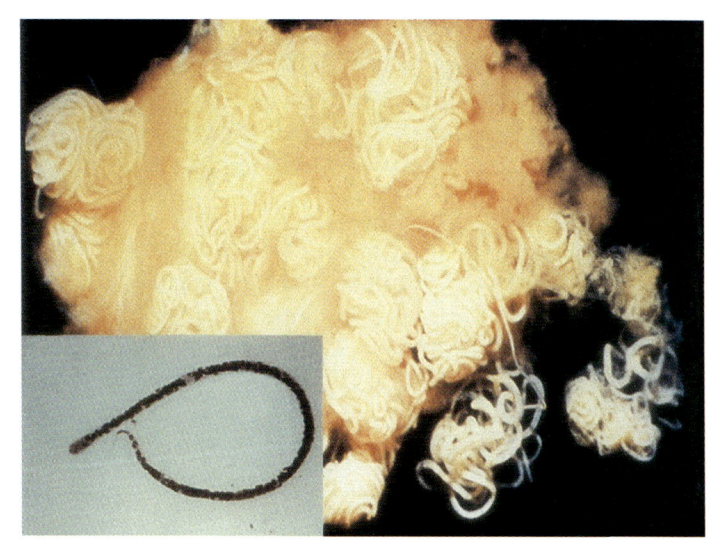

Figure 21-2 Adult worms of *Onchocerca volvulus* isolated from a fibrous nodule; *inset:* a microfilaria, as seen under a microscope. *(Photograph courtesy of Yankum Dadzie, MD.)*

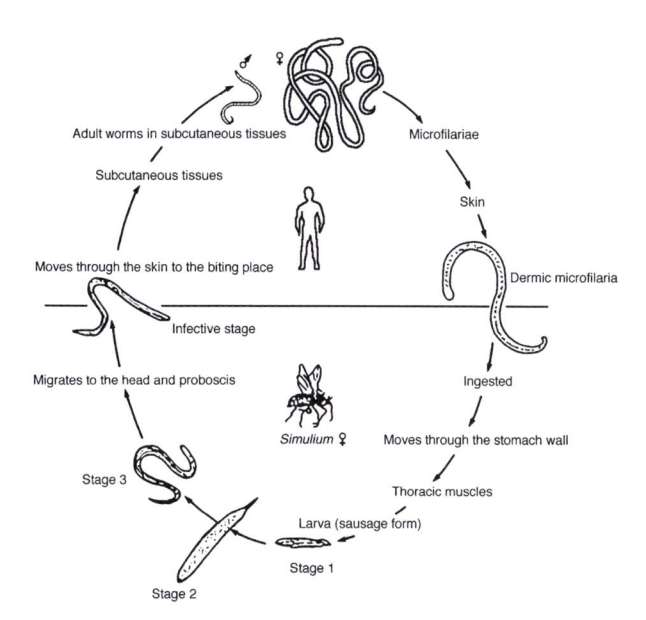

Figure 21-3 Life cycle of *Onchocerca volvulus*. A microfilaria, of L_1, ingested from the skin of an infected subject by a blackfly during a blood meal molts twice, through L_2 to L_3, in the blackfly over a period of 6–12 days. The L_3, or infective larva, is inoculated during a subsequent blood meal into another human being. In the human being, the L_3 molts twice through L_4 and L_5 to become an adult male or female worm. *(Courtesy of Yankum Dadzie, MD.)*

In Latin America, pioneering work done in 1915 distinguished the acute form of onchocerciasis, *erisipela de la costa*, from a more chronic manifestation. Reports on onchocercal eye disease, microfilariae in the globe, and changes in the fundus of the eye were first made in the early 1930s.

The first three tools to control onchocerciasis were discovered in the early 1940s: the insecticide *p'*-dichlorodiphenyltrichloroethane (DDT), applied against the vector, and the two drugs, the microfilaricide DEC and the macrofilaricide suramin. Unfortunately, all three agents turned out to be toxic. Today's effective control programs are based on recently developed approaches. These include environmentally safe insecticides, in particular the biological insecticide *Bacillus thuringiensis*, serotype H14; diagnostic tools, including DNA probes; and the safe drug ivermectin, the development of which was led by two American scientists, Mohammed Aziz and Bruce Greene.

Context

Onchocerciasis is not only a cause of blindness and health distress in remote rural populations without access to health care, but it is also a cause of misery, poverty, and premature death in the endemic communities. In such communities, over 10% of the total population or up to 50% of adults aged 30 years and over could be visually impaired. The blind, who are in their most productive and responsible years, are not only lost to the community labor force but also die at 3–4 times the rate of their normal-sighted counterparts of the same age. Until vector-control operations began in West Africa, communities such as these are known to have abandoned the fertile land along the rivers for fear of going blind and to have occupied less productive, arid land away from the rivers.

Onchocercal skin disease is a serious stigma in the endemic communities, and the affected are often ostracized. Individuals with onchocercal skin disease have low self-esteem, difficulty in finding marriage partners, and are often unable to hold public office. Onchocercal itching is a most bothersome symptom. These social ramifications add to the dimension of the burden already placed on a population subjected to the physical manifestations of onchocerciasis.

The World Health Organization estimates that 17.5 million people globally are infected, 99% of them in Africa and the rest in Latin America. About 270,000 are <3/60 and about half a million suffer visual disability. Upward of 120 million people live in the endemic areas and are therefore at risk of contracting infection.

Economic Impact

Cost of treatment

Current treatment of an onchocerciasis-affected individual prevents progression of the disease but does not cure it. People who have moved from an endemic to a nonendemic area or who have resided temporarily in an endemic area are effectively treated with a single annual dose of 150 µg/kg body weight of ivermectin for up to 10 years. As noted, ivermectin, produced by Merck & Co Inc, is given free of charge by the company for the treatment of onchocerciasis.

In endemic savannah areas, vector control by use of larvicides in OCP countries in West Africa is estimated to cost US$0.57 per person per year. Similar vector-control activities in forests are impossible because of logistics. The African Programme for Onchocerciasis Control (APOC), which covers Central and East Africa (see Fig 21-1), will spend, on average, US$0.40 per person per year during the 12 years in which it will operate to set up sustainable ivermectin distribution systems in endemic countries within its geographic scope. This program will treat 55 million people for as long as necessary to eliminate onchocerciasis as a disease of public health importance.

Cost of lost productivity

The economic impact of onchocerciasis in West Africa relates to labor loss and nonutilization of abandoned fertile land as a result of onchocercal blindness. In parts of Africa where onchocercal skin disease predominates, recent studies have identified labor loss, as well as a higher occurrence of children of affected parents dropping out of school, as additional economic effects of the disease.

On the positive side, cost–benefit analysis of OCP operations has shown an internal rate of return of 20%, a value highly comparable to any World Bank project in the productive sector. Similar studies of APOC produced an internal rate of return of 17%. Furthermore, onchocerciasis control has freed 25 million hectares (62.5 million acres) of fertile agricultural land in the OCP area. It is estimated that with simple, traditional agricultural methods, the freed land could be cultivated to feed 17 million people.

Pathogenesis and Immune Response

The filarial nematode *O volvulus* is the only known onchocercal species that infects humans. However, other species of filarial nematodes infect humans; these include *Wuchereria bancrofti* and *Brugia malayi*, which cause lymphatic filariasis and elephantiasis, and *Loa loa*, which causes loiasis.

A bite by the female infective blackfly vector, *Simulium* spp, may transmit several *O volvulus* L_3 larvae to the human host. Repeated bites result in numerous adult worms. The worms are often harbored in the fibrous nodules called onchocercomata, which are usually located at the bony prominences of the body but may also be in deep tissue. A single nodule measuring up to 1 cm in size may contain two or three females and one or two males. New nodules are frequently found around older nodules, and the adults are coiled in the nodules like a ball of string (see Fig 21-2). Although the nodules are usually painless, upon the death of the adult filarial worms, chronic inflammation is evident on histologic examination. Over their lifetime, adult female worms produce millions of mf, which migrate in the dermis and in the lymphatic channels of the dermis. The mf, which also are found in the lymph nodes, die after 6–30 months if not ingested by a feeding blackfly.

Our understanding of the complex host–parasite immune interaction is still evolving. *O volvulus*, like other filarial nematodes, has a number of characteristics that may explain its ability to avoid the host's immune response. Down modulation of cell-mediated responses has been observed in generalized onchocerciasis and may occur because of T-cell anergy caused by active suppressive mechanisms diminishing "proinflammatory" T-cell responses. The diminished antigen-specific lymphocyte activity is common in people with high levels of organisms who have little clinical skin reaction. Often a person with few demonstrable organisms has vigorous immune responsiveness and highly reactive skin disease.

Immune reaction is clearly an important phenomenon in onchocerciasis. In multiple studies, exposed individuals without parasitologic and clinical evidence of infection (ie, endemic-normal or putatively immune individuals) were found to display prominent cellular reactivity to *O volvulus* antigens. Indeed, these antigens induced substantial production of IL-2 and interferon-γ in peripheral blood mononuclear cells (PBMC) from endemic normals but not in those from patients with onchocerciasis. Because IL-2 induces CD4$^+$ T cells to produce IL-5, which in turn stimulates production of eosinophils capable of killing the parasite, these findings suggest IL-5 as a possible mediator of protection for the host against onchocerciasis and a determinant of different levels of infection intensity in different individuals. In contrast to this hyperresponsiveness to *O volvulus* antigens, the PBMC from patients with onchocerciasis clearly produced more of the "down-regulating" cytokine IL-10 than did cells from endemic normals.

Adult worms in encapsulated nodules induce little visible inflammatory reaction. It is hypothesized that the parasite may alter its extracellular cuticle surface with human proteins and surface-associated proteases to avoid human immune responses. Indeed, it is not clear whether the living parasite is capable of inhibiting the host inflammatory responses directly or whether the dead parasite releases new antigens that stimulate an inflammatory response. The pathogenesis of punctate multifocal stromal keratitis has been studied and shows inflammatory cells surrounding dead or dying mf. It appears that dying mf or adults induce anti-inflammatory host responses, which result in localized damage to the host tissue. What does seem clear is that the host's immune reaction to onchocercal infection is normally directed at containing or restricting inflammatory responses. It has been calculated that in lightly infected persons and in heavily infected adults, mf die at a rate of 20,000 per day and 500,000 per day, respectively, and some mechanism must exist to "contain" all the potential inflammatory reactivity.

Elevated levels of IgG, IgM, and IgE are common and result from polyclonal B-cell activation stimulated by the *O volvulus* infection and/or other simultaneous parasitic infection. The frequently occurring high levels of IgE may approach the levels found in tropical pulmonary eosinophilia syndrome. Only 10% of the high levels of IgE is directed against the parasite antigens. These high levels may contribute to the acute ocular inflammatory disease as a result of immediate hypersensitivity immune responses.

Although the mechanism and role of the antibody response in the eye remain unclear, anti–*O volvulus* antibody is usually present and has been demonstrated by immunofluorescence, complement fixation, and enzyme immunoassays.

Epidemiology

Surveys to Determine Prevalence/Incidence

In the past, population surveys to assess prevalence of onchocerciasis in endemic countries employed varying methods, lacked epidemiologic criteria for selecting communities for surveys, and did not always collect important data such as visual acuity. Recently, rapid epidemiologic mapping of onchocerciasis (REMO) using nodule palpation has been developed and used in APOC countries with good results. By convention, such surveys classify communities by endemicity levels, which are determined by the prevalence of mf-positive skin snips. A community is hyperendemic when its prevalence is ≥60%, mesoendemic when its prevalence is between 35% and 60%, and hypoendemic when its prevalence is below 35%.

OCP general survey results

When the OCP began in 1974, a crude prevalence of 62.7% infection with *O volvulus* was found, 2.8% with ≤6/60 vision and 2.7% with <3/60 vision (Fig 21-4). Recent crude prevalence values (1997–1998) have decreased dramatically. The rate of infection with *O volvulus* is 8.6%, the rate with vision of <6/60 is 0.7%, and with vision of <3/60 is 0.7% (Fig 21-5).

OCP ophthalmologic survey results

Ophthalmologic surveys were carried out in 13 villages in Burkina Faso, Côte d'Ivoire, and Ghana at the start of vector-control operations in 2716 persons and followed up 13 years later in 2673 persons. Age-specific analysis of the results demonstrated that onchocercal eye lesions of the anterior segment—that is, sclerosing keratitis and iridocyclitis—are significantly reduced with vector control, whereas eye lesions of the posterior segment—namely, chorioretinitis and optic nerve disease—undergo no statistically significant changes (Fig 21-6).

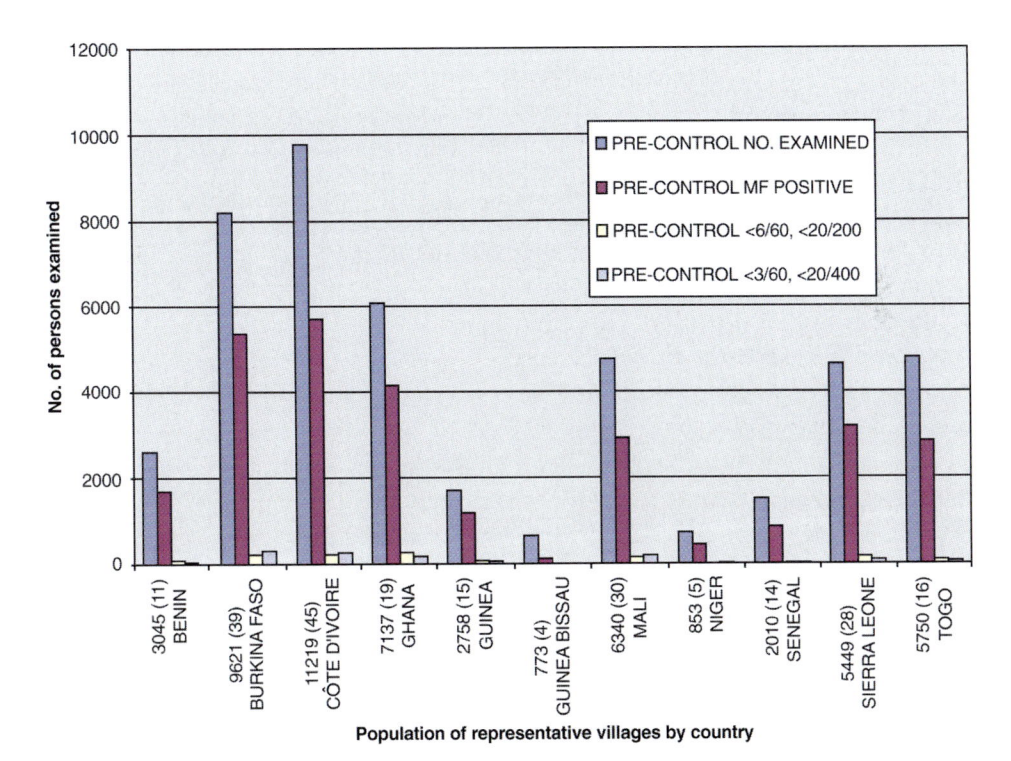

Figure 21-4 Distribution of epidemiologic parameters on onchocerciasis—that is, mf-positive individuals, visual acuity of 3/60–6/60 or 20/400–20/200, and visual acuity less than 3/60 or 20/400—in the populations examined in representative villages in 11 countries in the OCP before vector-control activities were begun. The abscissa shows names of the countries in which the examinations were carried out, the number of persons examined, and, in parentheses, the number of villages. *(Courtesy of Yankum Dadzie, MD.)*

242 • International Ophthalmology

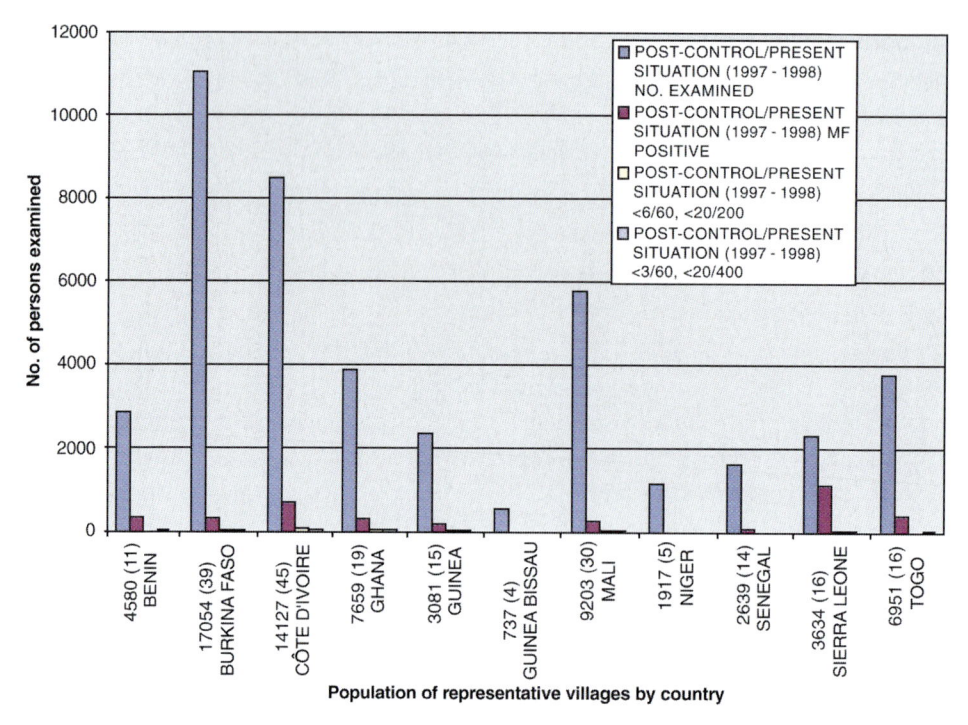

Figure 21-5 Distribution of epidemiologic parameters on onchocerciasis—that is, mf-positive individuals, visual acuity of 3/60–6/60 or 20/400–20/200, and visual acuity less than 3/60 or 20/400—in the populations examined in representative villages in 11 countries in the OCP 8–11 years after the vector-control activities were begun. The abscissa shows names of the countries in which the examinations were carried out, the number of persons examined, and, in parentheses, the number of villages. *(Courtesy of Yankum Dadzie, MD.)*

Survey results outside the OCP area

In the Taraba River Valley, Nigeria, the prevalence of <3/60 exceeded 20% in 6 communities, with 1 community recording a 71.9% blindness rate. The total sample, 2876 persons in 14 communities, was examined for eye lesions and tested for visual acuity using the tumbling E chart. Vision worsens as prevalence and intensity of *O volvulus* infection increases. High microfilarial loads were associated with severe eye damage and vision loss. These findings indicate that the Taraba River Valley could be one of West Africa's worst foci of onchocercal eye disease.

Risk Factors

The main risk factor for onchocerciasis is exposure to bites by infected female blackflies. This usually means living within an endemic community. The more infected bites, the more severe the disease. Because the habitat of the blackfly limits its dispersal from river banks, the closer a human settlement is to a highly productive vector *(Simulium)* river-breeding site, the more the inhabitants are exposed to infective vector bite and the higher the endemicity of infection in the community.

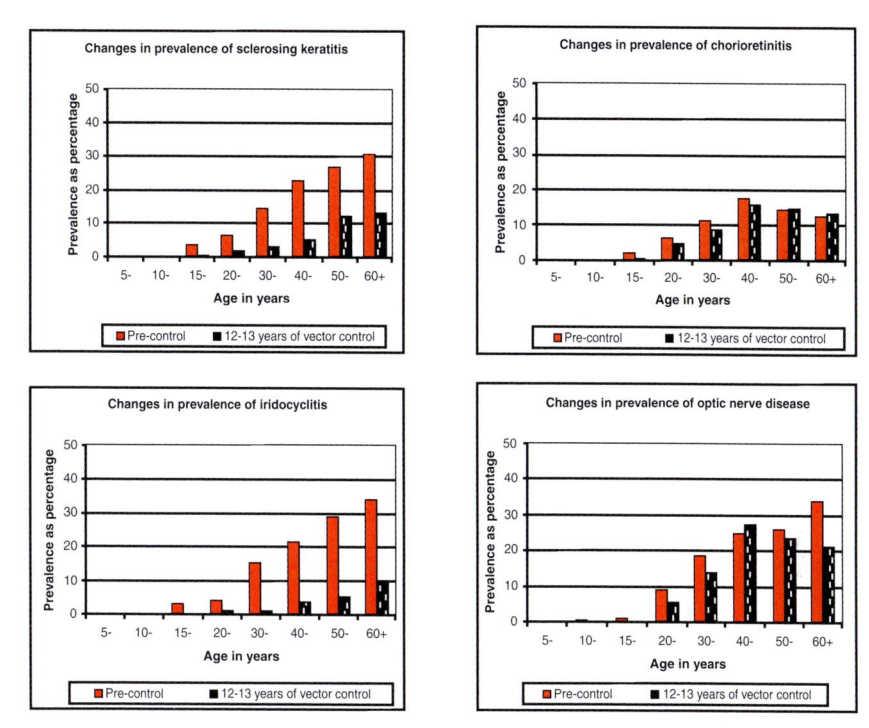

Figure 21-6 Comparison of age-specific prevalence of onchocercal eye lesions before the start of vector control in selected villages in three countries in the OCP and again 13 years later. *(Courtesy of Yankum Dadzie, MD.)*

Geographic and environmental factors

Geography and environment play a critical role in disease development and distribution. Geographically, the disease is limited to the tropics. In Africa, the area involved barely extends beyond 14° north and south latitude, as the vectors of onchocerciasis are adapted to high temperatures, and their reproduction is slowed as the ambient temperature becomes colder. In addition, two genetically distinct parasites are found in Africa, producing epidemiologically different disease patterns. A more severe form of the disease is found in savannah regions, where corneal vision loss from sclerosing keratitis predominates. Vision impairment occurs rarely in the forest zones, but when it does, it results from chorioretinitis and/or optic nerve disease. Environmental factors relating to hydrology influence the productivity of the preimaginal stages of the blackfly. Prevailing climatic conditions can influence its dispersal over and beyond its normal habitat. Although blackflies stay quite close to their breeding sites, they are known to travel up to 500 km if swept up by monsoon or harmattan winds.

Social factors

Social factors can play an important role, as they affect the exposure of the host to the biting blackfly. Farming, fishing, and fetching water from the river for daily use can greatly increase contact with the blackfly vector. The low number of people in rural areas means they are exposed to a high rate of fly biting. As the community develops socioeconomically, the population increases significantly; the human–fly contact decreases with an increased population exposed to the same numbers of flies. The result is a lower level of endemicity.

Diagnosis

A definitive diagnosis can be made when an *O volvulus* adult or mf are detected in an individual. This can be accomplished by visualizing an adult worm in an excised nodule or by visualizing mf in a skin snip under the microscope (see Fig 21-2) or during slit-lamp examination of the eye. A presumptive diagnosis may be made with the observation of typical nodules, skin changes, and ocular changes.

Antibody detection and polymerase chain reaction (PCR)–based assay offer improved sensitivity and specificity to skin snip diagnosis. A recombinant antigen, Ov-16, used in an enzyme-linked immunosorbent assay, has a sensitivity and specificity approaching 95% and is able to identify infection in the prepatent period. A PCR-based assay is highly sensitive in detecting the presence of parasite DNA in superficial skin scrapings. The skin scratch PCR assay has been found to be more sensitive in detecting low-density infections than microscopic examination of skin snips; it is also painless and reduces the risk of transmitting bloodborne infections.

Clinical Presentation and Findings

Onchocercal Nodules

Nodules are part of the clinical picture, with their distribution typically at the bony prominences of the body—that is, the rib cage, the trochanter, the knees, and occasionally the head. In Africa, head nodules are rare in adults and more common in children, but in the Americas they are found quite commonly in adults. The nodules are painless.

Lymphatic System

Regional lymph nodes may be palpable in areas of onchodermatitis. Microfilariae found in lymphatic channels and lymph nodes give rise to chronic inflammation. Occasionally, hanging groin may be found in highly infected individuals.

Skin Signs and Symptoms of Onchocerciasis

In the skin, pathologic changes resulting from acute inflammatory reactions are manifest clinically as itching and a visible papular rash and correspond to the active stage of inflammatory response of the host to dead mf. In Yemen, on the Arabian Peninsula, severe reactive dermatitis or onchodermatitis (called *sowda*) appears to be due to extensive plasma cell infiltrate. Sowda presents clinically as unilateral limb edematous swelling with intense pruritus, papular rash that is often pustular, hyperpigmentation, and local lymph node swelling. Hypertrophic skin changes have also been called *lizard skin*. Chronic tissue damage in the form of atrophy and hypopigmentation may be viewed as tissue damage resulting from cumulative inflammatory responses of the host to millions of dead mf over time. In chronic severe disease, especially visible on the shins, focal areas of increased pigmentation within areas of hypopigmentation may give an appearance of *leopard skin;* this finding has been used to assess the prevalence of onchocerciasis. A recent study has provided a new classification system based on clinical findings:

- Acute papular onchodermatitis
- Chronic papular onchodermatitis
- Lichenified onchodermatitis
- Atrophy
- Depigmentation

These entities may be found associated in the same subject (Fig 21-7).

Ocular Signs of Onchocerciasis

It has been postulated that mf get into the eyes by a number of different pathways. They may penetrate the cornea or the conjunctiva or get into the globe by way of the scleral channels through direct invasion. They may also enter the globe through the blood circulation. Once in the globe, mf migrate widely within it. A common early slit-lamp sign of ocular involvement is visible mf in the anterior chamber. The thin, 300-mm long, faintly translucent mf are seen moving in the aqueous fluid convection currents. Their numbers increase after face-down positioning. Dead mf may be seen in the cornea, on the lens, and in the vitreous. Living mf in the cornea are usually coiled and are best visualized with retroillumination and high magnification. Intraretinal mf are best seen using biomicroscopy with a contact lens and appear as small, highly refractile bodies with a greenish tinge, or with a fundus camera.

Keratitis

Punctate opacities about 0.5 mm in diameter are commonly visible in the superficial corneal stroma. A cellular infiltrate of lymphocytes, eosinophils, and edema surround the opaque dead mf. Later sclerosing keratitis begins with a limbal haze and may progress to an inferior, semilunar opacity and end as a total corneal opacity (Fig 21-8).

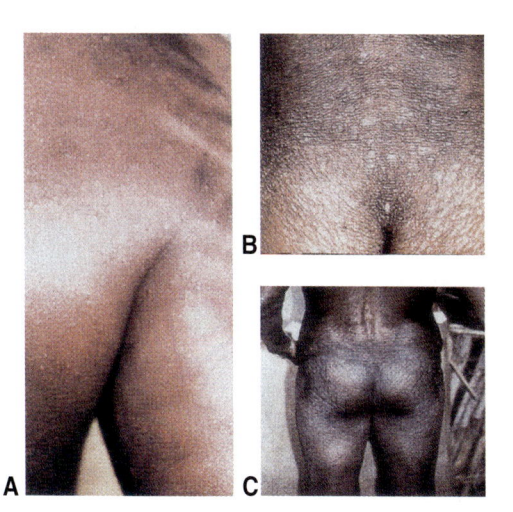

Figure 21-7 Different stages of onchodermatitis, as defined by recent classification of onchocercal skin disease: **A,** acute papular dermatitis; **B,** chronic papular dermatitis; **C,** atrophy. *(Photographs courtesy of Yankum Dadzie, MD.)*

Figure 21-8 Anterior uveitis with synechiae plus inferior semilunar opacity resulting from sclerosing keratits. *(Photograph courtesy of Yankum Dadzie, MD.)*

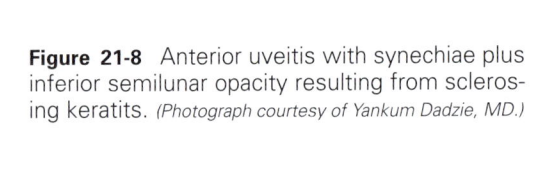

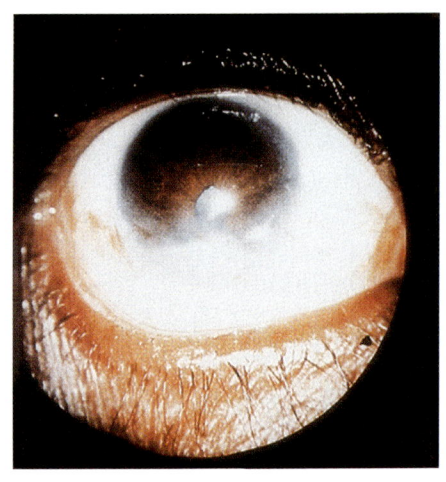

Anterior uveitis

It is possible to see hundreds of mf in the anterior chamber but no sign of uveitis. It is common to see mild, nongranulomatous uveitis when mf are in the cornea, anterior chamber, and/or iris. Chronic granulomatous uveitis and its complications of synechiae, occlusion of the pupil, secondary pupillary block glaucoma, and cataract may occur and are usually associated with mf in the ciliary body (see Fig 21-8).

Chorioretinitis

A wide spectrum of changes may occur, from focal retinal pigment epithelial changes with a visible intraretinal or subretinal mf in early disease to extensive chorioretinal atrophy in late disease. Advanced posterior segment disease includes retinal pigment epithelial atrophy, intraretinal deposits, later choriocapillary atrophy, subretinal fibrosis and pigment hyperplasia, and late-stage chorioretinal atrophy of the posterior pole (the so-called *Ridley's fundus*). Optic nerve disease may present as optic neuritis and end as optic atrophy (Fig 21-9). Typically, lesions of the anterior and posterior segments of the eyes are found associated with, but not necessarily at, the same stage of development.

Pathway to vision impairment

Onchocercal vision loss is commonly a result of either sclerosing keratitis or advanced chorioretinal disease with or without optic atrophy. Less commonly, vision loss is due to secondary glaucoma induced by uveitis or complicated cataract.

Visual field tests conducted systematically have demonstrated that onchocercal vision impairment due to visual field constriction to less than 10° (functional blindness) may increase the number of people who are blind by a third compared to that measured by visual acuity testing alone. Thus, an estimate of onchocercal vision impairment based solely on visual acuity measurement would be an underestimate.

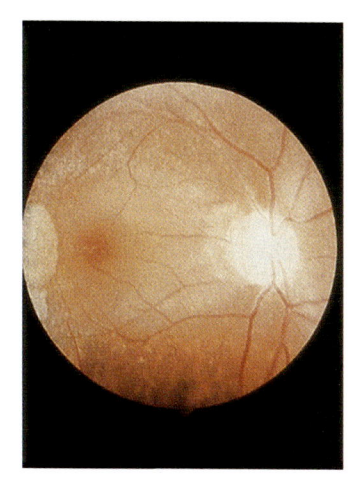

Figure 21-9 Fundus with temporal circumscribed confluent retinal pigment epithelium atrophy and optic atrophy with retinal vascular sheathing. *(Photograph courtesy of Yankum Dadzie, MD.)*

Prevention

No vaccination against onchocerciasis is available at present. Treatment of the community with ivermectin reduces the numbers of mf available for transmission and, hence, reduces the blackfly infectivity. The fewer the mf in a person with onchocerciasis—that is, the lower his or her infection load—the fewer the associated inflammatory complications. An individual going into an endemic area is advised to wear protective clothing that leaves few parts of the body exposed to an insect bite and to apply insect repellents to exposed skin. These protective measures are difficult to practice in the heat of the tropics.

Current Treatment Programs

Currently, treatment programs are in effect in the three major geographic areas endemic for onchocerciasis. The older West African OCP covers 11 countries, and the more recent Central and East African APOC covers the remaining 19 endemic African countries. The Onchocerciasis Elimination Program for the Americas covers 6 endemic countries in Latin America (see Fig 21-1). The Central and East African program and the American program use the strategy of large-scale ivermectin treatment of at-risk populations. The West African OCP, established in 1974, was originally based on vector control through use of larvicides. Since the advent of ivermectin in 1987, however, the West African OCP has changed its control strategy fundamentally. It now combines vector control with large-scale ivermectin treatment. This combination requires 12 years of control operations, whereas vector control alone requires 14 years to reduce the infection reservoir in the populations to zero levels. In addition, the OCP uses only large-scale ivermectin treatment of populations in certain zones in the program area.

Screening

Epidemiologic surveys of representative communities are carried out to identify areas and populations to be treated. Once a community or an area is identified as being in need of treatment, there is no reason to screen individuals further. All members of endemic communities undergo community-based treatment with ivermectin.

Vector Control

Although the initial results of vector control in the seven original West African OCP countries were encouraging, several problems developed. *Simulium* spp invaded the western and southern border areas of the OCP from outside the OCP. In 1986, the OCP expanded spraying (later combined with large-scale ivermectin treatment of populations) to include countries located at its western borders: Senegal, Sierra Leone, Guinea-Conakry, and Guinea-Bissau. It also extended the spraying beyond its original southern borders into the southern parts of Ghana, Côte d'Ivoire, Togo, and Benin.

Resistance to the initial insecticide, temephos, was another obstacle. The OCP overcame this by finding seven additional effective larvicides: pyraclofos; chlorphoxim; phoxim; permethrin; carbosulfan; *Bacillus thuringiensis*, serotype H-14; and etofenprox. These are currently applied in rotation.

The effectiveness of the vector-control operations is monitored by entomologic surveillance networks set up all over the program areas. Flies are caught daily and examined to determine their parity and infection level. The results are expressed as monthly and annual biting rates and monthly and annual transmission potential. The results of vector control in the original seven-country area of the OCP are extremely good. Prevalence rates have fallen to zero or near zero in 90% of the original area. Regular epidemiologic surveillance since larvicide application ceased 10–11 years ago has confirmed the absence of new infection. Vector control has also interrupted transmission in the border country areas of the West African OCP, except in Sierra Leone, where civil war has prevented control operations.

The OCP will terminate in 2002, when treatment will cease in most areas where the strategy of vector control or combined vector control and large-scale ivermectin treatment have been carried out. Such areas will begin a maintenance phase consisting of epidemiologic surveillance to detect and control recrudescence or remission of infection early if it occurs. Any recrudescence of onchocerciasis infection will be controlled through ivermectin treatment of the populations in the circumscribed area.

The environmental impact of the insecticide spraying is closely monitored, and thus far no significant impact on the nontarget fauna has been recorded. Although it has not been suitable for application in the forest zone, where forest galleries obstruct spraying of rivers from the air, OCP aerial spraying vector control has been cost effective though highly technical and expensive.

Chemotherapy

Diethylcarbamazine has been used for treating onchocerciasis since the late 1940s. It is an effective microfilaricide, but its use is associated with a severe adverse reaction known as the *Mazzotti reaction*. The use of DEC has therefore been abandoned. Suramin, a macrofilaricide, has also been used for over 5 decades. Because it is toxic and its use cumbersome, it has also been largely abandoned.

For the past 40 years, scientists have sought a safe drug for the treatment of onchocerciasis. The discovery and development of ivermectin was therefore an exciting and significant breakthrough.

Ivermectin is a macrocyclic lactone that has been used in veterinary medicine as an efficacious anti-ectoparasitic and anti-endoparasitic drug since the 1970s. Because it was observed to have a microfilaricidal effect in cows with bovine onchocerciasis, *O gutturosa*, a clinical trial in humans was initiated to test the efficacy of the drug against human onchocerciasis. After various clinical trials demonstrated the efficacy and safety of the drug, including to the eyes, as compared with DEC, ivermectin was registered in 1987 with the French regulatory board.

Ivermectin is given once a year at a dose of 150 µg/kg body weight. Large-scale treatment programs, however, apply height as a surrogate for weight, whereby individuals 90–119 cm tall take one 3 mg tablet; those 120–140 cm in height, two tablets; those 141–158 cm tall, three tablets; and anyone over 158 cm tall, four tablets. Certain categories of individuals are excluded from treatment: children younger than 5 years, pregnant women, mothers breastfeeding 1-week-old babies, and seriously ill patients. After the drug was registered, Merck offered ivermectin free of charge to anyone who needed it for as long as necessary. It set up the Mectizan Donation Program to oversee the donation and the Mectizan Expert Committee to review applications for the drug from large-scale treatment programs. Merck also donated tablets for use in clinics to treat isolated cases outside large-scale treatment areas.

The generous donation by Merck provided a number of nongovernmental organizations (NGOs) interested in the prevention of blindness with an opportunity to undertake large-scale treatment with ivermectin to prevent onchocercal blindness. It stimulated groups to organize distribution.

Since its registration in 1987, ivermectin has been used by the Central and East African and the American onchocerciasis control programs (see Fig 21-1). To overcome the challenge of large-scale delivery of the free drug to the communities that need it, the method of community-directed treatment with ivermectin (CDTI) has been developed. This method empowers each community to be in charge of its own treatment by selecting one or more of its members to be trained as the distributors of ivermectin. The communities also decide when they want to carry out their own treatment. They are responsible for organizing the treatment, including record keeping and reporting. The peripheral health system supervises and supports the activities and reports the outcome to the central health system. The Ministry of Health in each country is required to make regular reports on the progress of treatment activities to the programs concerned. Each ministry must account to the Mectizan Donation Program for the ivermectin used in the previous year at the time it is placing its next annual order.

The community-directed treatment method promises to be a sustainable approach that will enable the endemic countries to maintain treatment with ivermectin for as long as necessary to eliminate onchocerciasis as a public health problem. After 10–12 years of ivermectin treatment in the OCP, population coverage and compliance are still very good. Over 24 million people are treated with ivermectin each year in all the endemic areas, a truly outstanding result of the highly innovative donation program established by Merck in collaboration with WHO, the World Bank, and international and national NGOs and governmental agencies.

The enthusiasm of the population for their annual ivermectin treatment has also been recorded in many other endemic areas. The improvement in onchodermatitis, reduction in major symptoms of onchocerciasis, and the beneficial effect ivermectin has had on intestinal parasites are all positive features that have led to high community compliance. CDTI, which was developed originally for APOC, seems to have caught on well in the affected areas. Indications are that the ultimate goal of eliminating onchocerciasis as a disease of public health importance in the whole of the African continent and in the Americas is on course. Furthermore, a recent expert review shows that onchocerciasis is eradicable from the Americas, and the American program continues to work to that end.

Clinical Research Currently Under Way

Applied research has been the strength of the OCP, and various research institutions have provided invaluable support. The OCP has furnished environment-friendly insecticides and provided tools for monitoring the sensitivity of the *Simulium* vector to the larvicides. APOC developed the CDTI approach for ivermectin distribution. After 26 years of onchocerciasis control and intertwined operational research, many research questions have been answered. However, key knowledge remains elusive and several research issues are still being addressed.

The search for a macrofilaricide that could cure onchocerciasis is ongoing in the pharmaceutical industry and institutional research laboratories. The ideal macrofilaricide has been defined as a drug that is safe for use in mass treatment, devoid of the Mazzotti reaction, and given as a single oral dose.

There is concern that ivermectin resistance might occur, although no evidence of resistance exists after 15 years of use in humans for onchocerciasis. Nevertheless, a search is ongoing for a probe that can be used to detect resistance in the event of its occurrence.

A multicountry operational research effort to determine the parameters that will ensure the sustainability of community-directed treatment is ongoing. The African researchers are employing a common protocol for the study. This operational research includes behavioral science investigation into the attitudes of the communities during the course of the treatment. It also addresses the issue of the most effective way to ensure that ivermectin reaches the communities on time and regularly, for as long as necessary to carry out the treatment. Furthermore, operational research is being done to develop an instrument for enhancing the ability of communities to keep records correctly and to develop simple ways of monitoring the community-directed treatment.

Ivermectin, as a microfilaricide, eliminates mf from the community being treated but has only a limited effect on the adult worm population and its viability. Current methods for measuring prevalence do not give a true picture of the infection level of the community. Therefore, a search is under way for a tool to determine the endpoint of ivermectin treatment of communities, as was done with vector control.

Abiose A, Jones BR, Cousens SN, et al. Reduction in incidence of optic nerve disease with annual ivermectin to control onchocerciasis. *Lancet.* 1993;341:130–134.

Dadzie KY, Awadzi K, Bird AC, et al. Ophthalmological results from a placebo controlled comparative 3-dose ivermectin study in the treatment of onchocerciasis. *Trop Med Parasitol.* 1989;40:355–360.

Dadzie KY, Remme J, De Sole G. Epidemiological impact of vector control. II. Changes in ocular onchocerciasis. *Acta Leiden.* 1990;59(No. 1 and 2):127–139.

Elson LH, Calvopina M, Paredes W, et al. Immunity to onchocerciasis: putative immune persons produce a Th1-like response to Onchocerca volvulus. *J Infect Dis.* 1995;171: 652–658.

Garner A. Pathology of ocular onchocerciasis: human and experimental. *Trans R Soc Trop Med Hyg.* 1977;70:374–377.

Gibson DW, Duke BO, Connor DH. Onchocerciasis: a review of clinical, pathologic and chemotherapeutic aspects, and vector control program. *Prog Clin Parasitol.* 1989;1:57–103.

Murphy RP, Taylor H, Greene BM. Chorioretinal damage in onchocerciasis. *Am J Ophthalmol.* 1984;98:519–521.

Ottesen EA. Immediate hypersensitivity responses in the immunopathogenesis of human onchocerciasis. *Rev Infect Dis.* 1985;7:796–801.

PART V

Collaborative Research

Introduction

Research is the lifeblood of human advancement. If we are to reduce the incidence and severity of human blindness and visual impairment, studies focused on the specific disorders will need to be conducted. Although many of these investigations will take place in developing areas, where the majority of these disorders exist, the actual concepts involved will often originate in developed countries, where the appropriate academic personnel and funding exist.

In Part V, we present a number of actual studies that have been completed or are ongoing that exemplify how these investigations can be conducted. The recounting of my experience studying ophthalmia neonatorum in Kenya demonstrates how one can organize a prospective trial in a foreign country. This experience will, I hope, help future investigators conduct their own trials. Dr Alfredo Sadun's determination of the causes of the Cuban optic neuropathy epidemic reads like an exciting mystery thriller. Dr David Mackey's surveys and genetic analysis of glaucoma in Tasmania may help explain the pathogenesis of glaucoma in larger populations. Although the clinical features of different genotypes of sickle cell diseases differ among populations in various parts of the world, Drs Elaine Chuang and Alan Bird's Jamaican study is shedding light on the natural history of these diseases. Conducting excellent population surveys to define various associations of risk factors broadens understanding of the disease and targets conditions that require further study. The investigation of myopia in Hong Kong by Drs VanNewkirk, McCarty, and Taylor reports an important association between extreme myopia and vision impairment.

As the reader can discern, international collaborative research may take many forms. Some studies take the structure of a survey. Others are prospective investigations to clarify pathogenesis; these will become more common, especially as the science of human genetics continues to develop. Another research method is the prospective controlled and masked treatment trial.

What do all these investigations have in common? All are collaborations between an academic center in a developed country and a group of local investigators in the region of study. Usually, these collaborations begin with communication from the distant academic center to the local investigators, asking them to set up the study infrastructure. The study is then undertaken, results evaluated, and papers written. These collaborations must always be mindful of local customs, regulations, and sensitivities. The use of informed consent, which we take for granted in American studies, can be a challenge in foreign countries, not only because the language is different but also because the forms must be written using properly diplomatic wording. The transfer of supplies can also be difficult, as I found in one of my foreign collaborations, in which my entire first shipment of medications was stolen from the airport!

Dealing with foreign hospitals, medical schools, universities, ministries of health, customs for importation of supplies, and many other potential frustrations can confound the investigators. Why do it? Not only will the results be gratifying to the researchers, but much more importantly, the potential benefit to mankind is enormous.

The infectious causes of vision impairment discussed in this section have placed different burdens on the developing world than on the developed world. The current state of these diseases ranges from nearly eliminated to not yet fully appreciated—but with all of them, relatively simple public health measures may yield great benefits.

Sherwin J. Isenberg, MD

CHAPTER 22

Ophthalmia Neonatorum Research as a Paradigm for Conducting Studies in Developing Countries

Background

There are a number of reasons for conducting prospective research in developing countries. One reason is that the study conditions—onchocerciasis, for example—can be found only in these countries. A second would be to create a paradigm for studying disorders that exist in other developing countries. Among other benefits, this concept may serve to save money, make the study more efficient, or permit recruitment of more subjects. All of these potential advantages provided the reasoning for investigating a new technique to prevent ophthalmia neonatorum (conjunctivitis occurring within 30 days of birth).

In the 1880s, ophthalmia neonatorum was the main cause of blindness in European children. Prophylaxis, provided by antimicrobial eyedrops given at birth, decreased the incidence by more than 30 times by the turn of the century. Now, newer and more effective eyedrops may further reduce the number of affected infants. Because the current incidence of ophthalmia neonatorum in the United States is approximately 0.1% of births, it would take a great many births to properly study any medical intervention. However, in some parts of the developing world, where the incidence is more than 100 times greater, such a study could be done faster and in a more cost-effective manner.

Pilot Data

In a pilot study of 100 newborns in the United States in 1994, povidone-iodine ophthalmic solution was found to be more effective than erythromycin in reducing the number of bacteria on the human eye at birth. From birth to 24 hours later, colony-forming units were reduced 87% by povidone-iodine and 82% by erythromycin. Corresponding figures for species counts were 45% for povidone-iodine and 22% for erythromycin. More significant toxic reactions were caused by silver nitrate than the other two medications combined. Thus, povidone-iodine produced both fewer and less severe toxic reactions than silver nitrate.

Isenberg SJ, Apt L, Yoshimori R, et al. The use of povidone-iodine for ophthalmia neonatorum prophylaxis. *Am J Ophthalmol.* 1994;118:701–706.

Povidone-iodine has many potential benefits compared with the commonly used prophylactic eyedrops. Among these are its broad antimicrobial spectrum and lack of toxic reactions; its effect of turning the eye brown for 2 minutes, thus making the application evident to the health professional; and, importantly, its very low cost with wide availability. In light of these considerations, it was decided to study povidone-iodine for prevention of ophthalmia neonatorum in Kenya, where prophylaxis was not generally used and the disorder is quite prevalent (23% of all births without prophylaxis).

Laga M, Plummer FA, Nzanze H, et al. Epidemiology of ophthalmia neonatorum in Kenya. *Lancet.* 1986;2:1145–1149.

Mechanisms for Preparing a Foreign Study

Extensive planning goes into setting up a foreign study (Table 22-1). A foreign study requires an appropriate study site with proper investigators. In this case, a center was chosen that had not only an ophthalmic hospital but delivery rooms and a maternity center nearby. The ophthalmologists were well educated, dedicated to the project, and available to direct an excellent nursing staff.

For any large research project, funding must be obtained. The investigator should apply only to those agencies that will support research activity outside the United States or Canada. Prior to beginning the study, the infrastructure must be created. The Ministry of Health in the study country must be contacted to obtain all appropriate permits and consents. The supervising ophthalmologist of the study at the site can be of great value in dealing with the local government, university, and hospital. The organizing university (in the Kenya study, it was UCLA) must be consulted regarding informed consent issues. The Internal Review Board (or Human Subjects Protection Committee) of the university

Table 22-1 Algorithm for Planning an International Study

1. Prepare detailed outline of the investigation.
2. Seek an appropriate foreign study site.
   a. Effective physical site: clinics, operating rooms, and so on
   b. Dedicated physicians, nurses, and other staff capable of conducting the study and properly recording and transmitting data
   c. Any language barriers or local customs that might affect organization of the project?
3. Apply for and obtain funding.
4. Obtain appropriate permits and consents from Ministry of Health, university, and/or hospital at the foreign location.
5. Consult the organizing university regarding human subjects' protection issues. Documentation may or may not be needed from the organizing university.
6. In the foreign site, set up
   a. banking and money transfer arrangements
   b. protocols for shipping supplies and equipment
   c. methods for proper remuneration of study subjects, if needed
   d. methods for transferring data back to the organizing university

may indicate the forms that must be completed. It has been recognized that for many foreign research venues, informed consent may be obtained verbally rather than in writing. Some granting agencies demand this documentation before funding is given, but others do not.

> IJsselmuiden CB, Faden RR. Research and informed consent in Africa—another look. *N Engl J Med.* 1992;326:830–833.

It is important to develop a relationship with an appropriate local bank at the study site to permit easy transfer of funds on a regular basis from the grant fund account at the organizing university to a North American bank and then transferred, preferably electronically, to the local bank. The local bank will have to agree to provide monthly or quarterly account information to the principal investigator and organizing university to ensure a proper continuing flow of funds to pay expenses.

Medications and other supplies may need to be shipped to the study site. Some of these might come from the organizing university; other supplies can be shipped from a closer location (such as Europe) to save money. The study should be organized with the help of one principal investigator on site, other physicians as necessary, one supervising nurse, and other nurses working part time. The principal investigators from the organizing university should plan to visit the study site for at least a week to initiate the study and then annually until the study is completed.

In the Kenya study, povidone-iodine ophthalmic solution was compared with two control medications, silver nitrate ophthalmic solution and erythromycin ophthalmic ointment. The protocol dictated that the proper eyedrops be administered within 1 hour of birth. All infants who developed conjunctivitis were brought to a microbiological laboratory. We chose the microbiological laboratory that provided the most comprehensive culture services, even though it was located at a different hospital. The patients were transported to the hospital, where the cultures were taken and immediately processed. This approach prevented loss of cultures in transit. To ensure return of these children for follow-up, a gift of a baby blanket was given to the parents as a reward for their cooperation. This reward was greatly appreciated by the families and ensured a high level of compliance. The data were recorded on prepared data sheets by the on-site nurses and mailed periodically to UCLA, where the data were entered into a computer spreadsheet for later evaluation.

Findings

In the study of more than 3000 babies over 3 years, povidone-iodine proved to be more effective than the other two agents ($p < 0.01$) while being less toxic ($p < 0.005$) and far less expensive. Based on this study, povidone-iodine is now being used for ophthalmia neonatorum prophylaxis in hospitals in Kenya, Tanzania, Thailand, Congo, South America, and many other regions. The study, using Kenya as the "field laboratory," allowed us to investigate this disease much more rapidly than we could have in the United States. This model of treatment trial could be used to study other ophthalmic disorders.

CHAPTER 23

Epidemic Optic Neuropathy in Cuba

Background

History

An epidemic of blindness affecting as many as 50,000 patients in Cuba reached international attention in May 1993, when the Cuban government made a plea to the United Nations. We were fortunate to be one of the first investigators contacted, and on May 16, 1993, a team from the United States (Drs Alfredo A. Sadun and James Martone and Ms Lillie Reyes) met with Latin American representatives to the Pan American Health Organization (PAHO) in Miami, Florida.

Under special arrangements with the US State Department, the entire group flew directly to Havana, where we were received by the Cuban government. An impromptu press conference at the airport made clear that although the US media had largely ignored the epidemic, media from other countries around the world had not. Present at this and many future press conferences were CNN; European crews, including the BBC and Reuters; and Japan's NHK. These news agencies were well aware of the magnitude of the problem; they knew that Cuban authorities had been hard at work on it for the past year, using coxsackie enteroviral infection as a working diagnosis. Most of the 50,000 patients diagnosed with the disease had been admitted to hospitals in Havana for careful study.

Our group of clinicians performed systematic and detailed patient examinations while the PAHO epidemiologists carefully reviewed and analyzed the data already accumulated by the Cuban National Operative Group (NOG). This group consisted of about 1000 Cuban scientists and clinicians who had been investigating the epidemic for almost 1 year.

> Sadun A. Acquired mitochondrial impairment as a cause of optic nerve disease. *Trans Am Ophthalmol Soc.* 1998;96:881–923.
>
> Sadun AA, Martone JF. Cuba: Response of medical science to a crisis of optic and peripheral neuropathy. *Int Ophthalmol.* 1994–1995;18:373–378.
>
> Sadun AA, Martone JF, Muci-Mendoza R, et al. Epidemic optic neuropathy in Cuba: eye findings. *Arch Ophthalmol.* 1994;112:691–699.
>
> Sadun AA, Martone JF, Reyes L, et al. Optic and peripheral neuropathy in Cuba. *JAMA.* 1994;271:663–664.

Context

US embargo and loss of USSR support and aid

Since the Cuban missile crisis in 1962, Cuba had been economically sanctioned by a US-maintained embargo, which had also markedly constrained the importation of foods and some medicines into this island nation. However, the Soviet Union and communist Eastern Europe had, for many decades, subsidized or underwritten up to 85% of the Cuban economy. In 1990, dissolution of the communist bloc led to an economic crisis in Cuba, with severe shortages, especially in fuel and food. In addition, the US trade embargo was further enforced to preclude third countries from doing business with Cuba. The result in Cuba was severe food and medicine rationing. When we visited in 1993, the average adult was consuming only 1600 calories a day, and there were marked deficiencies in various vitamins and proteins.

> Barrett K. The collapse of the Soviet Union and the Eastern Bloc: effects on Cuban health care. Cuban briefing paper series. Georgetown University. 1993:2:1–4.
> Epidemic optic neuropathy in Cuba—clinical characterization and risk factors. The Cuba Neuropathy Field Investigation Team. *N Engl J Med.* 1995;333:1176–1182.

Bias toward virology and molecular biology

In 1986, Castro and the Cuban government built the Center for Genetic Engineering and Biotechnology near Havana. A reflection of Cuba's bold medical, scientific, and economic central plan, the center was, as we learned later, important to our investigation because it had created a scientific research bias toward virology and molecular biology. Cuba's commitment to research in these two fields was intended not only to garner international prestige but to help the Cuban economy through sales of vaccines to developing nations. Hence, the best and brightest of Cuba's medical scientists were brought into this well-funded political enterprise. Cuban medical science became dominated by the culture of molecular biology and virology.

Central policy decisions

Several central policy decisions (with dietetic implications), implemented by the Cuban government only 1 or 2 years before the beginning of the epidemic, may have had unintended consequences that affected the course of the epidemic. For example, in an effort to obtain as much foreign currency as possible (and a positive balance of trade), it was decided to export most of the rum made in the country; to ensure that this happened, rum became rationed in Cuba. When, in the middle of our investigation, we pointed to the considerable amount of rum consumed by our patients (often two to three bottles per week), Castro objected that this was impossible because he had limited consumption to one bottle per family per month. Other policies, pertaining to gardening and raising livestock, also influenced the diet of Cubans in the early 1990s.

Human Impact

By the middle of 1992, about 220 mysterious cases of blindness from optic neuropathy or peripheral neuropathy had been reported. Concern grew when, by the end of the year, the number had increased to 1000 cases. This concern turned into a national crisis when the numbers swelled to almost 50,000 cases by the middle of 1993. The fact that almost all cases involved adult men (there were no reports of patients under the age of 15 and very few cases of women or the elderly) was not only an epidemiologic curiosity but added to the enormous economic impact of the epidemic, as the disabled were, for the most part, family breadwinners. By the middle of 1993, almost 1% of all adult men in Cuba were completely disabled.

The economic impact grew when, as part of the national effort to understand and control this (possibly infectious) epidemic, it was decided to bring all patients to Havana for hospitalization. Given the difficulties of transportation in a society suffering extreme fuel shortages, this was not an easy task. In addition, the effort strained the bed capacities of each hospital, further adding to the economic devastation brought on by the epidemic.

Clinical Presentation and Findings

A typical patient with Cuban epidemic optic neuropathy (CEON) was a young man with a 3-month history of significant weight loss (about 20 lb), followed shortly thereafter by a 1–2 week period of bilaterally symmetric loss of central field (Fig 23-1) and visual acuity, often characterized as the lost ability to recognize faces. On examination, visual acuities were about 20/400 with severe dyschromatopsia. The fundus examination generally revealed a wedge-shaped defect of a selective loss of the nerve fiber layer in the papillomacular bundle (Fig 23-2). The adjacent superior and inferior nerve fiber layers were often swollen, especially near the optic disc. The visual field tests demonstrated central scotomata without peripheral field constriction (see Fig 23-1). In addition, CEON patients often had ataxia, hyperreflexia, decreased sensation to touch and vibration, and sometimes hearing loss.

Epidemiology

Surveys of Prevalence/Incidence

At the time, the total population of Cuba was slightly more than 10 million, of whom 3 million were adult men. In a period of 1 year, 1 of every 75 adult men developed symptoms of the epidemic. However, a disproportionate number of cases were being diagnosed on the western side of the island, especially near the province of Pinar del Rio, where the first cases of the epidemic were noted.

Risk Factors

Geographic

The concentration of cases lay in a west to east gradient, varying from over 1000/100,000 (in Pinar del Rio) to fewer than 10/100,000 in Santiago de Cuba in the eastern province (Figure 23-3). Indeed, it was once calculated that, on average, the epidemic spread east at the rate of approximately 26 kilometers per day. This was one of three major factors that prompted the NOG to suggest a viral etiology. The other two factors were the

264 • International Ophthalmology

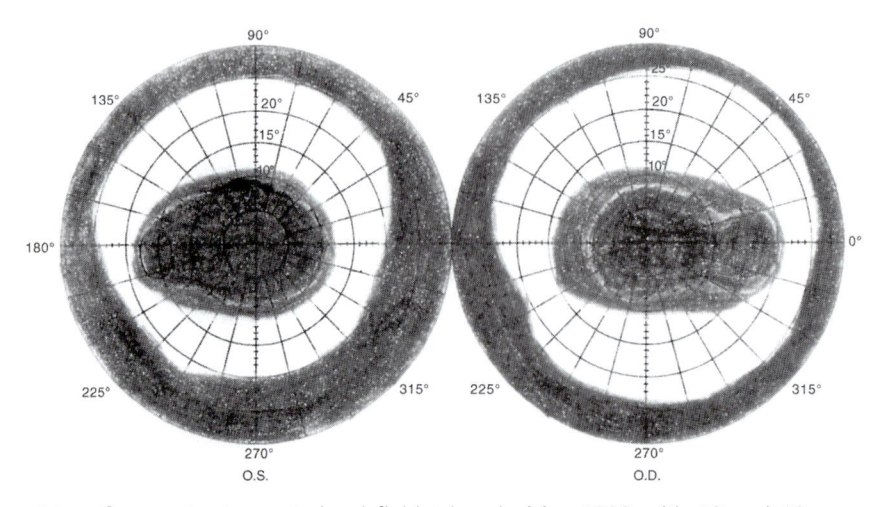

Figure 23-1 One-meter tangent visual field taken in May 1993 with 10 and 18 mm white targets. Bilateral cecocentral scotomata are demonstrated. *(Photograph courtesy of Alfredo A. Sadun, MD.)*

Figure 23-2 Fundus photograph (OS) taken at a patient's first visit in May 1993. Note vessel tortuosity and marked nerve fiber layer (NFL) swelling in arcuate bundles, with dropout of the papillomacular bundle. *(Photograph courtesy of Alfredo A. Sadun, MD.)*

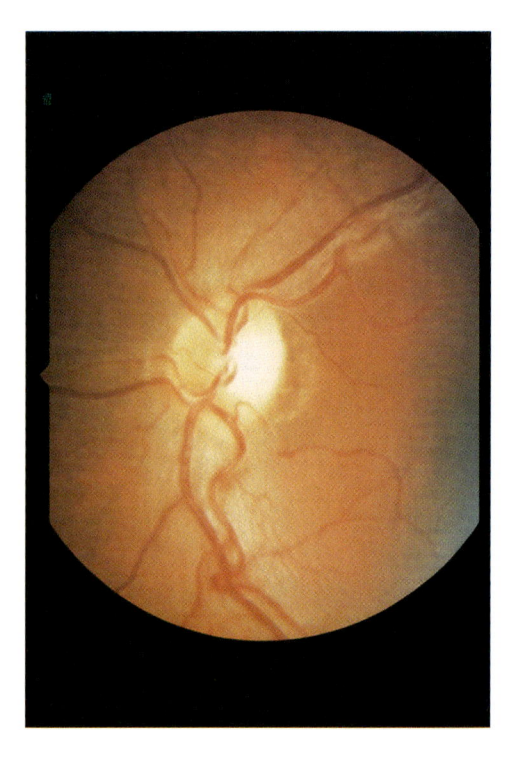

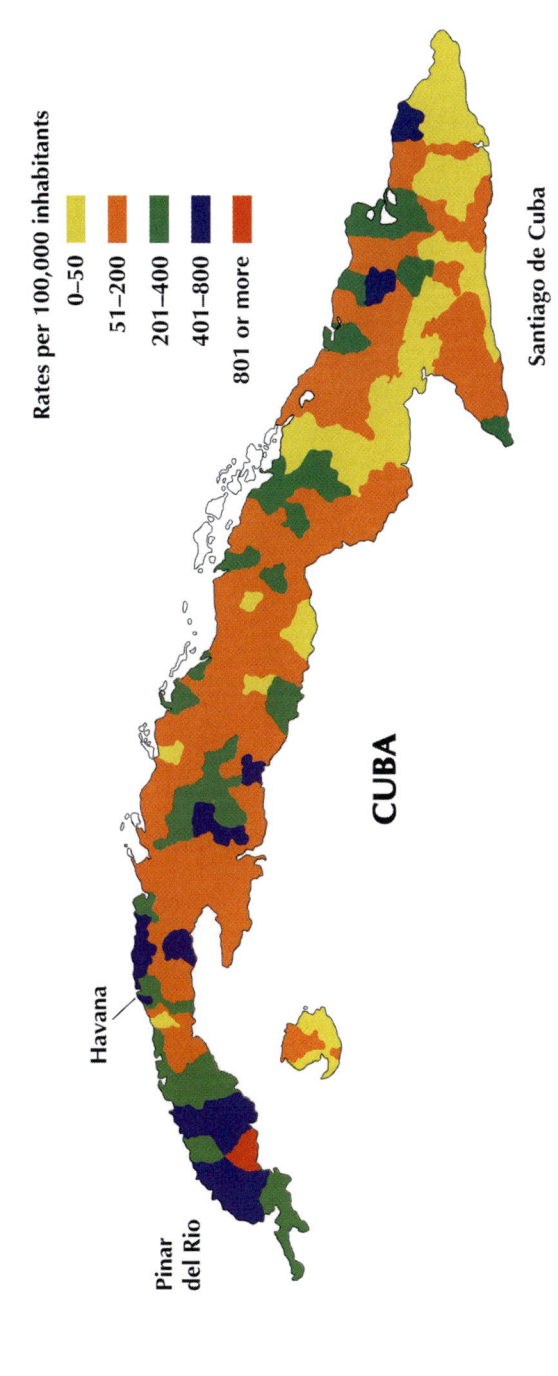

Figure 23-3 The concentration of cases lay in a west to east gradient, with the heaviest concentration in Pinar del Rio. *(Illustration adapted by Jeanne Koelling.)*

exponential increases in new cases and a NOG microbiology study in which 101 of 126 cerebrospinal fluid cultures were said to have grown coxsackie virus.

Contacts

Despite the three factors that suggested a viral etiology to the NOG, our group found the paucity of family contacts or group involvement to be a major factor mitigating against a viral cause for the epidemic. For instance, there were no significant outbreaks among the military, in orphanages, in boarding schools, or in retirement homes. In our own patient interviews, we found only one instance where two members of the same nuclear family were afflicted, and these siblings were not living together.

Habits

A number of risk factors associated with epidemic involvement were identified by our group and later confirmed by a CDC cohort study. Over 80% of our patients who were confirmed to have CEON were men; the average age was 39. Significant cigar smoking (more than 2 a day) or cigarette smoking (a pack a day) was found in 85% of the affected Cubans; most (65%) were cigar smokers. Eighty-five percent of those confirmed to have the epidemic form of optic neuropathy drank alcohol (defined as two or more drinks a day). Of those who drank alcohol regularly, most (53%) preferred rum and most (65%) consumed homemade brews of one type or another. However, the most striking risk factor may have been a diet deficient in calories, protein, and vitamins and possibly containing at least one form of toxin (cyanide). No patient with CEON was free of these risk factors.

Nutrition

Poor caloric intake was reflected in the weight losses recorded in our examinations of CEON patients. The lack of meat or fish in the diet was particularly striking. Ninety percent of our patients confirmed to have the epidemic form of optic neuropathy consumed meat, fish, or fowl less than once per month in the period preceding their visual loss. Green vegetables were also in short supply. The staple diet of most people was rice and potatoes and sometimes beans. Protein usually came in the form of soybean products, which were shaped to mimic meat patties. The consumption of cassava (a possible source of cyanide) was greater than usual; yet fewer than 10% of our patients ate cassava regularly. This diet produced vitamin deficiencies, especially in the class of B vitamins. Most particularly, folic acid levels were low for the general population, and 60% of our patients were found to be deficient in folic acid.

Pathogenesis

The clinical findings in CEON were very similar to those found in the relatively rare disorder of mitochondrial DNA called Leber hereditary optic neuropathy. However, there obviously could not have been a sudden and simultaneous occurrence of thousands of mutations to the mitochondrial genome. Nevertheless, we and others did check mitochondrial DNA with molecular biological analysis and found no primary mutations of

Leber. We suspected that, although a congenital mitochondrial disorder was unlikely, an acquired one might underlie the pathogenesis of this epidemic.

> Johns D, Sadun AA. Cuban epidemic optic neuropathy: mitochondrial DNA analysis. *J Neuroophthalmol.* 1994;14:130–134.
>
> Newman NJ, Torroni A, Brown MD, et al. Epidemic neuropathy in Cuba not associated with mitochondrial DNA mutations found in Leber's hereditary optic neuropathy patients. Cuban Neuropathy Field Investigation Team. *Am J Ophthalmol.* 1994;118:158–168.
>
> Nikoskelainen E, Hoyt WF, Nummelin K, et al. Fundus findings in Leber's hereditary optic neuroretinopathy. III. Fluorescein angiographic studies. *Arch Ophthalmol.* 1984;102:981–989.

The findings of our study, as well as those of subsequent investigations, suggested a complex interplay of nutritional and toxic issues that compromised, in particular, mitochondrial function (Fig 23-4). Deficiencies of vitamin B_{12} or the accumulation of cyanide from smoking or the consumption of cassava all can interfere with mitochondrial oxidative phosphorylation. However, we believe that the most common mitochondrial injury occurred as a result of folic acid deficiency aggravated by the consumption of chronic low doses of methanol found especially in homemade rum that has been aged for only a few weeks. The home-brewed rum that we analyzed contained almost 1.0% methanol. A morbid or lethal dose would be 15–30 mL of methanol, so the concentrations we found were too low to produce acute methanol toxicity. However, methanol metabolizes to formaldehyde and then to formate. The latter, if not detoxified by folic acid, will block mitochondrial oxidative phosphorylation and thus produce acquired mitochondrial impairment.

> Grant WM. *Toxicology of the Eye.* Springfield, Ill: Charles C. Thomas; 1962:340–348.
>
> Nicholls P. The effect of formate on cytochrome aa3 and on electron transport in the intact respiratory chain. *Biochem Biophys Acta.* 1976;430:13–29.
>
> Nicholls P. Formate as an inhibitor of cytochrome c oxidase. *Biochem Biophys Res Commun.* 1975;67:610–616.

Compromises of the mitochondrial energy production for cells might be compensated in certain tissues (as in extraocular muscle). However, neurons, especially those that are particularly long (such as those involved in peripheral neuropathy) or of small caliber (such as the papillomacular bundle contribution to the optic nerve) have particular constraints. Mitochondrial derangement may lead to ATP depletion as well as to the accumulation of reactive oxygen species. The former compromises axonal transport, even of the mitochondria themselves; the latter can induce apoptosis of retinal ganglion cells. In both cases, once a critical threshold is reached, a rapid die-off of small axons occurs, and the patient experiences decreased central acuity and dyschromatopsia and demonstrates a central scotoma.

The theory of a viral etiology proposed by the NOG and suggested by the exponential increases in cases, west to east geographic movement, and coxsackie growth in cerebrospinal fluid cultures had been pushed along by the culture of virology and molecular biology that dominated Cuban medical science. In the face of the new evidence, presented in May 1993, this theory was finally abandoned.

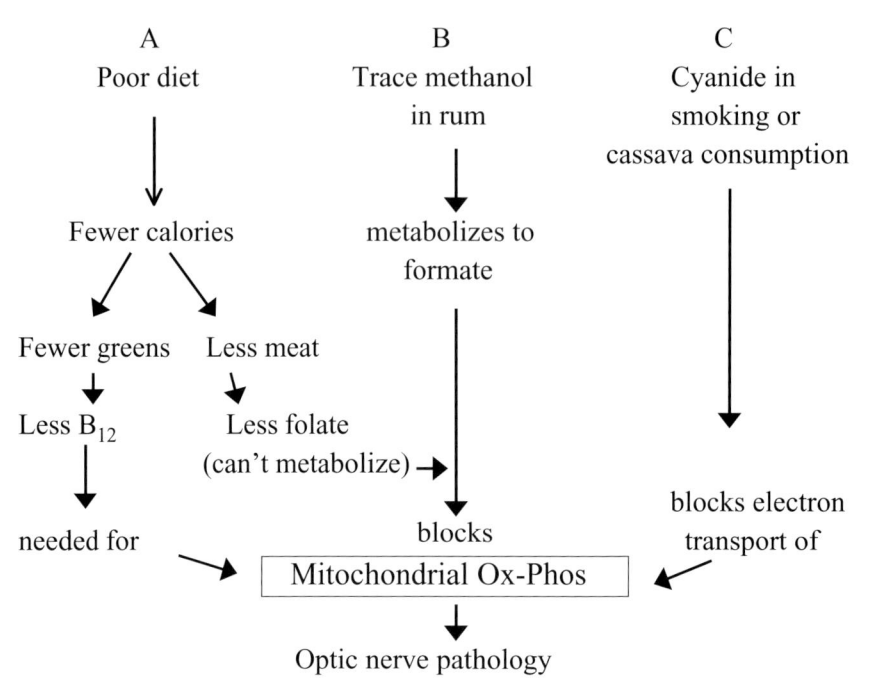

```
     A                    B                        C
  Poor diet         Trace methanol           Cyanide in
                        in rum              smoking or
                          ↓              cassava consumption
      ↓             metabolizes to
 Fewer calories         formate                   
   ↙      ↘                                       
Fewer greens  Less meat                            
    ↓          ↓                                   
 Less B₁₂    Less folate                           
    ↓      (can't metabolize) →                    
                                            blocks electron
 needed for        blocks                   transport of
         →  Mitochondrial Ox-Phos  ←
                    ↓
            Optic nerve pathology
```

Figure 23-4 A complex interplay of nutritional and toxic factors compromised mitochondrial function and led to optic nerve damage. *(Courtesy of Alfredo A. Sadun, MD.)*

Prevention

On departing from Cuba in May 1993, we and others suggested that vitamin supplementation, especially of folic acid and B_{12}, be provided to all the residents of Cuba. This was carried out with remarkable expedience, and by July virtually everyone in Cuba had been so treated. Efforts were also undertaken to discourage the consumption of home-brewed alcoholic beverages, which, by introducing methanol, further exacerbated the folic acid deficiencies. Prophylaxis by vitamin supplementation proved to be extremely efficacious, and diagnoses of new cases of CEON essentially stopped after August 1, 1993.

Current Treatment Programs

Vitamin supplementation was also offered to patients who had already suffered severe visual impairment from CEON. Surprisingly, these patients showed considerable improvement despite the permanent loss of the papillomacular nerve fiber layer and the temporal pallor noted on their optic discs. Among the patients that we first observed in May 1993 and then again after vitamin therapy in September 1993, the average before and after for visual acuities was 20/400 improving to 20/50 and for color vision 1 of 8 AO-HRR color test plates to 7 of 8 test plates seen correctly. Large absolute central scotomata had become smaller relative scotomata.

Research Currently Under Way

Histopathologic studies of an optic nerve from the one and only CEON patient who died (of unrelated causes) during her illness disclosed intra-axonal accumulations and vacuolations in axons just anterior to the lamina cribrosa.

An animal model of CEON has been developed in rats. The animals were fed a folic acid–deficient diet for about 13 weeks until their serum folic acid levels matched those found in CEON patients. The rats were then given several weeks of chronic, low-dose methanol injections, and their serum formate levels were monitored and found to be slightly higher than those found in CEON patients. Light microscopic examination of these rat optic nerves revealed similar histopathologic changes just anterior to the lamina cribrosa. Ultrastructural examination revealed evidence of morphologic changes in the mitochondria (in the retinal inner segments as well as in the optic nerve). We also found in the rat optic nerve decreased levels of ATP, indicating an energy depletion, as well as decreased levels of supraoxide dismutase (SOD-Mg) and glutathione, suggesting that reactive oxygen species, produced by the block in oxidative phosphorylation, may also play a role in retinal ganglion cell injury. Further studies of this type are currently under way.

Lessons Learned From This Epidemic

Several very basic lessons were learned in the process of investigating the cause of this epidemic of optic neuropathy in Cuba in 1993. Some of these lessons might be catalogued as follows:

- **Pathobiology:** Sometimes acquired pathology can mimic that which occurs genetically and this, then, suggests a common site of injury.
- **Epidemiology:** As they are classically taught, demographic data will help you understand where the risky behavior is. In the Cuban epidemic, middle-aged men were far more likely to be involved than women, the very young, or the very old. This reflected the habits of middle-aged men with regard to drinking rum (methanol) and smoking (cyanide).
- **Political**
  - Embargos may have unintended consequences.
  - Government policies (in this case rationing local consumption of aged rum) may also have unintended consequences.
- **Social**
  - Central planning may frustrate good instincts (as when the Cuban government encouraged its citizens to forsake low-calorie vegetable gardens for high-calorie beans and potatoes).
  - The existence of a privileged group (in this case biotechnology researchers) raises the voice of that group to the exclusion of other voices and, when you are a hammer, all of the world is a nail.

- **Neuro-Ophthalmology:** The special requirements of retinal ganglion cells and the peculiar anatomic features of the optic nerve head may make the optic nerve the "canary in the coal mine" for metabolic stress.

Sadun A. Acquired mitochondrial impairment as a cause of optic nerve disease. *Trans Am Ophthalmol Soc.* 1998;96:881–923.

Sadun AA, Martone JF. Cuba: response of medical science to a crisis of optic and peripheral neuropathy. *Int Ophthalmol.* 1994–1995;18:373–378.

Sadun AA, Martone JF, Muci-Mendoza R, et al. Epidemic optic neuropathy in Cuba: eye findings. *Arch Ophthalmol.* 1994;112:691–699.

CHAPTER 24

Glaucoma Inheritance Study in Tasmania: An International Collaboration

Background

Glaucoma is a leading cause of blindness and visual impairment in most countries; it is particularly common in African Americans. In developed countries, as many as 50% of glaucoma cases are undiagnosed. Strategies to eliminate glaucoma blindness need to focus on identifying undiagnosed glaucoma cases and facilitating early diagnosis and treatment for those at highest risk. Community-based glaucoma screening programs based on intraocular pressure, visual field, or optic disc assessment by optometrists, primary care physicians, and other community organizations have lacked sensitivity and specificity for diagnosing cases of glaucoma. The cost of screening and treating the disease is rising, but cost must be balanced against the economic burden of visual impairment and the impact on the individual's quality of life.

Epidemiologic studies have highlighted the importance of family history as a risk factor for glaucoma. To date, one gene for primary open-angle glaucoma (POAG) has been identified. The *GLC1A (TIGR/Myocilin)* gene has been associated with about 4% of POAG cases in numerous populations. Family and genetic strategies for glaucoma detection may be a more efficient way to achieve earlier and more complete diagnosis of the disease in the population. The identification of additional genes that cause glaucoma offers great promise.

> Fingert JH, Héon E, Liebmann JM, et al. Analysis of myocilin mutations in 1703 glaucoma patients from five different populations. *Hum Mol Genet.* 1999;8:899–905.
> Quigley HA. Number of people with glaucoma worldwide. *Br J Ophthalmol.* 1996;80:389–393.

Glaucoma Inheritance Study in Tasmania (GIST)

Population isolates are important tools in the identification of genes for diseases. Captive populations with a high standard of health care (ensuring at least 50% of cases of glaucoma are diagnosed) and comprehensive genealogy records (allowing pedigrees of glaucoma families to be identified) are the most suitable for genetic research. Island communities, such as Tasmania or Iceland, or culturally enclosed communities, as found in the French Canadians of Quebec or the Amish in the United States, provide such an environment.

The Glaucoma Inheritance Study in Tasmania (GIST) was designed to utilize these advantages in the Australian island state of Tasmania (population 470,000) to determine the genes that cause glaucoma, their prevalence and penetrance, genotype–phenotype correlations, gene–gene interactions, and responses to conventional treatment. Figure 24-1 shows the comparative size of the pedigrees and the diagnostic status of the family members in the GIST.

Another objective was to identify, for possible future early therapeutic intervention trials, a genetically susceptible population at risk of developing glaucoma. The GIST interviews enabled a comparison of the relationship between a reported family history of POAG and the actual family history as found by the GIST study. The accuracy of the reported family history and the GIST findings are shown in Table 24-1. The κ statistic of the agreement within 8 members of the GVic1 pedigree is shown in Table 24-2. In all cases, the reliability of family history data was greatest for immediate family members and worst for third-degree relatives.

As the Australian Blue Mountains Eye Study (BMES) has the most similar ethnicity, it was felt to be the most appropriate epidemiologic comparison study for predicting the number of glaucoma patients in Tasmania. The Blue Mountains study data, extrapolated to the total Tasmanian population, predicted 3571 cases of glaucoma, of whom half would be diagnosed.

Mitchell P, Smith W, Attebo K, et al. Prevalence of open-angle glaucoma in Australia. The Blue Mountains Eye Study. *Ophthalmology*. 1996;103:1661–1669.

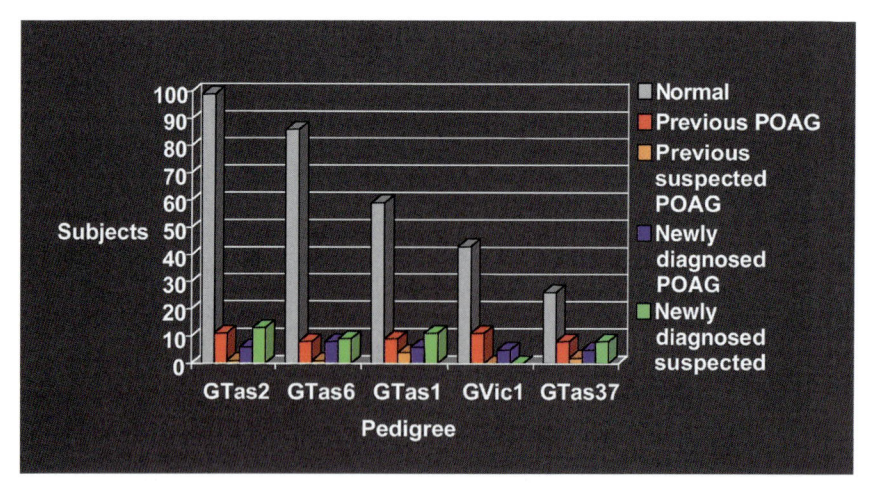

Figure 24-1 Comparative size of pedigrees and diagnostic status of family members. *(McNaught AI, Allen JG, Healey DL, et al. Accuracy and implications of a reported family history of glaucoma: experience from the Glaucoma Inheritance Study in Tasmania. Arch Ophthalmol. 2000;118:900–904. Copyrighted 2000, American Medical Association.)*

Table 24-1 **Agreement Between Family History of Glaucoma and Actual Diagnosis in 41 Participants**

Relationship	Accuracy, No. (%)	κ Statistic (SEM)
Parents	34 (84)	0.75 (0.10)
Siblings	19 (47)	0.26 (0.10)
Aunts/uncles	16 (39)	0.12 (0.14)
First cousins	15 (36)	0.14 (0.09)

(McNaught AI, Allen JG, Healey DL, et al. Accuracy and implications of a reported family history of glaucoma: experience from the Glaucoma Inheritance Study in Tasmania. *Arch Ophthalmol.* 2000;118:900–904. Copyrighted 2000, American Medical Association.)

Table 24-2 **Agreement Between Family History of Glaucoma and Actual Diagnosis Reported by 8 Members of the GVic1 Pedigree**

Relationship	Accuracy, No. (%)	κ Statistic (SEM)
Parents	8 (100)	. . .
Siblings	6 (75)	. . .
Aunts/uncles	7 (80)	0.75 (0.23)
First cousins	4 (50)	0.25 (0.33)

(McNaught AI, Allen JG, Healey DL, et al. Accuracy and implications of a reported family history of glaucoma: experience from the Glaucoma Inheritance Study in Tasmania. *Arch Ophthalmol.* 2000;118:900–904. Copyrighted 2000, American Medical Association.)

Study Methodology

From 1994 to 1996, with the cooperation of the 12 ophthalmologists in Tasmania, invitations to join the study were mailed to 3800 Tasmanian patients who had been investigated or treated for glaucoma over the previous 15 years. With extensive review of all the clinical notes of patients seen in all the ophthalmic practices in the state, it was possible to create a glaucoma registry for each ophthalmologist. In addition to mailing questionnaires directly to glaucoma patients, patient information posters and surveys were provided in ophthalmology clinics, optometry clinics, and pharmacies throughout the state. There was also local media publicity.

Participants provided information on their families. When numerous affected members were involved, the genealogy was extended by our research genealogist using a computerized family tree database. The largest, most severely affected glaucoma pedigrees came to our attention first and most frequently because of the numerous index cases. Using anterior segment evaluation, intraocular pressure measurement, Humphrey 24-2 visual fields (Humphrey Instruments, San Leandro, CA), and stereo optic disc photography (Nidek, Japan), volunteer ophthalmologists, trainee ophthalmologists, orthoptists, nurses, and students helped examine the affected and unaffected members of the larger families. We consider this an efficient strategy for diagnosing new cases at high risk of glaucoma.

In large glaucoma families—those with 13% of family members previously diagnosed with glaucoma or as glaucoma suspects—we identified another 16% of newly diagnosed glaucoma cases or suspects. DNA collected from blood or buccal mucosal swab was sent to collaborating laboratories at the University of Iowa, where they had recently identified the first locus for glaucoma, *GLC1A*. The addition of more families to their study helped narrow the gene interval and identify the *TIGR/MYOC* gene and the mutations in several families as well as a large number of individual glaucoma patients. Although some of this work could have been done at local laboratories in Australia, the scale and cost of this research and the very advanced facilities available in Iowa made collaboration the most efficient way to identify as many families with mutations in this gene as possible.

> McNaught AI, Allen JG, Healey DL, et al. Accuracy and implications of a reported family history of glaucoma: experience from the Glaucoma Inheritance Study in Tasmania. *Arch Ophthalmol.* 2000;118:900–904.
> Sheffield VC, Stone EM, Alward WL, et al. Genetic linkage of familial open angle glaucoma to chromosome 1q21-q31. *Nat Genet.* 1993;4:47–50.

By identifying genes within the families, particularly families with members having young age of onset of open-angle glaucoma, we were able to predict which family members were gene carriers and thus at high risk of glaucoma. A survey of patients in families with myocilin mutations showed that the majority wanted to know the results of their DNA testing. This contrasts with people at risk of untreatable disorders such as Huntington's chorea, where some choose not to have their carrier status revealed.

By knowing the entire population of patients being treated for glaucoma, it was possible to identify overlaps of families. This circumstance, where individuals had family members affected with glaucoma on both the maternal and paternal sides of their family, suggested that gene–gene interactions are involved in the expression of glaucoma. We were also able to assess the accuracy of individuals' recall of their family history of glaucoma, comparing this with the genealogic data. Even in larger pedigrees, 27% of previously diagnosed glaucoma patients were completely unaware of their family history of POAG.

Thorough data collection was possible in GIST because it involved a relatively small population; however, the conclusions from this study can be applied to much larger communities. The rate of diagnosis of glaucoma can be increased by asking individuals affected with POAG to find out if other family members are also affected. Taking a family history, however, does not end with the first consultation. Those with glaucoma should also inform all their relatives that those family members over the age of 40 years (earlier if an early family diagnosis of glaucoma was made) should be examined. Public authorities should inform the general population that people with a positive family history of glaucoma should be screened for the disease.

> Sack J, Healey DL, de Graaf AP, et al. The problem of overlapping glaucoma families in the Glaucoma Inheritance Study in Tasmania (GIST). *Ophthalmic Genet.* 1996;17:209–214.

Findings

After 7 years, the GIST project had identified over 1700 definite cases of glaucoma, half of whom had a family history of glaucoma. We created 350 pedigrees with multiple affected individuals; 11 of these pedigrees had mutations in the *GLC1A* gene (8 pedigrees had the Gln368STOP mutation), 3 pedigrees had Rieger syndrome with glaucoma, 1 pedigree had a mutation in *PAX6* with glaucoma, 4 pedigrees had congenital glaucoma, and 1 pedigree had Nail-Patella syndrome and glaucoma.

Mutation screening in the population allowed us to calculate the prevalence of myocilin mutation in glaucoma families. Examination and DNA testing of other family members allowed us to calculate the penetrance (the percentage of individuals with the gene who are affected) and establish the phenotype. The commonest mutation in myocilin, Gln368STOP, is found in over 1% of POAG patients. The age-related penetrance for ocular hypertension or POAG was 72% at age 40 years and 82% at age 65 years. Gln368STOP causes POAG with mean age at diagnosis of 52.4 ± 12.9 years and a mean peak intraocular pressure (IOP) of 28.4 ± 4.7 mm Hg, which is less severe than the other myocilin mutations.

Because our study examined an entire population, we discovered milder cases of glaucoma. Research performed at tertiary referral centers has a bias toward more severe disease. Community-based studies, such as the Rotterdam Eye Study, give a true picture of the full spectrum of glaucoma in families. The Rotterdam study established that the lifetime risk of a first-degree relative developing glaucoma was 22%.

Craig JE, Baird PN, Healey DL, et al. Evidence for genetic heterogeneity within 8 glaucoma families, with the GLC1A Gln368STOP mutation being an important phenotypic modifier. *Ophthalmology*. 2001;108:1606–1620.

Wolfs RC, Klaver CC, Ramrattan RS, et al. Genetic risk of primary open-angle glaucoma: Population-based familial aggregation study. *Arch Ophthalmol*. 1998;116:1640–1645.

Social Concerns

Numerous issues, such as transnational research, ethics involving local communities, subtle differences in the local language affecting the meaning of words on consent forms, and local laboratory concerns need to be considered with all such projects. Funding is a major concern, particularly where larger study groups are coming into smaller populations. In addition, national concerns need to be weighed against global advantages in the discovery of genes.

Future Treatment

GIST has established a cooperative population that will, once genes are identified, allow diagnostic investigations that are sensitive and specific enough to identify mildly affected gene carriers and enable therapeutic intervention. It has been organized to encourage cascade genetic screening in which individuals with glaucoma involve their families in order to identify other individuals with glaucoma and to investigate high-risk individuals (at least first-degree relatives of affected patients). Genetic research holds great promise. One can envision a time when accurate assessment of glaucoma risk can be made with a DNA test on a cheek swab. New drugs will be able to target genetic defects and therefore be safer and more effective.

CHAPTER 25

Natural History of Sickle Cell Retinopathy in Jamaica

Background

Sickle cell (SS) anemia was the first designated "molecular disease" (in 1949) and is but one of the hemoglobinopathies (specifically, a2bs2). The manifestations of this disease and its global impact are due to a single nucleotide base substitution in the gene for the b-globulin subunit of hemoglobin (Hgb). The sickle gene is found in all communities in which there has been historical exposure to malaria because heterozygotes are relatively protected from the most serious complication of plasmodium infection (Fig 25-1). The same mutation has occurred several times. Global morbidity and mortality are attributable

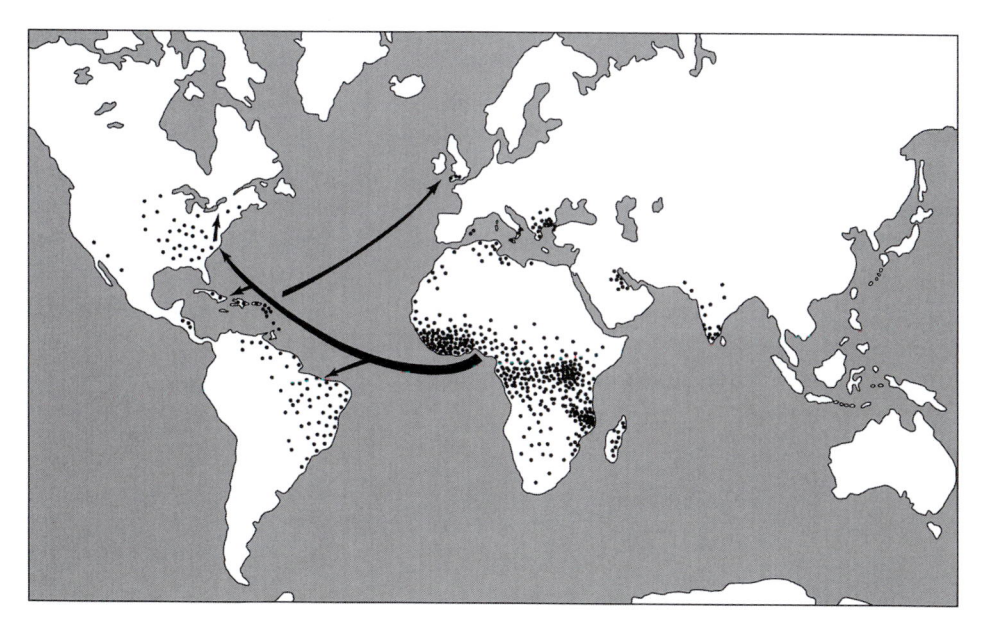

Figure 25-1 The distribution of sickle cell disease throughout the world, with arrows indicating the spread of the gene to the Americas and subsequently to Europe. The presence of the sickle gene in parts of the Mediterranean basin, Middle East, and India is not widely appreciated. *(Reproduced through the courtesy of Serjeant G.* Sickle Cell Disease. *1st ed. Oxford/New York: Oxford University Press; 1985:Fig 2.3, p 19.)*

to homozygous sickle cell disease (Hb SS), as well as to complex heterozygotes, including sickle-C (Hb SC), sickle thalassemia (Hb S beta-Thal), and others. Recent advances, newer strategies, and ongoing research include improved diagnosis and management of sickling complications, manipulation of intracellular red cell Hgb molecules (eg, inhibition of Hgb S polymerization, induction of Hgb F), bone marrow transplantation, and gene therapy.

All categories of ocular involvement are sequelae of the same sickling and vaso-occlusive processes occurring elsewhere in the body. For comprehensive coverage of ocular complications of sickling hemoglobinopathies, refer to BCSC Section 2, *Fundamentals and Principles of Ophthalmology,* and Section 12, *Retina and Vitreous.* Other than sequelae of hyphema and elevated intraocular pressure, visually important manifestations of sickling primarily involve the posterior segment—most importantly, proliferative sickle retinopathy (PSR)—via vitreous hemorrhage and traction or rhegmatogenous retinal detachment.

This chapter discusses past and current studies of sickle cell retinopathy and emphasizes the importance of disease evaluation in prospective studies of the natural history of sickling hemoglobinopathies. Few good studies exist of this natural history. The seminal work, under the guidance of Prof Graham Serjeant at the Sickle Cell Unit at the University of the West Indies, has provided most of the reliable data available. Clinical practice attracts complications. Only the most severe cases are seen by physicians, and in general the severity of disease is less than is commonly believed.

Epidemiology

Recent studies of genetic markers and linkage patterns explain the geographic distribution and variations observed in sickle cell diseases. Furthermore, the clinical features of different genotypes of sickle cell diseases differ among populations derived from Equatorial Africa, Italy, Greece, the Indian subcontinent, or Saudi Arabia. For example, it is widely believed that crises with Hb SS are much more common in the African and Caribbean Diaspora than in Saudi Arabia, but hip necrosis and ocular changes are equally common to the two groups. Variation in the severity of systemic clinical course and ocular disease occurs among different genotypes. Sb+ thalassemia and SC disease are associated with infrequent painful crises and little end organ damage, but PSR development is more common than with Hb SS. In addition, the disorders may be ameliorated in the presence of the high persistent fetal hemoglobin gene.

Natural History of Sickle Retinopathy

Sickle cell diseases are associated with intermittent retinal arteriolar occlusion, which may or may not proceed to permanent loss of peripheral capillary perfusion. As demonstrated in Jamaican children, vaso-occlusive events may be common but also totally reversible. With advancing age in some individuals, there is an overall progression of arteriolar occlusion, with extensive remodeling of the peripheral vasculature and sequelae of ischemia (Fig 25-2). Angiographic studies have shown that the "sea fans" of PSR arise from arteriovenous anastomoses at the border of avascular retina (Fig 25-3). Goldberg's 1971 five-stage classification provides a logical pathophysiology upon which to visualize the progression of sickle retinopathy, but the classification does not include the earliest initiating and modulating events. (See BCSC Section 12, *Retina and Vitreous*.)

Findings From Jamaica

Understanding of the natural history of the sickle retinopathies has been limited, perhaps in part because of socioeconomic and demographic aspects associated with populations affected by sickling hemoglobinopathies. Since the early 1970s, the Medical Research Council in England has funded studies of sickle diseases in a large Jamaican cohort, including the extent and natural history of ocular involvement. Consecutive sickle patients (314 SS and 173 SC) and hemoglobin AA controls were identified and recruited via umbilical cord blood analysis at birth.

Data from this cohort include annual fundus examinations from the age of 6 years, with fluorescein angiography and angioscopy. These data have allowed assessment of the development of the peripheral retinal vasculature in sickle cell diseases. The presence of acute obstructions (see Fig 25-2), peripheral lesions, hemorrhage, and posterior displacement of the angiographic border and others have been tabulated annually. Most importantly, a particular peripheral capillary vascular pattern showing capillary stumps or bifurcations (see Fig 25-3) has been determined to correlate with the highest risk of sea fan development. The process of autoinfarction of these proliferative vascular growths has also been observed to play an important role in eliminating continued active vasoproliferation.

By 1998, SS subjects in the Jamaican study had been reviewed for a median of 18.2 years and SC subjects for 20.0 years. Forty-seven cases had PSR, 40 with SC disease and 7 with SS disease. Sickle C subjects had a PSR incidence of 29% and SS subjects, a PSR incidence of 3%. Incidence increased with age in both genotypes and was the same for males and females. Of the 47 with PSR, 29 were unilateral and 18 were bilateral. Of 39

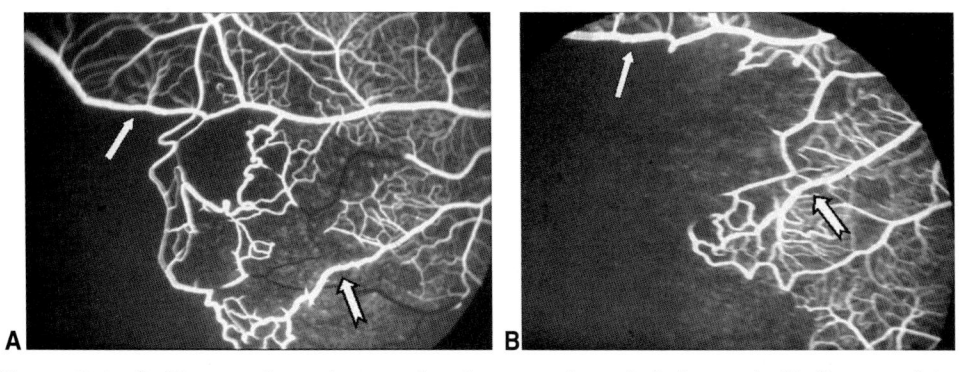

Figure 25-2 A, Fluorescein angiogram showing recently occluded vessels. **B,** One year later there was loss of peripheral capillaries. The arrow and notched arrow show the same vessels. *(Photographs courtesy of Elaine L. Chuang, MD.)*

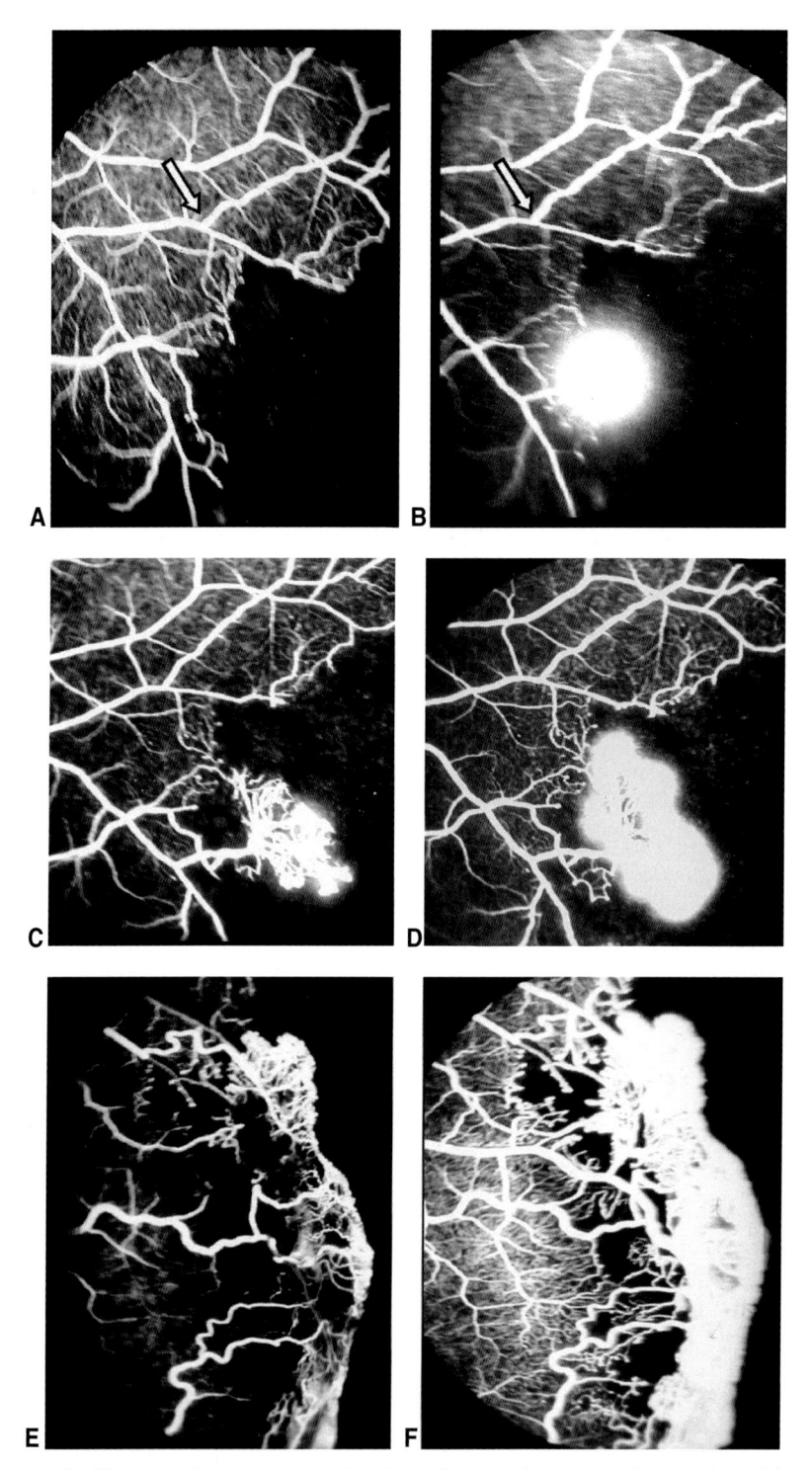

Figure 25-3 A, Fluorescein angiogram showing closure of the vascular border with an edge that does not have qualitatively normal characteristics, type 2A. **B,** One year later there was a small proliferative lesion that grew **(C, D, E, F)** during the subsequent 2 years. *(Photographs courtesy of Elaine L. Chuang, MD.)*

in whom more than two observations of PSR were available, it regressed in 11, remained stable in 13, and progressed in 15 (see Fig 25-3), males exhibiting more severe PSR than females. Patients with unilateral PSR have a 17% probability of regressing to no PSR and a 13% probability of progressing to bilateral PSR. Those with bilateral PSR have a 2% probability of regressing to a unilateral PSR state and a 2% probability of regressing to no PSR. PSR severity increases at an increasing rate, with this effect more marked in SC patients. Only two eyes had permanent depression of visual acuity as a result of retinal detachment consequent to PSR. It is evident that progression is not inevitable although, because vision loss in sickle cell disease generally occurs after 30 years of age, the most relevant combined data derived prospectively from this natural history study may not be available as yet.

Treatment and Prevention of Visual Loss

Past therapies applied to eyes with PSR have included diathermy, cryotherapy, photocoagulation of sea fan feeder vessels, and sectoral and circumferential scatter photocoagulation. A controlled trial of peripheral scatter photocoagulation showed that treatment reduces the incidence of vitreous hemorrhage. Yet no patient in the trial had permanent vision loss. The basis for treatment has been an assumed uniformly high risk of vision loss after the development of PSR, which has not been demonstrated. In fact, established PSR, especially in older SC patients, has been observed frequently and is uncommonly associated with vision loss. This is most likely due to spontaneous regression of active sea fans.

Photocoagulation carried out in ischemic, thin peripheral retina carries a significant risk of retinal hole formation. Furthermore, treatments such as feeder vessel coagulation have been complicated by choroidal neovascularization and vitreous hemorrhage in addition to tractional and rhegmatogenous retinal detachment. Until better definition of high-risk factors for significant loss of vision is achieved, the development of PSR should not be considered an absolute indication for therapy.

The low prevalence of vision loss from sickle cell diseases, at least in Jamaica, implies that large numbers of patients would need to be treated (probably at an early age) to achieve benefit to a few. Many would be treated unnecessarily. The argument that the Jamaican experience cannot be extended to sickle cell retinopathy in countries with different climates or different haplotypes is not supported by studies in Saudi Arabia and England, whose data were identical to Jamaican data. Extended experience may allow prevention to be focused on those at greatest danger of vision loss by documenting the natural history over longer periods and by determining more specific risk factors for vision loss due to sickle cell disease.

Clarkson JG. The ocular manifestations of sickle-cell disease: a prevalence and natural history study. *Trans Am Ophthalmol Soc.* 1992;90:481–504.

Farber MD, Jampol LM, Fox P, et al. A randomized clinical trial of scatter photocoagulation of proliferative sickle cell retinopathy. *Arch Ophthalmol.* 1991;109:363–367.

Goldberg MF. Classification and pathogenesis of proliferative sickle retinopathy. *Am J Ophthalmol.* 1971;71:649–665.

Penman AD, Talbot JF, Chuang EL, et al. New classification of peripheral retinal vascular changes in sickle cell disease. *Br J Ophthalmol.* 1994;78:681–689.

Serjeant GR, Serjeant BE. Management of sickle cell disease; lessons from the Jamaican Cohort Study. *Blood Rev.* 1993;7:137–145.

Serjeant GR, Serjeant BE. *Sickle Cell Disease.* 3rd ed. Oxford/New York: Oxford University Press; 2001.

CHAPTER 26

Hong Kong Myopia

Background

Myopia has long been recognized as a significant ocular disease in China. In 1936, the prevalence was estimated to be as high as 65% of adults. Recently, the prevalence of myopia among Hong Kong Chinese between the ages of 19 and 39 years has been reported to be 71%. In a study of Hong Kong university students, the prevalence of myopia was as high as 90%.

The Hong Kong Vision Study (HKVS) was developed to collect data that would assist in the appropriate design of a larger study of eye disease in Hong Kong. The goal was to collect data that would be comparable to studies in the United States and Australia that had used similar methodology. Refer to Chapter 4 in this volume.

Collaboration was key in developing methodology for the Hong Kong study. The Centre for Eye Research Australia (CERA) provided a survey manual protocol from the Melbourne Visual Impairment Project (VIP) and on-site training in both English and Cantonese to the team of investigators. The CERA programmer, who was a native of Guangdong Province, China, and fluent in Cantonese, translated the questions from the Melbourne study into Cantonese for the Hong Kong study research manual. A coinvestigator of the Hong Kong study and professor at the Hong Kong Polytechnic Institute retranslated the questions to ensure that the meaning was accurate in the local dialect. The immediate goal was to learn if survey methods developed in the United States and Australia were applicable to collecting reliable data on a Chinese population of Hong Kong when translated into Cantonese. The prevalence of eye diseases and risk factors found in the pilot study would be helpful in estimating the appropriate sample size and the size of the effect a study might detect, the confidence with which that effect might be considered, and the standard deviation of the population being studied.

Although the Rotterdam Eye Study, a cross-sectional population-based study of eye disease, reported myopic choroidal degeneration as an important cause of vision impairment, the Hong Kong study's myopia findings appear significant and different from those of any previously reported population-based study of eye disease. Elsewhere in Europe, myopia is registered as the cause of 5% of the blindness in Denmark and approximately 15% of that in Germany.

> Klaver CC, Wolfs RC, Vingerling JR, et al. Age-specific prevalence and causes of blindness and visual impairment in an older population: the Rotterdam Study. *Arch Ophthalmol.* 1998;116:653–658.

Livingston PM, Carson CA, Stanislavsky YL, et al. Methods for a population-based study of eye disease: the Melbourne Visual Impairment Project. *Ophthalmic Epidemiol.* 1994;1: 139–148.

Van Newkirk MR, McCarty CA, Martone JF, et al. Methods for the Hong Kong Vision Study: a pilot assessment of visual impairment in adults. *Ophthalmic Epidemiol.* 1998;5:57–67.

Pathogenesis

The debate regarding the etiology of myopia consists of arguments favoring genetic factors versus those favoring environmental factors. In Hong Kong, 70%–80% of medical students have myopia compared with 20%–30% of youths in rural Guangdong province. Myopia and educational attainment have a strong relationship.

Genetic influence in myopia is circumstantial but strong; parental history of myopia appears significantly more important than a child's near activities. A study of myopia in Singapore military personnel found a strong association with parental myopia (odds ratio [OR] 3.6) and high myopia (OR 5.2).

Seet B, Wong TY, Tan DT, et al. Myopia in Singapore: taking a public health approach. *Br J Ophthalmol.* 2001;85:521–526.

Clinical Presentation and Findings

Myopia is an important risk factor for several eye diseases. The incidence of rhegmatogenous retinal detachment among myopic patients is reported to range from 0.7% to 6%. This predisposition may occur because of an increased rate of vitreous liquefaction and posterior vitreous separation. High and extreme myopia can be associated with degenerative or pathologic changes. The most frequent pathologic findings associated with high and extreme myopia are myopic configuration of the optic nerve, 37.7%, and posterior staphyloma, 35.4%, whereas subretinal neovascularization, Fuchs spot, and lacquer cracks are much less common.

Curtin BJ. *The Myopias: Basic Science and Clinical Management.* Philadelphia: Harper & Row; 1985:61–113.

Grossniklaus HE, Green WR. Pathologic findings in pathologic myopia. *Retina.* 1992;12: 127–233.

Findings From the Hong Kong Vision Study

The prevalence of myopia ($\geq$0.5 D) in the Hong Kong study was 41.1% (146/355). The prevalence of myopia in the urban cohort of the Visual Impairment Project ($\geq$0.5 D) was 22.5% (569/2533). The prevalence and degree of myopia in the comparable studies are shown in Table 26-1.

The difference in these proportions between the Hong Kong study and the urban cohort of the Visual Impairment Project was highly significant—that is, $\chi^2 = 28.83$, $P < .00001$.

Table 26-1 **Prevalence and Degree of Myopia in Comparable Studies**

Study	Low Myopia (−0.5 to −5 D)	High Myopia (−5.25 to −10 D)	Extreme Myopia (≥10.25 D)
Hong Kong Vision Study	38% (108/355)	8.2% (29/355)	2.5% (9/355)
Visual Impairment Project, urban cohort	21% (532/2533)	2% (29/2533)	0.3% (8/2533)

Of the 9 participants in the Hong Kong study with extreme myopia, 3 women and 2 men had bilateral moderate visual impairment (<20/60) due to myopic choroidal degeneration. The women ranged in age from 46 to 70 years and the affected men, from 67 to 77 years. Their refractive errors ranged from −10 D to −22 D. Axial lengths were measured with A-scan biometry in 6 (67%) of these 9 participants. Surprisingly, the 70-year-old woman participant with high myopia and advanced peripapillary chorioretinal atrophy involving the macula had an axial length of 23.9 mm. Axial lengths in the other participants ranged from 28.4 mm to 32 mm. Three of the 9 participants with extreme myopia had unilateral visual impairment due to myopic choroidal degeneration. In all, 8 (89%) of the 9 participants with extreme myopia suffered from myopic choroidal degeneration and visual impairment affecting at least one eye. The major difference in the data of the Hong Kong study compared with that of other population-based studies is the frequency of high and extreme myopia and myopic choroidal degeneration.

> Van Newkirk MR. The Hong Kong vision study: a pilot assessment of visual impairment in adults. *Trans Am Ophthalmol Soc.* 1997;95:715–749.

The World Health Organization compilation of data from surveys performed in 29 provinces of China reported that chorioretinal diseases caused 7% of profound blindness. It is not possible to know from these data whether myopic choroidal degeneration is included in chorioretinal diseases. The diagnostic methodology of these surveys apparently did not include indirect ophthalmoscopy or fundus photography, which might explain a failure to diagnose myopic choroidal degeneration. Because the exact description of that chorioretinal disease is not included, no comparison can be made with the data from the Hong Kong study. Although it is not possible to make accurate predictions from the data of this study, further detailed study of extreme myopia in China is indicated.

> Thylefors B, Négrel AD, Pararajasegarani R, et al. Available data on blindness (update 1994). *Ophthalmic Epidemiol.* 1995;2:5–39.

In the Netherlands, the Rotterdam study observed 32 participants with profound vision impairment (<20/400). Of these, 2 (6%) had myopic choroidal degeneration. In addition, 23% of the younger age group (55–74 years) participants were observed to have moderate and severe vision impairment (>20/400 and <20/60) caused by myopic choroidal degeneration. Of all participants in this study with moderate and severe vision impairment, 11 (6%) of 192 eyes were impaired by myopic choroidal degeneration.

Prevention

Prevention of high and extreme myopia would have beneficial effects worldwide. Unfortunately, however, no preventive measures are available at this time. Although some case reports of the beneficial effects of atropine, scleral reinforcement, bifocals, and contact lenses are in the literature, no supportive evidence from well-designed, randomized, controlled clinical trials exists. Further, although topical pharmacologic agonists such as apomorphine, a dopamine receptor agonist, appear to retard the induced scleral growth in the form deprivation animal model, no data are available in humans.

> Iuvone PM, Tigges M, Stone RA, et al. Effects of apomorphine, a dopamine receptor agonist, on ocular refraction and axial elongation in a primate model of myopia. *Invest Ophthalmol Vis Sci.* 1991;32:1674–1677.

Conclusion

The success of this pilot study confirms that a well-designed methodology is transferable to different cultures, languages, and environments. The results of the Hong Kong Vision Study indicate that the sampling, recruitment, and data collection methods are feasible in Hong Kong and that further efforts to complete an eye disease prevalence study are warranted. Similar applications of this methodology may be feasible in other languages and cultures. If so, it would enable more accurate comparisons of survey data among different populations of the world.

PART VI

Effective Health Care Delivery Systems

Introduction

Most of the chapters in this part describe programs developed in different parts of the world that provide clinical care to help decrease the prevalence of eye diseases. Several of the chapters identify cataract blindness as a major cause of visual impairment in their region. The data have been derived from thoughtful and well-organized epidemiologic studies. The authors describe how these studies were used to focus on the elimination of the problem by prevention, research, and medical and surgical approaches. Projects established to provide medical and surgical care continuously evaluate their results for acceptable outcomes. The institutions described are by no means the only ones that provide excellent and much needed services to their regions, but they are good examples of how much can be achieved with limited resources.

Chapter 27 describes the Aravind Eye Care System. This model was established by Dr Venkataswamy and his family and further developed in recent years. It utilizes highly refined clinical care procedures that maximize the use of financial resources, thus allowing the funding of an "equitable development model" to provide care regardless of patients' financial resources. Chapter 28 describes the L.V. Prasad Eye Institute. The institute was modeled after those in developed nations, but its goal is to meet local needs—in this case, the needs of a poor and overpopulated state in India. Chapter 29 describes the Kikuyu Eye Unit in Kenya, Africa. In this program, limited resources are channeled to provide care in a large, overpopulated, and geographically diverse area. Chapter 30 addresses eye-care programs in Brazil and Peru. The authors point out the importance of identifying the needs of the population in the region. Unique features include using existing health care facilities throughout the region and employing local private practice ophthalmologists to provide needed care in the public health sector. The program highlights the need to involve the international community in providing much needed financial resources. Chapter 31 presents The Fred Hollows Foundation system of cataract management, which emphasizes that surgical intervention is not the endpoint; rather, results must be assessed and surgical quality maintained and improved. The system has developed ways of overcoming financial obstacles by using training modules, supply and equipment manufacturing, and cost-recovery mechanisms. Finally, Chapter 32 discusses the growing importance to developing nations of eye banking and corneal transplantation. The Eye Bank Association of India (EBAI) is a successful model of such a comprehensive eye banking and corneal transplantation system in the developing world.

There are common trends in these regional programs. First, the problems are identified through well-done epidemiologic and public health studies. The programs all provide clinical care in economically impoverished areas that are overpopulated and geographically widespread. They highlight the need to have eye-care units staffed by local health care workers. Funding is provided by a combination of local and international programs. Finally, they all emphasize the importance of continued evaluation of the ongoing programs to determine and improve the quality of care they provide.

Eduardo C. Alfonso, MD

CHAPTER 27

The Aravind Eye Care System

Background

Blindness and visual impairment are major causes of disability in India, affecting a very productive segment of the country's population. Epidemiologic data regarding the prevalence and etiology of blindness in India differ from source to source but nevertheless demonstrate a significant cause of disability and loss of productivity. The World Health Organization (WHO) estimates the prevalence of blindness (VA <3/60 in the best eye) in India to be approximately 1%. The percentage of blindness due to cataract is approximately 50%. Accordingly, approximately 4.9 million individuals in India are considered to be blind from cataract.

> Jose R, Bachani D. World Bank-assisted Cataract Blindness Control Project. *Indian J Ophthalmol*. 1995;43:35–43.
>
> Thylefors B, Négrel AD, Pararajasegaram R, et al. Global data on blindness. *Bull World Health Organ*. 1995;73:115–121.

Conservative estimates (excluding those under 35 years of age who are blind from cataract) published at the beginning of this decade indicated that roughly 3.8 million people in India would become blind from cataract annually. To prevent the number of cataract blind from increasing, it would be necessary for eye surgeons in India to perform a minimum of 3.5 million sight-restoring cataract operations each year; others have suggested that this number may need to be as high as 5 to 6 million.

> Limburg H, Kumar R, Bachani D. Monitoring and evaluating cataract intervention in India. *Br J Ophthalmol*. 1996;80:951–955.
>
> Minassian DC, Mehra V. 3.8 million blinded by cataract each year: projections from the first epidemiological study of incidence of cataract blindness in India. *Br J Ophthalmol*. 1990; 74:341–343.
>
> Venkataswamy G. Combating cataract [editorial]. *Indian J Ophthalmol*. 1995;43:1.

Cataract surgery is an extremely cost-efficient method of medical intervention, especially when compared with others, such as cardiac bypass surgery. It is therefore prudent to consider large-scale cataract intervention, as this inexpensive procedure has an excellent chance of quickly and fully restoring a patient to productivity as a member of society. The economic burden of blindness in India for the year 1997 was estimated at Rs. 159 billion (US$4.4 billion). At this time, there is no foreseeable decrease in this figure, and, indeed, it may continue to increase. As competition for limited government resources and international assistance grows, the need for the widespread promotion of financially self-sustaining eye-care systems is increasing. Without such efforts, the social and economic burden of the blind in India may soon reach unmanageable levels.

> Shamanna BR, Dandona L, Rao GN. Economic burden of blindness in India. *Indian J Ophthalmol.* 1998;46:169–172.

Significant progress has been made in combating blindness and visual impairment in India. The Aravind Eye Care System in Tamil Nadu, India, is one such effort that has achieved great success in the battle to reduce the burden of blindness on the subcontinent. Established by Dr Venkataswamy and his family after his mandatory retirement from the local government hospital, the first Aravind Eye Hospital opened in Madurai in 1976. Since then, Aravind has grown from an 11-bed hospital with three doctors to a comprehensive system of five major hospitals with nearly 2500 beds. In 25 years, over 71 million patients have been seen as outpatients, and roughly 3 million patients have undergone surgery. The quality of surgery is high, annual profits surpass US$1 million, and, presently, close to 75% of all patients are provided with free eye care. The Aravind Eye Care System has effectively achieved *sustainable provision of services* while maintaining its orientation toward serving the poor.

Along with the increasing volume of patients has come the expansion of Aravind's facilities from a single hospital into a network of five hospitals, situated in Madurai, Theni, Tirunelveli, Coimbatore, and Pondicherry. Aravind's medical staff, which has also expanded rapidly, currently comprises 75 ophthalmologists, 70 residents, and 30 fellows training in the various specialty clinics. Because the spirit of the hospital is based on appropriate utilization of staff, a team of 560 ophthalmic paramedics and 540 ancillary staff complement the medical staff.

The Equitable Development Model

The Aravind Eye Care System has realized these accomplishments through the creation and implementation of the *equitable development model* of quality eye-care services. As one approach to fighting blindness in low-income countries, the equitable development model relies on maximizing quality and efficiency to create demand and improve supply. By continuously reinvesting excess revenue back into the system to increase service capacity, the equitable development model provides resources to maintain an equitable service orientation while building capacity without outside investment. According to this model, a properly managed eye hospital can create revenue in excess of expenditures and can use that profit to subsidize services to individuals otherwise unable to pay. Similarly, excess revenue and production capacity can be used to improve and expand existing services.

Understanding the Model

The equitable development model of sustainable eye-care services, as conceived at the original Aravind Eye Hospital in Madurai, is founded on the concept of cost recovery from cataract surgery and, more recently, on the sales of intraocular lenses, sutures, and pharmaceuticals as well. Once an efficient surgical system is created, cost-recovery techniques may be used to generate enough revenue from cataract surgery and other operations to cover operating costs. This requires increasing productivity, decreasing costs, and lowering prices. With increasing volume, the cost per procedure decreases, making it more attainable for the poor. The efficiency of the surgery is based on a unique, extensive system of eye camps that brings patients to a high-volume, efficiently run hospital system, where eye evaluations and surgical care are then provided. Extensive business-based quality assurance processes are carried out to ensure excellent quality care at all levels.

Number of Surgeries

Although the use of excess revenues to finance services to the poor is commendable, many ophthalmologists consider it unrealistic to expect user fees in resource-poor settings to exceed the cost of providing services. In fact, it has been demonstrated that other health services oriented toward serving the poor are rarely able to recover much more than 20% of their costs.

Eye-care delivery, especially refractions and cataract surgery, may be exceptions because each is usually a one-time intervention; the odds of success are excellent; patients usually perceive a rapid noticeable difference; and minimal time is lost from daily schedules. This difference is communicated to other residents in the same village, who then increase the demand for service.

The uniqueness of cataract-oriented eye care is its exceptional level of cost-effectiveness. Many public health programs aimed at prevention fail because people are often unwilling to pay for preventive services. In contrast, people are very willing to pay for a cure. Most chronic and acute diseases are costly to treat or are untreatable, and cost and treatment regimen can vary substantially from patient to patient. As a result, creating financially sustainable health services is generally difficult, if not impossible—unless services to the poor are not included. Cataract-based eye services are different, offering low-cost curative treatment and rehabilitation services for which people are generally willing to pay.

By creating a solid financial framework centered on the provision of cataract surgery, eye-care programs can make high-quality surgery affordable to the poor while, at the same time, generating a profit. In doing so, services can be strengthened and expanded without the need for outside capital. Therefore, it is essential to change the mentality and practice of ophthalmologists and eye-care professionals by emphasizing the importance of low-cost, high-volume, high-quality eye care. By practicing and promoting the equitable development of sustainable eye-care programs, eye hospitals can establish permanent services with the potential for eliminating the backlog of treatable blindness that has, thus far, been so difficult to combat.

> Green D. *Financial Sustainability for High Quality, Large Volume, Sustainable Cataract Surgery Programmes.* Quality Cataract Surgery Series. Madurai, India: Aravind Eye Hospitals and Postgraduate Institute of Ophthalmology; Lions Aravind Institute of Community Ophthalmology; Seva Foundation; 2000.

Clinical Services

The core processes that drive most activities in Aravind are "demand-generated" systems for high efficiency in service delivery, quality assurance, and financial viability.

Demand Generation

Aravind works on a two-tier service model—those who pay and those who receive free services. This system allows relatively richer patients to subsidize the cost of services for some disadvantaged groups. Aravind's marketing system works by combining consistent service with large volumes that reduce the cost of each operation. To reach patients who need eye care and get them into the system, Aravind uses rural eye screening camps. Each geographic district is assigned to a camp organizer (an Aravind staff member), who, in turn, finds a local community partner to organize the camp. The community partner publicizes the eye camps with posters and banners. On the appointed day, the team of doctors and paramedics screen patients at the camps, transporting to the base hospital those who need operations. Those who need spectacles receive them that day at an affordable price. Patients with complex conditions, such as glaucoma or retinopathy, which require relatively sophisticated interventions, are referred back to the base hospital.

Free eye screening camps are conducted every day of the week, held in villages that cover a population of 30–35 million people. During the year 2000, a total of 1548 camps were conducted in which 426,350 patients were examined and 93,519 patients received free surgery.

While in the community, the medical team also educates the population in proper eye care. Other community projects include screening for diabetes-related eye disorders; community-based rehabilitation; integrated education for blind children; eye screening at schools; and treatment of children suffering from refractive errors, strabismus, and vitamin A deficiency. The benefits of community involvement act as a catalyst, bringing wealthier patients from various communities to the paying hospital. If the wealthier patients come for care, poorer patients will then follow.

The hospital uses counselors to alleviate the fears and doubts of anxious patients. The counselors are women selected from the same rural community served by the hospital; they receive 2 years of intense training. Effective counseling at the hospital and the camps has increased the number of patients who come for surgery. In addition to allaying fears, counseling helps patients accept surgery as a reasonable option, have realistic outcome expectations, and comply with instructions. It has also resulted in increased patient satisfaction.

All the hospitals in the Aravind system conform to local social and cultural standards. They are open longer hours to accommodate agrarian workers. Walk-ins are welcome and the fee structure offers an affordable range of prices to paying patients and free service to poor patients (Figs 27-1 and 27-2).

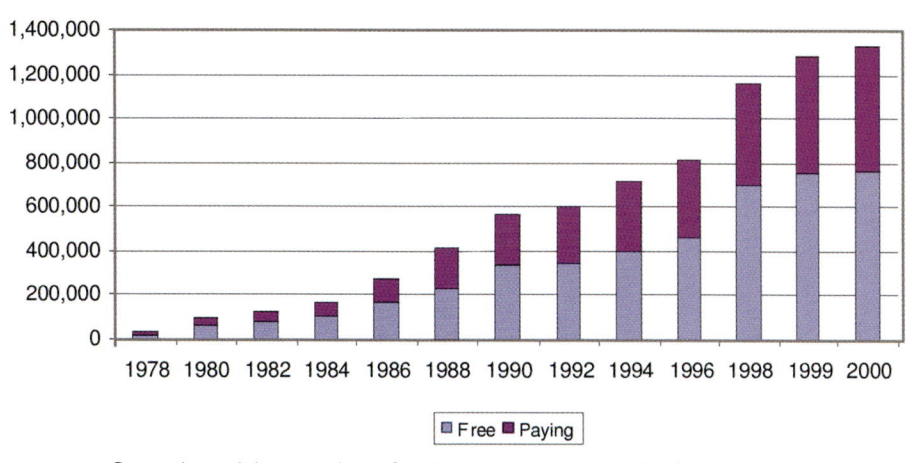

Figure 27-1 Outpatient visits: number of patients who are seen for free and number who pay. *(Courtesy of Alan L. Robin, MD.)*

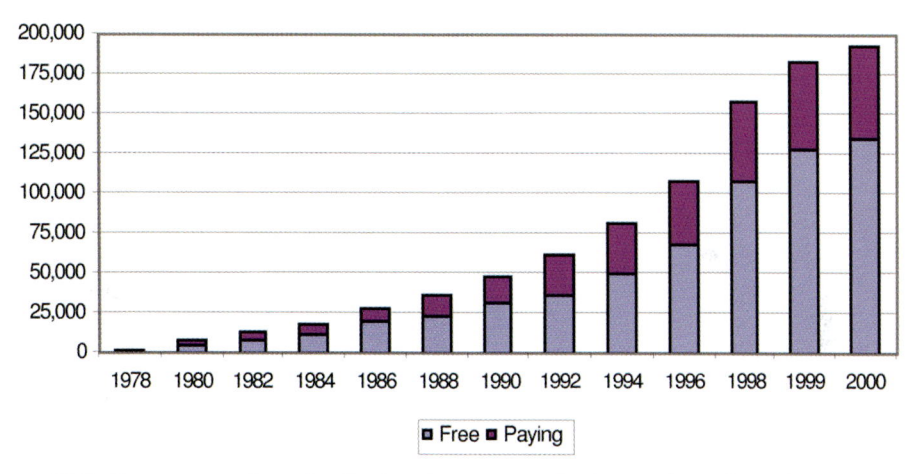

Figure 27-2 Surgery: number of patients who are seen for free and number who pay. *(Courtesy of Alan L. Robin, MD.)*

Understanding Sustainability and Cost Recovery in Eye Care

The equitable development model of eye-care services requires careful planning and management based on the foundations of sustainability and cost recovery. Using four overarching themes—local ownership and fiscal self-sufficiency, social marketing, economies of scale, and efficient services—equitable development in eye care can become a reality.

Local Ownership and Financial Self-Sufficiency

A common problem of hospital administration is the source of funding and the use of funds received from that source. Whether capital is filtered down from a ministry of health or an outside agency, the receipt of funding from outside the specific activities of the eye hospital itself can be restrictive and may cause many administrative difficulties. Large international donors such as the World Bank generally require that allocated money be spent according to a strict and rigid schedule. This gives little incentive for creative solutions aimed at bringing long-term sustainability.

It is clear that dependence on outside funding sources is limiting and may inhibit the development of sustainable organizational capacity. Nevertheless, hospitals oriented toward serving the poor are seldom able to free themselves from their reliance on outside donor agencies. The implementation of cost-recovery mechanisms is one way by which eye hospitals can become self-financing and avoid this problem. By achieving self-sufficiency in this way, the control of financial resources is handed down to local authorities. Equitable development of eye-care programs encourages local doctors and administrators to achieve program ownership by defining their needs and objectives and putting them into action. Giving these community leaders control of financial resources vests them with the authority to bring about meaningful and long-lasting change.

Social Marketing

Marketing enables global corporations to successfully promote the sale and use of their products. Companies build name recognition based on a standardized image of the quality of their goods, thus effectively promoting their purchase. A good example of this is McDonald's. One can expect the "same" hamburger from this company whether one is in Chicago or Hong Kong.

By establishing unique and valued identities for brand name goods, marketing techniques create demand among targeted consumers for specific products. The use of marketing techniques need not be limited to the promotion and sale of material goods, however. Hospitals and health systems, including those specializing in eye care, can promote sound health behavior with the proper use of social marketing practices. This concept was discussed in a 1993 Harvard Business School Case Study:

> Tell me, can cataract surgery be marketed like hamburgers? Don't you call it social marketing or something? See, in America, McDonald's and Dunkin' Donuts and Pizza Hut have all mastered the art of mass marketing. We have to do something like that to clear the backlog of 20 million blind eyes in India. We perform only one million cataract surgeries a year. At this rate we cannot catch up. . . . Why can't we bring eyesight to the masses of poor people in India, Asia, Africa, and all over the world? (Rangan VK. The Aravind Eye Hospital, Madurai, India: In Service for Sight. Harvard Business School Case 593-098. Harvard Business School, Cambridge, MA; 1993.)

Eye hospitals can successfully encourage the use and sale of their services by changing consumer behavior through the science of social marketing. By increasing the acceptability of desired behaviors in specific target audiences, eye hospitals can effectively create a demand for their services that would otherwise be lacking.

To be successful, social marketing requires that hospitals adopt a consumer orientation. Satisfied patients will advertise a good hospital for free by spreading word of the treatment they received to friends and family.

What does it take to develop a good hospital like this? First, an appropriate location for the facility must be carefully selected. Hospitals must be convenient not only to the patients they serve but to eye-care professionals as well, for a location must be able to retain competent personnel in order to be viable. A little market research can help determine an appropriate site. The demographic indicators of a particular region can point to a suitable location for a hospital that combines the potential for income generation with an orientation toward serving the poor.

To attract and retain customers (particularly those willing to pay), a hospital must not only be efficient and maintain a level of excellence, it must also transmit this perception of quality regarding its services. The use of intraocular lenses (IOLs) in all cataract surgeries is one way to satisfy customers and convey that quality service is provided. Cataract surgery with IOL implantation greatly improves the visual outcomes of patients while eliminating the need to wear aphakic glasses postoperatively. By eliminating a patient's need for glasses, which are often lost or broken within the first year after surgery, hospitals can improve patient satisfaction. This, in turn, may lead to increased advertising of services by satisfied patients and a corresponding increase in demand from new patients. The perception of quality by the patient gives the service a real value and allows the hospital to charge a fee when a patient's income allows. This, in turn, makes the patient part of the team and somewhat accountable for the results, in terms of showing up for appointments, taking medications as directed, and returning for follow-up.

Many hospitals oriented toward serving the poor are reluctant to charge for services, wary that it will render programs inaccessible and inequitable. However, the equitable development model of sustainable eye care proposes that, by understanding a population's capacity to pay, a hospital may charge appropriate and affordable prices for eye care *and* keep services financially accessible to the poor. Aravind has determined that 1 month's income is an acceptable charge for cataract surgery and is not a deterrent to care.

Reducing the cost of surgery to a level roughly equivalent to what the majority of a population is willing to pay allows a hospital to charge for services without fear of creating programs exclusively for the rich. Target populations, as distinguished by income level, can then be segmented by several distinct fees for services. A plan that fits local parameters is recommended, as in the following:

> Various fee schedules employed experimentally or in routine practice can be examined to gain insights into consumer ability and willingness to pay. The problem with this approach is that findings from one setting are not necessarily applicable in another location, where attitudes, socioeconomic conditions, and available sources of health care may be quite different. . . . Apart from rigorously scientific approaches to setting fees, we should not underestimate the experience gained by providers as to what is likely to be acceptable in the local setting; perhaps the matter is not as mystical as it would appear. (Reinke WA, et al. Management of Health Systems in Developing Countries. Lecture notes, p 10. Johns Hopkins School of Hygiene and Public Health, Baltimore, 2000.)

A simple three-tiered pricing structure, in which services are priced at above cost, around cost, or free, has been implemented in eye hospitals in India, Nepal, Egypt, and Malawi. These tiered pricing structures allow revenue to be generated from those who can afford to pay while maintaining free services for the poor. By providing small benefits such as beds, private rooms, and separate waiting areas for patients who are willing to pay for care, hospitals can structure their services so as to encourage patients to discern a distinction in quality and voluntarily select the highest priced services they can afford.

Economies of Scale

Eye programs emphasizing cataract surgery have a distinct advantage in that a standardized, replicable approach to surgery may be taken without sacrificing service quality. By dividing labor appropriately and organizing treatment procedures into an efficient, systematized process, surgery of replicable quality can be performed at higher volumes per surgeon. As Aravind ophthalmologist and chief medical officer Natchiar observes,

> One surgeon can perform approximately five extracapsular [cataract] extractions with insertion of posterior chamber intraocular lenses per hour . . . assisted by three scrub nurses, one orderly, one circulating nurse, and one nurse to sterilize instruments. (Green D. *Financial Sustainability for High Quality, Large Volume, Sustainable Cataract Surgery Programmes.* Quality Cataract Surgery Series. Madurai, India: Aravind Eye Hospitals and Postgraduate Institute of Ophthalmology; Lions Aravind Institute of Community Ophthalmology; Seva Foundation; 2000:16.)

Increasing volume per surgeon while maintaining a hospital's fixed costs allows the per-unit cost of surgery to be minimized. Known as *economies of scale*, mass production approaches to eye care lessen the average cost per surgery in order to maximize profit, thus making per-unit cost one measure of efficiency in eye care. By reducing per-unit cost via increases in volume, while maintaining quality, eye-care services can be provided equitably and satisfactorily to the masses of individuals with cataract blindness in low- and middle-income countries. The key to economies of scale is efficiency that drives and helps improve quality.

Systems for Highly Efficient Service Delivery

Increasing the utilization of eye-care services is by itself a major challenge that is facilitated by maintaining efficient and high-quality service delivery. This is accomplished by increasing capacity and efficiency through appropriate systems.

The Aravind systems are designed to optimize the balance between resources and patient load. Systems and practices that increase efficiency are introduced. Conversely, systems or procedures that do not contribute to clinical outcome, patient satisfaction, or efficiency are considered wasteful and are modified or dropped. The staffs are involved in decision making, thus enhancing their motivation and encouraging good team practice. The systems that have helped Aravind to maximize the process are as follows:

- Standardization
- Division of labor
- Quality assurance
- Financial viability
- Balance of resources
- Architectural layout and work flow

- Adoption of newer technologies
- Information and review system
- Attitude and patient care

Standardization

Aravind follows a standard operating procedure for all clinical activities. Focus is given to better instrumentation, training of paramedical staff, and patient flow because all of these contribute to increasing efficiency and quality of care. The standard operating procedures are periodically reviewed against outcomes, new technologies, new instrumentation, and patient expectations.

Division of labor

Appropriate utilization of staff is of paramount importance. Clinical ophthalmic tasks include diagnosis and treatment. In many settings, an ophthalmologist does the entire range of clinical tasks including routine ones because of the limited number of staff. If physicians focus on what they do best—decision making and surgery—they can be more efficient and have greater job satisfaction. At Aravind, ophthalmologists are not required to do tasks such as refraction or routine administrative work. Paramedical staff are trained to perform many routine and specialized tasks, from assessing visual acuity to A-scan biometry and computerized visual field analysis.

Similarly in surgery, many of the preparatory steps are allocated to a trained nurse. By the time a surgeon sees a patient on the table for cataract surgery:

- The patient has been screened and found to have cataract
- No other ophthalmic diseases that could interfere with cataract have been identified
- Other medical problems have been evaluated
- Preoperative medical testing has been completed
- An appropriate IOL has been chosen
- The eye has been adequately dilated
- An appropriate block has been performed
- The patient is on the table and draped
- A surgical prep has been performed
- Surgical instruments are sterile and ready for use

Such preparation significantly increases the volume of surgery an ophthalmologist can perform. Systems are designed and continually reevaluated to ensure an efficient flow of patients either in the field or in the hospital. For example, in the operating room, the surgeon is provided with two surgical setups. This practically eliminates the waiting time between surgeries. Table 27-1 illustrates the surgical (extracapsular cataract extraction

Table 27-1 Output per Hour Under Different Scenarios

Number of Tables	Assisting Nurses	Circulating Nurses	Instrument Sets	Surgeries per Hour
1	1	1	1	1
1	1	1	3	3
2	2	1	6	6

[ECCE]/phacoemulsification with PC-IOL) output per hour under different scenarios for a single well-trained surgeon using one microscope and one phacoemulsification machine. The same types of principles are applied across all activities at the Aravind system to maximize resource utilization.

As a result of these systems, Aravind has developed efficient systems of patient care. An Aravind doctor can perform 20–30 cataract surgeries within 3 to 4 hours. An average ophthalmologist in India performs about 350 cataract surgeries per year, whereas an Aravind surgeon performs about 2000 such surgeries—with no apparent compromise in quality. In fact, quality might be increased because repetition appears to improve technical skills.

Quality assurance

Processes that ensure quality of care are integral to the Aravind system. Computers are used to analyze many aspects of patient care, including surgical complications and outcomes. In monthly meetings, these data are used to evaluate performance and services and plan for improvement. A more advanced complications and outcomes monitoring system has recently been developed for cataract surgery in which the individual surgeon gets details of complications, a complication score and how it compares with past performance, and the hospital's average and best outcome. Postoperative infection rate is closely monitored and for the year 2000 was 0.04%.

Monthly patient satisfaction surveys and weekly review of patient suggestions and complaints are carried out.

Financial viability

Aravind has paid close attention to developing administrative expertise for long-term viability. Medical and other staff receive a fixed salary linked to their overall performance—not to patient load. Paying patients pay close to market rates, and the inpatient facility offers a variety of comfort levels for varying fees. For instance, in the paying sector, the patient pays an equivalent of about US$1 for a comprehensive eye examination. The cost of a cataract operation including an IOL varies from US$60 to US$275, depending on the choice of rooms, procedure (ECCE or phacoemulsification), and the IOL (rigid or foldable). In the free hospital, patients receive free services but are required to pay US$11 for the same surgery to cover the cost of supplies such as the IOL and the discharge medication. Thus the core activity of patient care, cataract surgery, is entirely self-sufficient both for operating and capital costs.

Lions Aravind Institute of Community Ophthalmology (LAICO): Expanding Infrastructure

Today, the Aravind staff faces the daunting challenge of spreading the equitable development model of sustainable eye care throughout India and the rest of the world. As Dr Venkataswamy, Aravind's founder, noted in a Harvard Business School case study in 1993:

> My goal is to spread the Aravind model to every nook and corner of India, Asia, Africa; wherever there is blindness, we want to offer hope. Tell me, what is this concept of fran-

chising? Can't we do what McDonald's and Burger King have done in the United States? (Rangan VK. The Aravind Eye Hospital, Madurai, India: In Service for Sight. Harvard Business School Case 593-098. Harvard Business School, Cambridge, MA; 1993.)

To help achieve this lofty goal, the Lions Aravind Institute of Community Ophthalmology (LAICO) was founded in the early 1990s "to help eye hospitals strengthen their capacity to offer effective and sustainable eye-care programs." LAICO provides a wide variety of services, including educational and training courses and clinical education programs, and conducts research projects in both systems management and clinical ophthalmology. The most significant service activity of LAICO involves the hospital development programs in Asia and Africa. These outreach programs involve a collaboration between participating hospitals and LAICO staff (both natives of the area and other Indians who have moved into the area) to create comprehensive eye hospital development strategies. The initial focus is on eye hospital infrastructure using the equitable development model used at Aravind. LAICO hopes to build successful management systems in eye hospitals in developing countries that provide the volume and quality of care found at Aravind.

In-House Technology

One of the most unique and innovative aspects of the Aravind Eye Hospital system is its focus on appropriate technology through the development of local capacity. In June 1992, Aravind established Aurolab, its own IOL factory. By manufacturing IOLs of Western quality and specifications at reduced cost, Aurolab has allowed further reductions in the unit cost of cataract surgery. In 1998, Aurolab expanded its production capacity by manufacturing and supplying suture needles and offers these at affordable prices. Today, Aurolab manufactures IOLs, suture needles, spectacle lenses, and pharmaceuticals, and it has plans to begin producing low vision aids. All of the surgical supplies meet European quality standards and Aurolab IOLs also have attained United States FDA approval.

By manufacturing quality consumables in-house, Aravind has minimized its reliance on Western imports and greatly reduced the unit cost of surgery. The Fred Hollows Foundation has established comparable IOL manufacturing capabilities in Eritrea and Nepal with considerable success. Previously, the high cost of ophthalmic consumables represented a major barrier to the delivery of quality eye care to the poor. This development of local manufacturing capacity represents a practical solution to the problem and identifies a major area of productive activity that has been relatively ignored to date. Efforts are now under way to establish group purchasing organizations (GPOs) to extend consumable price reductions to other eye hospitals in low- and middle-income countries. Using economy of scale, GPOs provide a mechanism by which groups of hospitals can purchase supplies in bulk at reduced cost. With expanded and sustained efforts to minimize the cost of ophthalmic equipment and consumables, eye-care professionals can dramatically reduce the cost of eye care, making access more equitable and quality vision restoration services possible for the poor.

Challenges in the Scaling-up Process

The equitable development model of sustainable eye-care services has been successfully demonstrated by the Aravind Eye Care System, but it remains to be seen if the strategy can achieve comparable results given dissimilar circumstances in other areas of the world. One of the principal assumptions underlying the paradigm is that ophthalmologists, regardless of their qualifications and the setting in which they operate, will be able to consistently provide high-volume, high-quality eye surgery. Regardless of innovations in management, sustainable services will not be possible until a cadre of properly trained ophthalmologists and paramedical staff are available. Surgical personnel not only must be taught the skills to perform operations efficiently and effectively, they must believe that making changes in the way they practice is beneficial to them and the communities they serve. A lack of human infrastructure may prove to be the biggest difficulty in spreading the equitable development model.

A second big challenge facing equitable development in eye-care programs concerns the ability of communities to successfully finance eye-care services. The translation of population-based economic data into pricing strategies for cataract surgery is a pillar of cost-recovery theory in ophthalmology. It is the basis for pricing structures in the Aravind Eye Hospital system in India and the Lumbini Eye Hospital in Nepal and has been successful in predicting the population's willingness to pay in both cases. Nevertheless, the model has not been successfully transcribed outside of Southeast Asia, and it is debatable that populations will have the economic resources to finance their own care. Moreover, it is not certain that populations will be willing to pay as much for eye care (namely, 1 month's income according to the paradigm) in Africa as they do in Southeast Asia, regardless of the availability of resources. The willingness of a community to change the way it gets medical care must be viewed in terms of knowledge, cultures, and individual perceptions. No one can predict how new intervention programs will be accepted in different regions and cultures.

Despite lingering questions, the equitable development model of sustainable eye care, which has the potential to greatly diminish the burden of blindness in India, may be viable in similar developing countries. Universally, the public sector is faced with limited resources, and cost-recovery schemes for services rendered seem necessary. By continuing to implement and evaluate pilot projects in cataract-endemic areas of the world, the potential impact of the equitable development model of sustainable eye care can be assessed and documented. As ophthalmologists and other eye-care professionals gain a better understanding of the strengths and weaknesses of the current model, the provision of equitable and sustainable eyecare services will continue to improve. Even if full financial sustainability is not possible in all programs oriented toward serving the poor, sustainability planning will encourage improvements in quality and efficiency beneficial to any hospital.

> Green D. *Financial Sustainability for High Quality, Large Volume, Sustainable Cataract Surgery Programmes.* Quality Cataract Surgery Series. Madurai, India: Aravind Eye Hospitals and Postgraduate Institute of Ophthalmology; Lions Aravind Institute of Community Ophthalmology; Seva Foundation; 2000.

L.V. Prasad Eye Institute

Background

Although the finances and degree of training necessary to provide state-of-the-art health care has increased throughout the world over the past few decades, the real challenge in health care has been to establish institutions that are responsive to the dynamic needs of the communities in which they exist. In many countries, as public funds dwindle, alternative funding mechanisms involving the private sector are on the rise. The challenge for providers interested in the health of the entire community is to extend care both to those who can and those who cannot afford it. To address these global issues, new systems of health care must be developed. Developing a methodology to transform outmoded patterns of thinking into dynamic approaches to the health care needs of a community is the greatest challenge.

The L.V. Prasad Eye Institute

The L.V. Prasad Eye Institute (LVPEI), an ophthalmologic institute in Hyderabad, India, demonstrates some lessons that can be applied when establishing specialized health care facilities in countries with comparable challenges. Hyderabad, the capital of Andhra Pradesh, is centrally located in southern India. With its 70 million people, Andhra Pradesh is a typical state with respect to its ethnic diversity, economic strength, prevalence of health care, and level of literacy. Information furnished by the state health department indicates that there are about 2050 hospitals and dispensaries and a doctor-to-population ratio of 1:1250. Doctors in all specialties and subspecialties practice in both the public and private sector. There are about 40,000 hospital beds and a bed-to-population ratio of 1:1750. The average life expectancy for someone born today in Andhra Pradesh is 65 years. In India as a whole and in Andhra Pradesh in particular, despite a large number of trained physicians, medical standards are poor. There are few industries in the state, and the economy is largely subsistence agriculture. Recently, Hyderabad has become a major center for information technology and is becoming a major force in biotechnology. In spite of this, the unemployment rate is between 30% and 40%.

In 1983, the idea of establishing a system of high-quality, comprehensive eye care for all patients, regardless of ability to pay, was conceived by Dr Gullapalli N. Rao, then an associate clinical professor of ophthalmology at the University of Rochester Medical Center in the United States. The idea became a reality in 1986, and the L.V. Prasad Eye

Institute opened in 1987. Despite the limitations of the environment in which it was established, the Institute has developed a model of health care delivery that is medically up-to-date and strategically relevant to the needs of the patient population. Today, LVPEI has a staff of 360, including 16 full-time salaried ophthalmologists, 2 internists, 6 part-time anesthesiologists, 20 optometrists, 10 basic scientists, 5 directors, and 30 administrators. Structurally, it is run as a nonprofit organization, encompassing service, training, research, community eye health, rehabilitation of the blind, and product development.

LVPEI caters to a population of 100 million. It is one of three major referral facilities for comprehensive clinical ophthalmology services in the country. Annually, about 150,000 patients are seen at the Institute and about 20,000 surgical procedures are performed (Figs 28-1 and 28-2). In addition, the two rural satellite clinics at Mudhol in Adilabad district and Toodukurthy in Mahaboobnagar district handle approximately 25,000 outpatients and perform 3500 surgeries annually (Fig 28-3). In LVPEI, 30% of all patients are from Hyderabad, 30% are from the state of Andhra Pradesh, 39% are from throughout the rest of India, and the remainder are from other countries. Patients range from neonates to the elderly, and the diseases run the gamut of ophthalmic disorders. Specialists in all major ophthalmic subspecialties, supported by laboratory services and anesthetists, are available to provide care. The Institute has state-of-the-art equipment to treat the entire range of eye disorders.

Overview of Challenges

The difficulties overcome in the effort to establish the Institute can be classified into three areas: financial, programmatic, and personnel. Initial challenges included raising funds, establishing a facility at which comprehensive eye care could be delivered effectively, and employing appropriately trained personnel to conduct patient care. As the Institute matured, the board of directors agreed to conduct epidemiologic and clinical investigations, establish an eye bank, develop training programs for all categories of eye-care personnel, design a rehabilitation program for the visually impaired and blind, and create outreach programs for rural underserved communities.

Finances

The bulk of capital expenditures, including start-up funds, expansion, and equipment purchases, were made possible through donations and grants. Ongoing expenses include payroll; physical facilities; medical and research supplies; utilities and maintenance; insurance; and funding for research, outreach, and rehabilitation.

Donations

Initial funds were raised in 1984 through a foundation established in the United States. A movie producer, L.V. Prasad, donated US$1 million and land. Currently, donations comprise 20% of the Institute's funds (33% national, 66% international). LVPEI has a small fund-raising staff to identify and develop contacts with philanthropic institutions and individuals. Given its commitment to indigent patients and its success as an educational facility, the hospital receives donations of equipment from corporations eager

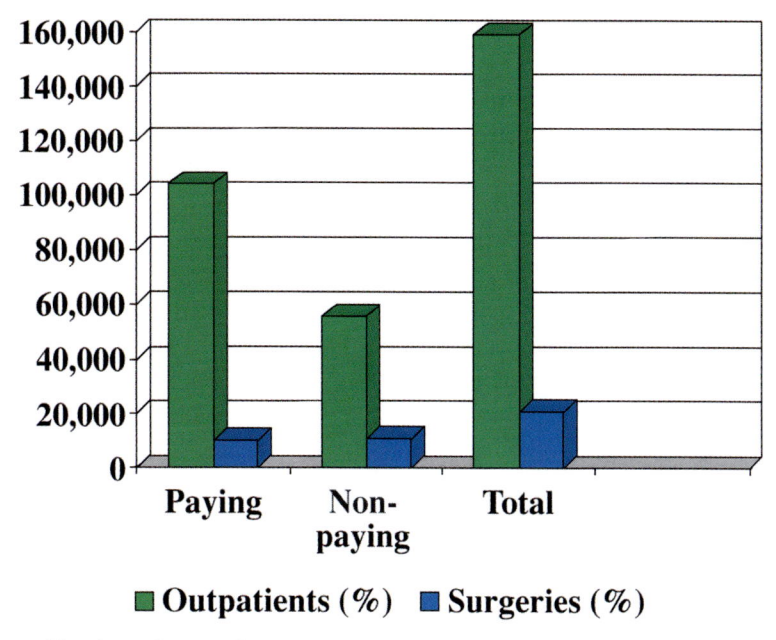

Figure 28-1 Number of outpatients seen and surgeries performed at the main institute in Hyderabad, April 1999–March 2000. *(Courtesy of Gullapalli N. Rao, MD.)*

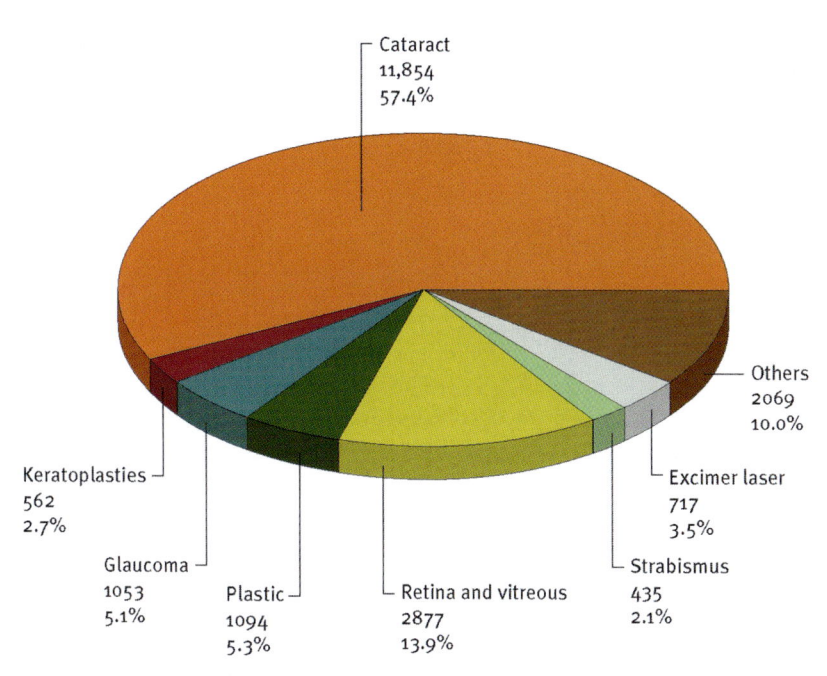

Figure 28-2 A total of 20,661 surgical procedures were performed during the period April 1999–March 2000. *(Courtesy of Gullapalli N. Rao, MD.)*

- Cataract: 11,854 (57.4%)
- Others: 2069 (10.0%)
- Excimer laser: 717 (3.5%)
- Strabismus: 435 (2.1%)
- Retina and vitreous: 2877 (13.9%)
- Plastic: 1094 (5.3%)
- Glaucoma: 1053 (5.1%)
- Keratoplasties: 562 (2.7%)

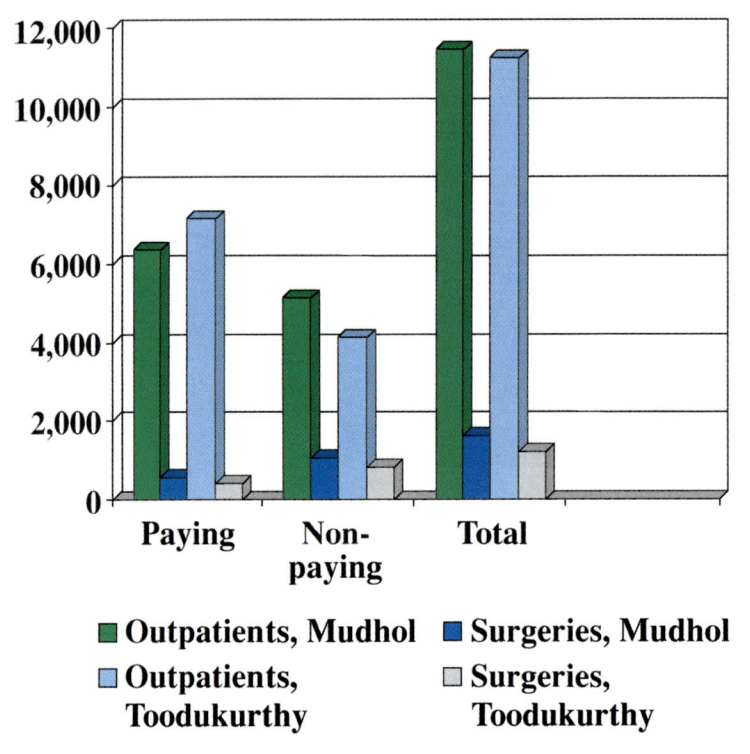

Figure 28-3 Number of outpatients seen and surgeries performed at the rural satellite eye centers, Mudhol and Toodukurthy, India. *(Courtesy of Gullapalli N. Rao, MD.)*

to showcase their instruments during the Institute's training programs. Approximately 25% of equipment is donated, 50% is obtained at or below cost, and 25% is purchased at market value.

Fees

Although private and corporate health insurance may be available through employment, health care is an out-of-pocket expense for 95% of patients due to the high unemployment rate in Andhra Pradesh. Based on current levels of billing, fees generate 60% of the Institute's income. Given the existing fee schedule, a 1:1 ratio of nonpay to pay patients sustains patient care, as well as at least 50% of research, training, rehabilitation, and outreach expenditures. Paying patients are classified according to four tiers of financial ability. Inability to pay is based on eligibility for government ration cards, and hospital staff is authorized to change a patient's status to nonpay at any time. The fee schedule has not been changed in 5 years.

Grants and public monies

Although the Institute actively solicits donations, to maintain administrative autonomy, governmental and international development funds that invite mandates and bureaucracy are not accepted. LVPEI's programs of research, rehabilitation, and rural outreach compete for and receive grants from many international organizations involved in eye care and eye research. Although grants provide 20% of the Institute's annual revenues, these divisions of the Institute are not yet self-sufficient and require approximately 50% of the Institute's fee-generated income.

Programmatic Focus

Basic science research

Although the staff of LVPEI was involved informally in collaborative research from the beginning, a formal division of basic science research was established in 1997 (Table 28-1). The division presently depends on funding from other sources, such as patient care, clinical research grants, and donations, but the Institute's administration actively encourages the division to apply for grants and become financially independent.

Eye bank

In 1987, when the Institute opened its doors, there was no immediate regional source of tissue for corneal transplants. The challenge was to establish the protocols and guidelines necessary for the procurement, preservation, and distribution of donated tissue. After 3 years of work and consultation with Tissue Banks International in Baltimore, Maryland, a program satisfying international standards of eye banking was established in Hyderabad at LVPEI. The challenges and solutions encountered in this effort are the basis of a formal course that the Institute offers in eye banking. The Institute conducts regular public awareness rallies to educate the local population about the importance of donating eyes for corneal transplantation and maintains statistics of organ donorship.

Personnel training

Medical and paramedical training is not standardized in India, and the latest innovations in ophthalmology are practically limited to textbook descriptions for many students. The Institute conducts programs to train residents in ophthalmology and in a host of paramedical ophthalmic specialties. LVPEI is a major center of continuing medical education in ophthalmology in the developing world, given its state-of-the-art equipment and American-trained physicians. Over 7000 eye-care professionals have benefited from its short-term (1–3 months) and long-term (1–2 years) training programs and seminars over the past 12 years. The training for ophthalmologists is in the form of subspecialty fellowships and short-term courses in skills enhancement. Other training programs include those for ophthalmic technicians, nurses, and eye bank personnel, and for eye-care

Table 28-1 Current Ongoing Basic Research Projects at L.V. Prasad Eye Institute, Hyderabad, India

Major Basic Research Project	Department
Mapping of genes in inherited glaucoma and retinoblastoma	Genetics and Pathology
Molecular characterization of *Acanthamoeba* species	Microbiology
Apoptosis in human corneal epithelial cells following HSV	Virology
Enzymatic studies in mycotic keratitis	Mycology
Delaying cataract onset using locally available foods	Biochemistry

management. Expenses for these programs are defrayed through grants from corporations and international nongovernmental development organizations such as Sight Savers International (United Kingdom) and Orbis International (United States).

Rehabilitation of the blind and visually impaired

In 1991—for the first time anywhere—LVPEI developed a rehabilitation center for the visually impaired on the campus of an ophthalmologic hospital. This program enables adult and pediatric patients to become self-sufficient in their daily living activities (Table 28-2A and B). Parents of blind children are taught to facilitate the normal development of their children. This training is offered on an outpatient basis. Over 48 parents received this service in 1999. The center networks with international organizations to develop an integrated education system for visually handicapped children in public schools. The long-term goal of this division is to establish a series of rehabilitation and vocational training programs for the state that involve other disabilities.

Services in underserved areas

The Institute has initiated several strategies to develop comprehensive coverage for eye care in many underserved areas of the state through the establishment of a separate division. The two major components are the Urban Slum Programs and Rural Outreach Programs (Table 28-3A–C).

The Urban Slum Program is carried out through a vision screening center located in an underserved area of Hyderabad, where a full-time optometrist provides basic refraction and screening services. Last year, approximately 5000 patients were screened at the center. In addition, this center also provides school screening and a community-based rehabilitation program.

The Rural Outreach Program has developed satellite eye centers in remote underserved rural areas to provide comprehensive eye care, including treatment, prevention, and rehabilitation, to a community of 500,000 people. The recognized need for such centers originated within the community itself, and a major philanthropist donated the land and contributed a small grant toward setting them up. This satellite group includes

Table 28-2 A. Services Provided at the Centre for Sight Enhancement, L.V. Prasad Eye Institute, Hyderabad, India

Service Provision	July–December 1997	January–December 1998	January–December 1999
Patients seen	311	1084	1329
Low vision devices dispensed	410	1452	1997

B. Services Provided at the Centre for Rehabilitation of Blind and Visually Impaired, L.V. Prasad Eye Institute, Hyderabad, India

Service Provision	July–December 1997	January–December 1998	January–December 1999
Patients seen	431	1000	1382
Rehabilitation services provided	445	1593	4722

Table 28-3 A. Outpatients and Surgeries at Rural Eye Centre, Mudhol, Adilabad, 1999

Patient Statistics (%)	Paying	Nonpaying	Total
Outpatients	6337 (55.4)	5099 (44.6)	11,436
Surgeries	548 (35.0)	1018 (65.0)	1566

B. Outpatients and Surgeries at Rural Eye Centre, Toodukurthy, Mahaboobnagar, 1999

Patient Statistics (%)	Paying	Nonpaying	Total
Outpatients	7132 (63.5)	4099 (36.5)	11,231
Surgeries	385 (32.4)	803 (67.6)	1188

C. Outpatients Seen at Urban Vision Screening Centre, Ramnagar, Hyderabad, and Surgeries Performed for Referred Patients at L.V. Prasad Eye Institute, Hyderabad, 1999

Patient Statistics (%)	Survey	VST*	Others	Total
Outpatients	3123 (64.3)	256 (5.3)	1474 (30.4)	4853
Surgeries	298 (63.7)	28 (6.0)	142 (30.3)	468

* VST = Vazir Sultan Tobacco Industries, which supports the Vision Screening Centre.

several eye hospitals and the private clinics of individual ophthalmologists. Over 20 programs are presently covered through this strategy. Personnel employed in this program are selected from youth residing in the communities being served.

In addition to providing eye care, these satellites collect epidemiologic information for community eye health planning in Andhra Pradesh and the rest of India and for improving the capacity of these hospitals and clinics to give better quality service and become financially self-sustaining in underprivileged areas of the state and country, as well as study outcomes after surgery. The best models for delivering eye care to the community come from areas where work from this division is undertaken.

Maintaining Quality

Training and performance review

LVPEI has a rigorous program of personnel training and performance review to promote high-quality, patient-oriented service. The Institute promotes continued development of the professional staff by supporting their participation in medical conferences abroad. Risk management and peer review are accomplished through incident reports, mortality and morbidity statistic reviews, and random patient record reviews. Complications are noted and incident reports are completed by the staff. Retrospective analyses of major medical problems are undertaken annually in order to compare institutional outcomes with international standards.

Delivery of care

Patient processing at the Institute is especially sensitive to the needs of the visually impaired. Corridors and walkways are free of impediments and furnishings; "greeters" welcome and escort all patients from their arrival to the completion of their visit. It is a patient-oriented flow: The patient enters a "visiting room," to which all caregivers come. The patient's chart remains in the room so that written communication among members of the team is facilitated. Paying and nonpaying patients are handled in the same manner but are routed through different sections of the facility.

Data collection and implementation of change in patient care

At LVPEI, epidemiologic studies are under way to determine the major ophthalmologic trends of the region. Outcome studies evaluate patient compliance and the effectiveness of patient education after written discharge instructions are reviewed with patients by the nursing staff. Weekly surveys show that compliance by inpatients with discharge instructions is 70%. Positive and negative aspects of the hospital experience are also investigated to make necessary improvements (75% of inpatients and 25% of outpatients return surveys).

Conclusion

In less than 15 years, L.V. Prasad Eye Institute has developed into a world-class eye-care organization in a developing country situation. The critical factors in this development appear to be clear programmatic focus, a well-defined strategic plan, dedicated personnel, and an excellent global support network. LVPEI has succeeded in becoming a model that embodies excellence and equity in eye care in line with the aspirations of global VISION 2020—The Right to Sight program.

CHAPTER 29

Kikuyu Eye Unit

Background

In the 1880s, Presbyterian missionaries in Kenya were dying from malaria at a high rate in their station near the coast. In the 1890s, they moved up to high ground in the area of the Kikuyu tribe, where there was no malaria. The Kikuyu Hospital was founded on its present site in 1894 and today is still the property of the Presbyterian Church of East Africa. A management committee formed from church members and the hospital senior staff runs the hospital. The eye unit, part of the general hospital, was begun in 1978 with funding from Christoffel-Blindenmission (CBM) of Germany, a nongovernmental organization (NGO). Most capital improvements have been made possible by CBM. Since its founding, the Kikuyu Eye Unit (KEU) has tried to provide eye care in all the subspecialties and has gone into the field to do surgery in very basic conditions (Fig 29-1). It is now the largest eye center in Africa outside of South Africa.

Epidemiology

Kenya has a population of 30 million, with 3 million living in the capital city of Nairobi. As 30 of the 45 Kenyan ophthalmologists work in Nairobi, the ratio of ophthalmologists

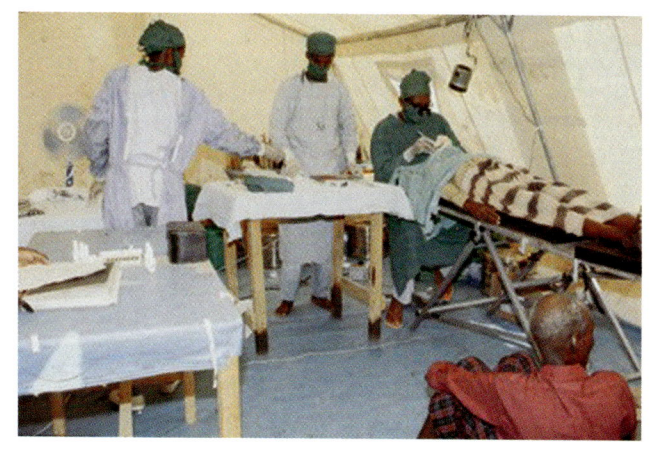

Figure 29-1 Operating in a tent in Dadaab Refugee Camp, in East Africa. *(Photograph courtesy of Mark Wood, MD.)*

to residents in the city is 1:100,000. This means that the ratio of ophthalmologists to the rural Kenyan population is 1:1.8 million. The VISION 2020 global initiative goal is 1 ophthalmologist per 500,000 people.

Half a million patients are examined per year in the country and about 7500 cataract surgeries are carried out, mainly with intraocular lenses (IOLs). There is a backlog of 80,000 patients blind from cataract. The leading cause of blindness in Kenya is cataract (45%), followed by trachoma (16%) and glaucoma (12%). Trachoma is found in the remote areas of northern Kenya. The disease is more common and prevalent in the neighboring country of Sudan. Trauma is common as well and occupies much of ophthalmologists' time and resources. Most ocular trauma results from unsupervised children playing with sticks and stones. Corneal perforations are common, especially in the arid areas of "the bush," where thorn trees frequently injure people herding stock or gathering wood. Onchocerciasis is not seen in Kenya but is common in the surrounding countries of Congo and Sudan.

Ophthalmic Infrastructure

Ophthalmic services in Kenya are coordinated by the Ministry of Health through the National Prevention of Blindness Committee. The Kenya ophthalmic program is headed by the chief government ophthalmologist, and statistical data are collected by the Kenya Society for the Blind.

Government salaries are low, and ophthalmologists rely on their private practices to make a living. There are 10 zones within the country; these roughly follow the provincial administrative boundaries. An ophthalmologist is assigned to each zone. There are also 70 clinical ophthalmic officers, who are posted to provincial and district hospitals.

The University of Nairobi, situated at the Kenyatta National Hospital, is the national referral center. The KEU is the other tertiary referral center. Training for residents and clinical ophthalmic officers is centered at the Kenyatta National Hospital.

Structure of the Kikuyu Eye Unit

The Presbyterian Church of East Africa Kikuyu Hospital is 20 kilometers from Nairobi. The Eye Unit has six examining rooms, all equipped with slit lamps. The outpatient clinic sees 250 to 350 patients per day (75,000 per year). An ophthalmologist runs the daily clinic with the help of clinical officers. A wide variety of diseases is seen, often in advanced stages. Many patients have been blind from cataract for years. Glaucoma patients present late, when they are already blind and treatment is not possible. Retinoblastomas often have extended beyond the globe and produce massive proptosis. Patients with congenital cataracts may have their first ophthalmic assessment at the age of 15 years. The prevalence of diabetes is increasing and its pathology is also usually advanced.

A whole range of other eye diseases is seen in the clinic. There is no subspecialty backup, so the clinic doctor must deal with each case to the best of his or her ability. Patients come long distances for their first ophthalmic assessment and wish to be treated before they journey back. A separate surgical team is available daily in the operating theater to provide treatment for these blind patients who have traveled far from their homes.

The ward has 72 beds, half for men and half for women. A routine cataract patient spends 2 nights in the hospital. Patients are referred from the whole of East Africa and occasionally from West Africa. The hospital offers all services except neurosurgery, CT scanning, and MRI, which are available in Nairobi. Laboratory services are basic, but, again, more comprehensive service is available in Nairobi.

The operating room is large and contains four operating tables (Fig 29-2). This setup allows one consultant surgeon to supervise the other surgeons-in-training or clinical assistants. It is fully equipped for all types of surgery, including vitreoretinal, orbital, lacrimal, penetrating keratoplasty, and oculoplastics.

The low vision department is in a separate building connected by a corridor and has a daily clinic that is run separately from the eye clinic. The optical department is equipped with five lanes for refraction; one has an automatic refractor. The optical shop and workshop are rented to an optical business, whose main outlet is in Nairobi. A contract between the optical company and the Eye Unit allots 15% of optical income to the Eye Unit. The price of glasses is negotiated between the two. Spectacles can be purchased for US$4, but a whole range of more expensive frames is available.

Within the hospital, a 12-room hostel is available for students, who come from all over Africa and abroad for training in ophthalmology.

Eyedrops are produced in the eye unit laboratory by a technician. This laboratory makes 20 different types of eyedrops from imported powders and dispenses 85,000 bottles annually.

A records department keeps patient files on computer; the accounts department is also computerized.

Personnel

The director of the KEU is a Kenyan national. Four ophthalmologists who have had 3 years of postgraduate training at the University of Nairobi Kenyatta National Hospital work in the KEU. In addition, four clinical officers who are ophthalmic assistants are trained in surgery. The clinical officers undergo 3 years of general medical training followed by a year in ophthalmology at the Kenyatta National Hospital. An additional year of training in cataract surgery with lens implantation is available. The clinical officers do most of the screening in the clinic and the routine cataract surgery in the operating theater.

Other clinic personnel include two medical clinical officers and an orthoptist/low vision therapist. The low vision clinic has four therapists trained at KEU. This low vision therapist training program is in the process of gaining formal approval from the Ministry of Education. There is no formal optometry training in Kenya. One optometrist of Indian origin, who trained at L.V. Prasad Eye Institute, Hyderabad, India, works in the KEU with one optometry assistant.

The number of students at KEU varies. There are usually 2 cataract surgeons-in-training (clinical officers), 1 postgraduate ophthalmologist from the University of

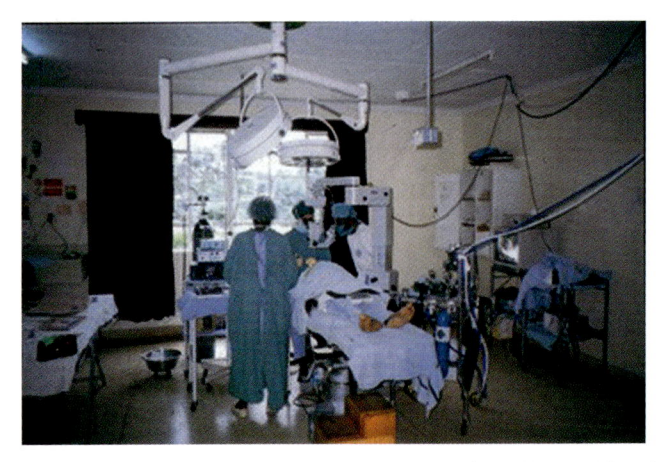

Figure 29-2 Operating theatre in the Kikuyu Eye Unit, part of the Kikuyu Hospital near Nairobi. *(Photograph courtesy of Mark Wood, MD.)*

Nairobi, 2 low vision therapists, 12 eye workers (training to provide screening in outreach programs), and 4 nurses training in the operating theater.

Services by Department

Outpatients

Daily refraction and low vision clinics run concurrently. Because no appointment booking system is available, patients arrive at the clinic and wait. They are seen on a first-come, first-served basis. The clinic closes after the last patient is seen. Because many patients come a great distance to the KEU, follow-up examinations are often not possible.

Surgery

East Africa has very few subspecialty services. The Kikuyu Eye Unit provides vitreoretinal surgery (300 cases per year), corneal transplants (60 cases per year), and oculoplastic surgery, including orbital and lacrimal surgery. The South Florida Eye Bank and the Eye Bank of Missouri send corneal graft tissue. KEU was a country leader in IOL surgery 10 years ago and now runs a program to retrain ophthalmic surgeons who are changing from intracapsular surgery to extracapsular cataract extraction (ECCE) with IOL. Although a phaco machine is available, phacoemulsification is not offered because of the cost of consumables.

Cataract surgery is performed using a manual technique with a linear or continuous curvilinear capsulorrhexis (CCC) and placement of the lens in the bag. At KEU, cataract surgical techniques continue to evolve; lately, the staff has begun using small incision tunnel techniques. Congenital cataract is a common referral at KEU. Intraocular lens surgery has been performed for some years on children with this condition because other methods of aphakic correction were not practical. The KEU congenital cataract surgical technique consists of a CCC with the vitrectomy cutter, lens placement in the bag where possible, with an anterior vitrectomy and posterior capsulotomy. YAG laser is available for treating posterior capsule opacification and iridotomy. A diode laser is used in the operating room and the outpatient clinic for retinal photocoagulation.

Low vision clinic

The low vision clinic was established to deal with childhood blindness and still works predominantly with children. This program is financed by CBM and is the only one in East Africa. There are 7 schools for the blind in Kenya and 19 other schools that have integrated programs for visually impaired children. All these schools are visited regularly by staff from KEU.

Optical department

The optical department refracts 17,000 patients per year and dispenses 12,000 pairs of spectacles. Although this KEU service is provided at a much lower cost than optical services in the private sector, the department is profitable, and the profits are shared with other KEU departments.

Diabetes clinic

The general hospital provides a daily diabetes clinic. All patients with diabetes are screened for diabetic retinopathy in the Eye Unit, and 400 photocoagulation treatments for diabetic retinopathy are performed each year.

Teaching

The National Prevention of Blindness Committee and the University of Nairobi use the KEU staff and facilities to give students in their programs surgical experience and practical training.

Residents spend 6 weeks of their course at KEU, mainly learning cataract surgical skills. Clinical officers learn IOL surgery and refraction. Because there is no recognized optometry school in Kenya, KEU started a 3-month course in refraction for ophthalmic clinical officers, taught by the KEU optometrist. The ophthalmic clinical officers are taught retinoscopy and how to prescribe spherical equivalent lenses. The KEU low vision therapists train assistants for the low vision schools in Kenya. Primary school teachers are taught basic low vision screening techniques at KEU. The ocular pharmacy laboratory trains technicians to reconstitute the imported powder for topical ophthalmic medications. Also, nurses are taught to screen for basic eye diseases, and a course in surgical nursing is offered twice a year.

Fortunately, KEU attracts world-renowned specialists to teach the unit's ophthalmologists and the ophthalmologists from local programs. Moorfields Eye Hospital in London has provided specialists for over 12 years. Specialists in vitreoretinal surgery and oculoplastics come on an annual basis and spend a week operating and teaching. Moorfields also provides ocular pathology services for specimens shipped from KEU. The Australian Embassy recently donated a surgical wet lab, which improves the training of surgeons in current microsurgical techniques.

Research

Research is done in an African context. Clinical research has included studies on IOLs in children, the prophylactic effect of povidone-iodine for ophthalmia neonatorum, penetrating keratoplasty, and assessing the quality of cataract surgery, all published in international journals. The Ophthalmic Society of East Africa meets once a year and publishes a journal. Staff members from KEU participate in these activities.

Outreach

Outreach is a major activity of KEU. A surgical team is in the field every week and serves villages within reasonable distance by road. The outreach techniques used at Aravind Eye Hospital in Madurai, India, and at L.V. Prasad Eye Institute in Hyderabad, India, are being studied and applied in the East African region. Patients seen in outreach clinics less than 100 km from KEU are transported by hired bus to KEU for surgery. This is more efficient than transporting a surgical team to the villages. In addition, surgery in the eye operating room at KEU is of a higher quality. As has been shown in India, the greater the surgical volume, the lower the fixed costs per cataract.

Air transportation is needed to take the team further into the field to areas such as northern Kenya, Somalia, and southern Sudan (Figs 29-3 and 29-4). This service is provided by Mission Aviation Fellowship, which has professional pilots and a large single-engine aircraft that can lift a payload of up to 1000 kg. Flights to Somalia and Sudan can take up to 5 hours and require a stop to refuel. A KEU team of six includes three surgeons who can perform as many as 500 surgeries per week in remote facilities. The team spends up to a week in hospitals, refugee camps, churches, or schools. Serving these underserved regions is not without risk to the team due to political or cultural violence. Tents may be the only shelter for the operating rooms. All equipment, including lights, generators, operating tables, trolleys, and consumables, has to be flown in.

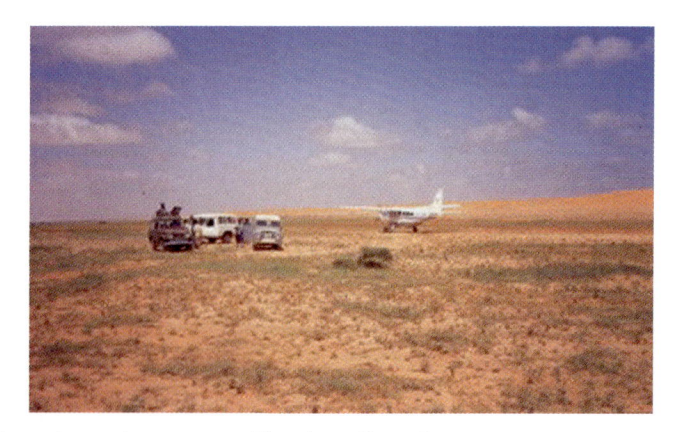

Figure 29-3 Armed security escort at Haradere, Somalia. *(Photograph courtesy of Mark Wood, MD.)*

Finance

KEU earns 75% of its operating budget from patient fees and the sale of spectacles (Table 29-1). New ways are being explored to generate more revenue and become totally independent of outside funding. This means creating higher output to reduce fixed costs per case and exploring the market for better-priced consumables. Patients pay 4500 Ksh (US$50) for cataract surgery with an IOL. Good-quality lenses from India cost US$7 and consumables with the lens cost roughly US$16. This charge to the patient covers most of the cost that the hospital incurs and includes accommodation for 2 nights in the hospital. Patients who cannot pay are provided for by an established fund.

Private patients are accommodated in the system with visible benefits for the extra cost. Private patients pay 25,000 Ksh (US$312).

Christoffel-Blindenmission provides about US$180,000 per year, which goes for salaries, consumables, and capital expenses. The training programs are fully funded by CBM. The original buildings are nearly 100 years old and were built by the Presbyterian Church of East Africa and Asian benefactors. More recently, EZE (Evangelische Zentralstelle fuer Entwicklungshilfe), an organization of the German Protestant church, matched funds from CBM to build the wards, the operating room, and the refraction examination lanes. Several governments with embassies in Kenya, including Canada, Japan, Australia, and Austria, have provided funds for buildings and furnishings. A new waiting area for patients is being built this year from CBM funds. Charitable organizations such as Help Aged, Simavi, and Plan International, as well as individuals and local initiatives, such as

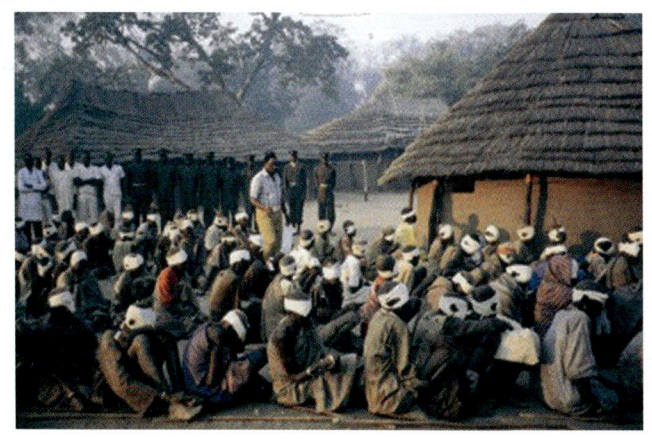

Figure 29-4 Postoperative ward rounds in Billing, southern Sudan. *(Photograph courtesy of Mark Wood, MD.)*

Table 29-1 KEU Audit, 2000

	Kenya Shillings (KSH)	US$
Income	50,915,471	636,443
Expenditures	47,096,258	588,703
Net Surplus	3,819,212	47,740

the Christmas craft fair, Kenya Charity Sweepstake, and schools and service clubs, have all helped to buy equipment, pay patient fees, and sponsor eye camps. These fund-raising activities require that proposals be written and many meetings held with donors.

Christoffel-Blindenmission

Apart from the input by local governments, CBM is the most important agency in ophthalmology in Africa. Outside Germany, CBM is known as Christian Blind Mission International. It is the largest aid organization for visual disabilities in the world and has input into the World Health Organization and the International Association for the Prevention of Blindness. Finance for KEU's capital developments rely on this source. CBM has about 60 projects in East Africa (Fig 29-5). It has built hospitals near the capital cities of Nairobi, Kenya (KEU); Kampala, Uganda (Mengo Hospital); and Dar es Salaam, Tanzania (CCBRT Disability Hospital).

Conclusion

Although KEU is not comparable to eye units in the developed world, it is a leader in comprehensive eye care in the region. Ideas and methods from the developed world are being introduced where possible, and KEU has been at the forefront of these local developments in East Africa.

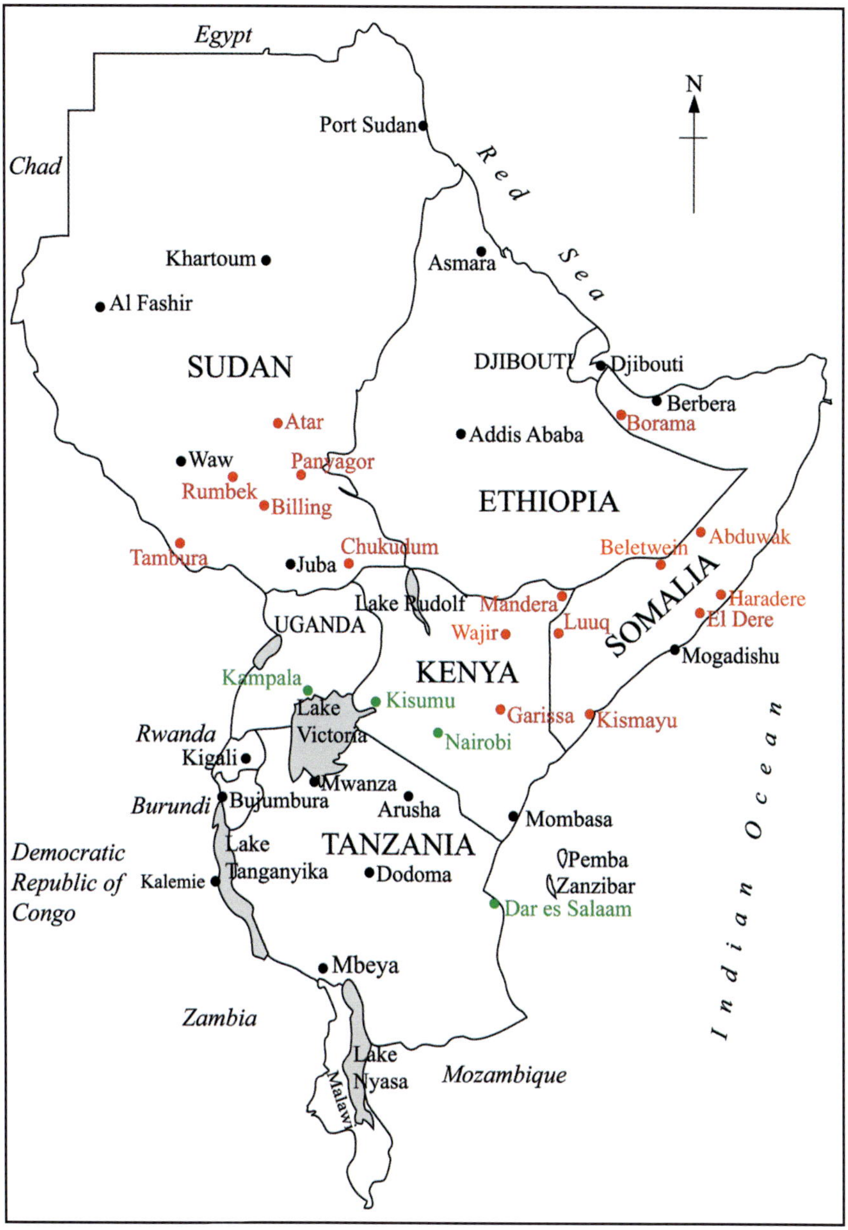

CHAPTER 29: Kikuyu Eye Unit • 319

Figure 29-5 Eye hospitals built by CBM (shown in green) and KEU outreach camps sponsored by CBM (shown in red). Flights to the outreach camps are organized by Mission Aviation Fellowship. *(Courtesy of Mark Wood, MD.)*

CHAPTER 30

Cataract Care in Brazil and Peru

Background

Cataract-free zone (CFZ) projects were established in 1986 to define vision impairment in selected communities of Brazil and Peru. In addition, programs to address the increasing problem of avoidable vision impairment due to cataract and uncorrected refractive error were started in selected regions of these countries. In 1989, the good results of the CFZ projects in Brazil and Peru led to the creation of CFZ projects in nine additional Latin American countries.

Brazil

Magnitude of the Problem

In Brazil, an estimated 0.4%–0.5% of the population has vision that is <20/400. With a total population of 160 million, the estimated number of people with vision <20/400 is approximately 640,000–800,000. Brazil is a large country with continental dimensions, and the economy and quality of health care vary greatly among different regions. In more developed areas, the estimated prevalence of blindness (<20/400) is as low as 0.25%. In poorer, or less developed, areas, the estimated prevalence of <20/400 vision is 0.75%.

Most CFZ programs and projects use visual acuity of <20/100 in the better eye as the definition of vision impairment. The common causes of vision impairment differ between children and adults. The most important causes of vision impairment for adults in Brazil are cataract, uncorrected refractive error, glaucoma, and retinal diseases. For children, the common causes of vision impairment are congenital cataract, infection (especially toxoplasmosis), uncorrected refractive error, and retinopathy of prematurity. Approximately 50% of the known cases of congenital cataract in Brazil are caused by infections, with rubella the most common cause. Other important worldwide causes of vision impairment such as trachoma, onchocerciasis, and vitamin A deficiency are endemic only in localized areas of South America.

Cataract causes 40%–50% of the cases of vision impairment in Brazil. It is estimated that 500,000 patients need cataract surgery each year. Uncorrected refractive error accounts for another 40% of vision impairment. Other causes include glaucoma, retinal disorders (diabetic retinopathy, age-related macular disease), and corneal infections.

Backlog of Unoperated Cataract

There is a large backlog of patients with cataract in Brazil. The reasons for the backlog include fear of the surgery, logistical barriers, inability to pay, social causes, and religious beliefs. The majority of people in Brazilian CFZ projects with vision impairment due to cataract (69%) report that financial difficulties are the principal reason they have not had surgery done. However, there are other reasons, including the patient's impression that he or she has adequate vision (even though vision is less than 20/100 in the better eye), poor access to ophthalmologists (usually because of distance), lack of friends or family to provide transportation, and the fear of becoming blind due to cataract surgery.

Getting an appointment to see an ophthalmologist is a great challenge. The public health system is prepared to receive these patients in only a few public health clinics. The distances between patient and clinic may be great. After the first ophthalmic assessment determines that cataract surgery is indicated, a hospital appointment takes some months. An average of seven visits to the eye clinic is required before a patient has cataract surgery. Getting back and forth to the clinic is a major barrier for many patients.

As in other countries, the prevalence of cataract increases with age in Brazil. It is projected that the population over 50 years of age will increase 4 times by the year 2020. This means the number of people blind from cataract will increase in a similar proportion unless the health care system dramatically increases the cataract surgical rate.

Public Health System and Available Eye Care

The public health system in Brazil is free for the entire population. It is estimated that only 30% of the population can afford private health insurance, leaving 112 million people who depend on the public health care system. The annual budget for public health is US$10 billion, or approximately US$90 per person. Developed countries like Japan, Canada, and France spend US$1000–1500 per person per year on health care.

Brazil has about 8000 ophthalmologists (1:20,000 people). The vast majority of these—perhaps as many as 95%—practice in the cities; people who live in rural areas travel to the city closest to them for eye care. In the past 3 decades, the population has shifted so that two thirds or more now live in urban areas.

More than 50% of Brazilian ophthalmologists perform cataract surgery. In most cases, use of the facilities (equipment and operating rooms) and staff dedicated to cataract surgery is inefficient. A rational and more effective application of resources is needed to increase the number of patients and thus reduce the cost per surgery. Once cataract surgical services can accommodate more patients, the number of appointments available for eye care in the public health posts must be increased.

Most private hospitals provide health care services for the 48 million people with private health insurance. However, many of the private hospitals also provide contract services for the public system. Approximately 3500 ophthalmologists participate in the cataract program of the public system. Both systems must improve efficiencies in the use of human and material resources.

Personnel Training

One way to increase efficiency is to train more technicians and staff. Campinas, one of the most developed cities in Brazil, has two university hospitals and a large number of public health centers. The University of Campinas (UNICAMP) pioneered a 2-month course for ophthalmic technicians with high school diplomas in 1990. This course is now offered 4 times a year and has trained about 400 people, virtually all of whom work in cities. Only 10% of these technicians work for the national program. In addition, a 2-day course for currently employed ophthalmic personnel designed to improve basic ophthalmic skills has been attended by almost 2000 eye-care workers.

Cataract-Free Zone Projects: Peru and Brazil

In 1986, the cataract-free zone project was started in Chimbote, Peru, and Campinas, Brazil. The first phase was to determine the number of people blind from cataract in each city and the accessibility to cataract surgery in those cities, and a door-to-door census was carried out. The results in both cities were similar: 50% of vision impairment was caused by cataract. Soon after the census, 133 patients in Chimbote and 97 patients in Campinas had cataract surgery. Of the 97 patients in Campinas, 85% achieved 20/40 vision. After the census and the implementation of an improved process that enabled patients to receive an ophthalmic assessment near their home and undergo surgery within 30 days, the cataract surgical rate increased from 58% to 82% in these cities.

CFZ projects clearly showed that reducing cataract blindness was possible. They also helped Peru and Brazil understand what was needed in terms of cataract care. The original door-to-door survey method, for example, was found to be costly, especially in terms of personnel and time.

Recently, other CFZ projects have used a "self-test" for visual acuity screening, with a retest at health centers to select which patients are to be examined (Fig 30-1). A complete CFZ operational method, including every detail of the campaign, was determined prior to testing. The self-vision test consisted of a Snellen 0.2 line (20/100) of print and was distributed widely within the CFZ. People who failed to recognize the 0.2 acuity line when wearing glasses were asked to go to a public health center.

The local health center, which also conducts the annual national immunization program, was used for visual acuity screening and for a first assessment by an ophthalmic technician (Fig 30-2). A trained ophthalmic technician measures the visual acuity in those people who have failed the self-test. Anyone with visual acuity less than 0.2 (20/100) in the better eye is sent the same day by bus or van to an eye examination center to be examined by an ophthalmic team that includes ophthalmologists, ophthalmology residents, medical students, nurses, and technicians. A 40-member ophthalmic team provides ophthalmic assessment for the number of people failing the screening test per 100,000 population. The eye examination center uses equipment borrowed from the university, including a slit lamp, indirect and direct ophthalmoscopes, A-scan biometry, and autokeratometer/refractor. The team carries out these assessments working 1 weekend in each region or city. Their visit is preceded by mass media announcements of the importance of visual acuity tests.

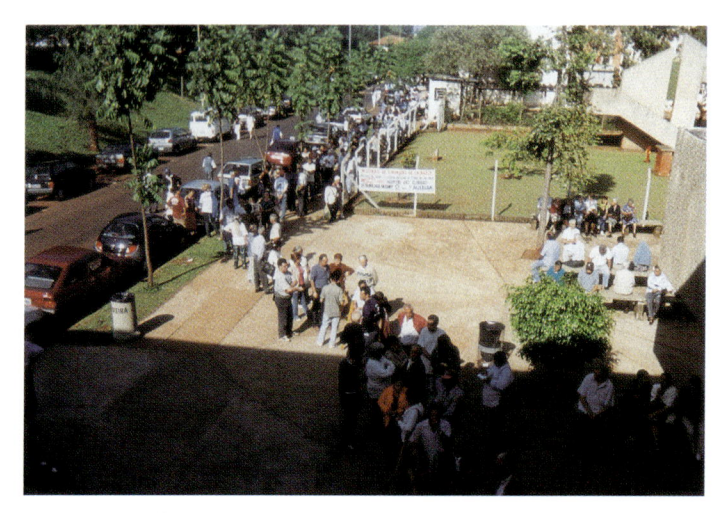

Figure 30-1 Waiting line of a CFZ project in Campinas, Brazil. *(Photograph courtesy of Newton Kara José, MD.)*

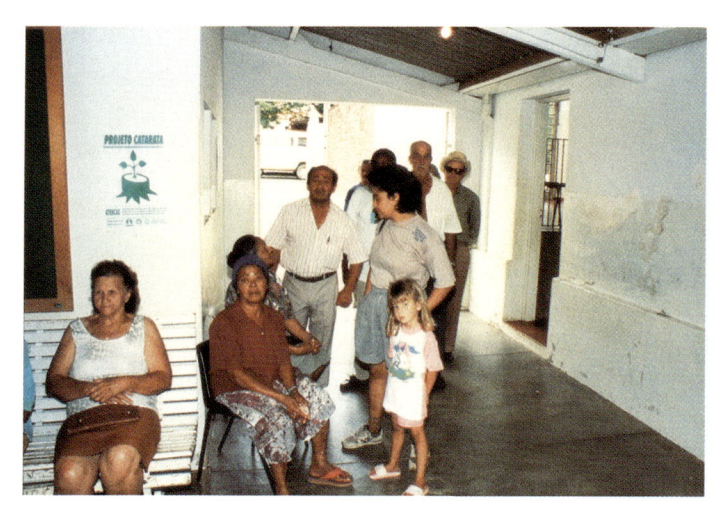

Figure 30-2 Patients waiting to be examined at a health clinic in a CFZ project in São Paulo State, Brazil. *(Photograph courtesy of Newton Kara José, MD.)*

Peru

Since 1986, many CFZ projects have been carried out in Peru with the support and active participation of the involved communities. Each project begins with selection of a community based on a number of factors: projected number of patients needing surgery, distance from a health center, and other logistical concerns (Fig 30-3). Then a technician from the selected community is sent to the Instituto Nacional de Ojos (National Institute of Ophthalmology) to be trained in activities related to primary eye care. Upon returning to the community, the technician begins to screen potential cataract patients. An ophthalmology resident from the National Institute of Ophthalmology goes to the com-

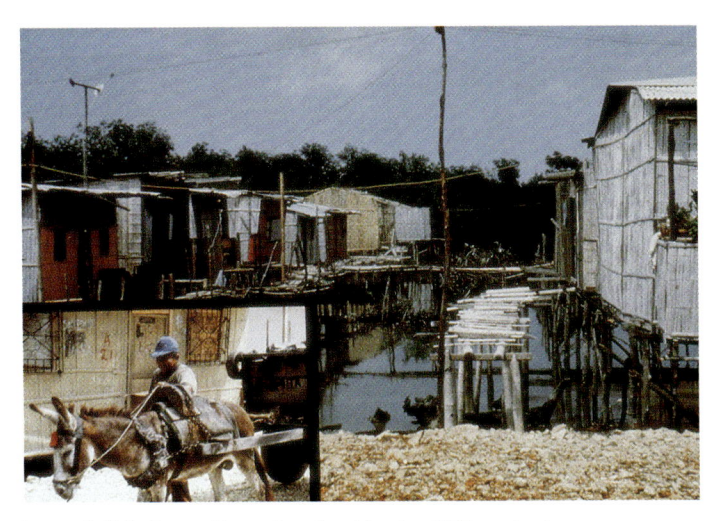

Figure 30-3 Area of Chimbote, Peru, involved in the CFZ project. *(Photograph courtesy of Francisco Contreras, MD.)*

munity to examine those selected by the technician. One week later, a surgical team, including a third-year resident and an ophthalmologist from the National Institute of Ophthalmology staff, come to the community to perform the surgeries (Fig 30-4).

The surgical procedures are performed in the community health center of the ministry of health or occasionally in established local surgical facilities. The ophthalmology resident remains in the area for 1 week providing postsurgical follow-up care. Most projects also have follow-up eye examinations 3 months after surgery by the staff of the National Institute of Ophthalmology.

The Peruvian Society of Ophthalmology has established the Group of Prevention of Blindness. This group organizes workshops and seminars to increase the cataract surgical rates and to improve and evaluate the results of the surgeries.

An effort has been made in Peru to increase the number of ophthalmologists involved in community CFZ campaigns by recruiting ophthalmologists and health auxiliaries and training them in the operational methods used in CFZ projects.

Brazil

CFZ projects have reduced barriers to cataract surgery for people in the selected communities in Brazil. Usually surgery is booked within 30 days of the first ophthalmic assessment, compared to 7 to 10 clinic visits at regular health centers in Brazil.

The results of 10 years of CFZ projects involving the State University of Campinas (UNICAMP) include 74 projects that have screened a total of 3,075,600 people. Of the 405,048 people over 50 years of age and considered at risk of cataract, complete eye examinations, including visual acuity measurement, refraction, biomicroscopy, indirect ophthalmoscopy, and applanation tonometry, were performed in 11,462. Uncorrected refractive errors were found to cause vision impairment in 5447 (47.52%) of the patients. These people received lens prescriptions and, in most cases, free glasses. Symptomatic cataract was observed in 2704 patients (25.23%). Another 23% had cataract coexisting

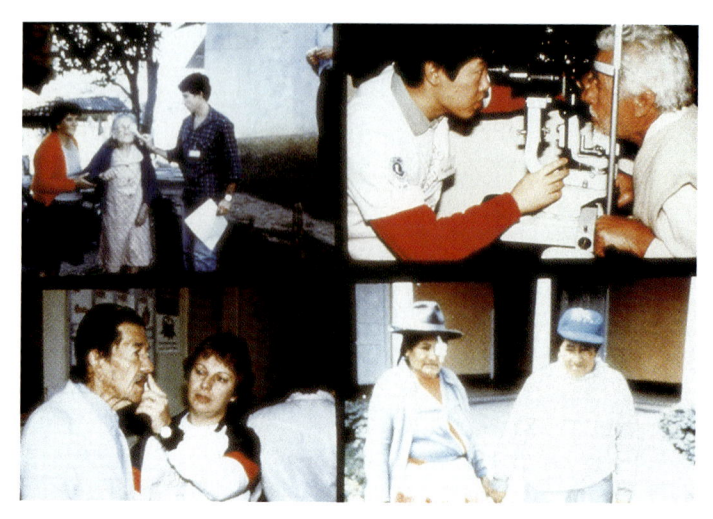

Figure 30-4 Health care workers and patients in the CFZ project in Chimbote, Peru. *(Photograph courtesy of Francisco Contreras, MD.)*

with other eye diseases. The remaining 5.65% had other eye diseases causing impaired vision.

Patient compliance and follow-up attendance is a major problem in patients with vision impairment. A survey at a UNICAMP glaucoma clinic showed that 67% of the patients are lost to follow-up. Poverty is a major barrier to patients with uncorrected refractive error. Another study found that 30% of those who received a prescription for glasses did not fill the prescription because of financial limitations. Glasses may cost up to 37% of an individual's salary. Since 1994, UNICAMP has operated a dispensing shop to provide glasses at low or no cost to the majority of patients who receive prescriptions. This shop is subsidized in part by the national health system, the hospital budget, and donations from the optical industry.

More than 35,000 cataract operations have been performed in Campinas at the outpatient operating rooms, the university hospital, and the satellite units in the last 10 years. UNICAMP serves as a referral center for 4 million people living in 90 cities. The opening of two satellite units has provided a secondary level of eye-care services capable of treating 94% of the population's eye-care needs. Since 1989, one of these units, located in the city of Divinolandia, has improved access to eye-care treatment for 14 cities. This satellite system is an example of the efficient and sustainable service working within the public health system. Here, third-year residents, working with a staff ophthalmologist and trained allied health personnel, attend and treat most common eye problems, including performing surgery from 7 AM to 7 PM 5 days a week.

The CFZ model of selecting patients for surgery has spread to most parts of Brazil since the program began.

Surgical Techniques

Extracapsular cataract extraction (ECCE) technique is the most common cataract surgery in Brazil and Peru. Phacoemulsification is performed by less than 25% of surgeons. For much of South America, the use of phacoemulsification is limited by the necessity to learn new surgical techniques, the initial capital cost of the equipment, and the disposable costs in every case. Currently, it may be more appropriate to continue using the extracapsular technique as standard because of the limited budget of the health system. Close to 100% of patients in Brazil receive a posterior chamber IOL.

National Campaigns

In 1998, a Brazilian national campaign for the prevention of blindness via cataract surgery was coordinated by the Brazilian Council of Ophthalmology. As a result of the work of 2000 ophthalmologists, about 30,000 patients had their vision restored either by surgery or by correction of refractive errors with free glasses. In 1999, due to the success of the 1998 campaign and a better understanding of population needs, the minister of health agreed to support a new project to increase the number of cataract surgeries. The patients were examined either during CFZ weekend projects or during routine examinations in health centers. In some communities where there was a waiting list of patients, those people waiting in line were examined and treated. More than 3500 private practice ophthalmologists performed 142,000 cataract surgeries in 1999. In the public sector, about 250,000 cataract surgeries were done in 1999, a 215% increase over the previous 2 years.

The results of this large campaign show what can be accomplished by communities, the government, and ophthalmologists working as a team. Most of these ophthalmologists are not employees of the public system. Although they do not receive payment for the eye examinations, assessment, and selection of cataract patients, they are reimbursed for each surgery. In the cataract campaign of 2000, payment for each surgery was about US$220, which covered the IOL, other consumables, and a surgeon's honorarium.

Supporting Organizations and Agencies

CFZ projects in Brazil and Peru have had assistance from a number of organizations and agencies. These include the National Eye Institute of Bethesda, Helen Keller International, Brazilian Lions Clubs, Peru Lions International, Operation Eyesight Universal, SEE International, the State University of Campinas (UNICAMP), Consejo Nacional de Salud de Peru, community associations, service clubs, religious groups, and other universities.

Additional assistance has come from the Peruvian Ministry of Health; the Instituto Nacional de Ojos; and, in rural areas, Operluce and Oprece Eye Clinic of Lima, Peru.

Future Programs

In order to effect a long-term solution to the problem of vision impairment and to use the available resources optimally for the entire population, a long-range national program is needed to replace these individual campaigns. In Brazil, these campaigns have been useful in decreasing the number of people with vision impairment due to cataract in localized areas of the country and in showing the necessity of establishing a broad nationwide eye-care program. A national ophthalmic program is expected to be implemented to provide eye care, mainly cataract surgery, refraction and glasses for children and adults, treatment of diabetic retinopathy, and low vision services. The program is to include a quality-control system for monitoring these services.

As 70% of the Brazilian population cannot afford a private health plan, most of the population depends on the public health system. The budget for this system for the 2000 campaign was US$50 million, a significant amount of money in Brazil, which has provided adequate funding to accomplish meaningful eye-care delivery objectives.

Conclusion

Cataract-free zone projects have increased the number of cataract surgeries, reduced the barriers to eye care, improved utilization of eye-care services, and restored vision to hundreds of thousands of people in Central and South America. National programs are needed to further reduce barriers to the surgery. Such programs should encompass the educational, logistic, and efficiency aspects of eye examinations and surgery. Refraction and low-cost glasses should be included. Efficient measures must be implemented to reduce the backlog of visually impaired people. Education on the prevention of blindness, improving access to cataract surgery, and correcting refractive error are important ways to reduce the number of people with vision impairment.

> Angra SK, Murthy GV, Gupta SK, et al. Cataract related blindness in India and its social implications. *Indian J Med Res.* 1997;106:312–324.
> Contreras F. Cataract-free zone in Latin America. *Am J Ophthalmol.* 1990;110:203–204.
> José NK, Contreras F, Campos MA, et al. Screening and surgical intervention results from cataract-free-zone project in Campinas, Brazil, and Chimbote, Peru. *Int Ophthalmol.* 1990;14:155–164.
> Kara José N, Almeida GV, Alves MR, et al. Campanha Nacional de prevenção de cegueira e reabilitação visual do idoso. *Rev Med, São Paulo.* 1997;76:293–328.
> Kupfer C. Worldwide prevention of blindness [editorial]. *Am J Ophthalmol.* 1983;96:543–545.
> Leite Arieta CE, José NK, Carvalho Filho DM, et al. Optimization of a university cataract-patient care service in Campinas, Brazil. *Ophthalmic Epidemiol.* 1999;6:113–123.
> Négrel AD, Minassian DC, Sayek F. Blindness and low vision in southeast Turkey. *Ophthalmic Epidemiol.* 1996;3:127–134.
> Senne FMB. Resultado da criação de um banco de óculos e laboratório óptico no serviço satélite de oftalmologia da Unicamp em Divinolândia, SP. *Arq Bras Oftalm.* 1994;57:225.
> Steinkuller PG. Cataract: the leading cause of blindness and vision loss in Africa. *Soc Sci Med.* 1983;17:1693–1702.
> Thylefors B, Négrel AD, Pararajasegaram R, et al. Global data on blindness. *Bull World Health Organ.* 1995;73:115–121.
> Tielsch JM, Javitt JC, Coleman A, et al. The prevalence of blindness and visual impairment among nursing home residents in Baltimore. *N Engl J Med.* 1995;332:1205–1209.

CHAPTER 31

Cataract Management in Developing Countries

Background

Worldwide, it is estimated that 180 million people are visually impaired. Of these, some 45 million are blind, 80% avoidably so. Cataract is a major cause of avoidable blindness, accounting for about 50%. More than 90% of the unoperated backlog of those who are blind with cataract is found in the developing nations. In these countries, the majority of cataract blind—sometimes over 90%—live in rural areas. It is here that the impediments to the delivery of good-quality cataract surgery are greatest.

With an increasing and aging world population, if the present number of cataract surgeries is maintained, the number of cataract blind will double in the next 20 years. However, the International Agency for the Prevention of Blindness/World Health Organization's collaborative global initiative, VISION 2020—The Right to Sight, aims to eliminate preventable and curable blindness by 2020. Cataract intervention is a priority.

> Brian G, Taylor H. Cataract blindness—challenges for the 21st century. *Bull World Health Organ.* 2001;79:249–256.
> Resnikoff S, Pararajasegaram R. Blindness prevention programmes: past, present, and future. *Bull World Health Organ.* 2001;79:222–226.

Too frequently, the overwhelming number of cataract blind has engendered the view that surgical intervention in itself is sufficient. However, an intervention that fails to restore vision, whether because of poor patient selection, surgical complication, or uncorrected significant refractive error, may just as well have not occurred. Such a result is worse than doing nothing: It consumes resources and is an opportunity lost. The aim must be to increase the number of surgeries completed and, simultaneously, to improve the vision outcome.

Ophthalmologists from developed countries, as "medical tourists," operating on a few selected cases in developing countries, may meet the need for good-quality surgery but frequently create more problems for the local medical services than they solve. For example, community expectations may be raised, creating conflict between the community and resident health care workers, who lack the skills and resources to meet the raised expectations after the "medical tourists" have departed. The important aspects of preoperative patient selection and postoperative care may be overshadowed during a short visit by these ophthalmologists by time devoted to the transfer of surgical skills. The resident health care workers may be ill-prepared to recognize or manage postoperative complications, which usually lead to adverse outcomes. An efficient exchange of ideas among "medical tourists," resident health care workers, and patients requires fluency in the local language or the presence of a competent translator. The surgical act is only a small part of any successful, sustainable cataract blindness initiative.

Any intervention, for cataract or the other major blinding conditions, must be seen in a broad context: health as a development tool, development aid, health project management, and so forth. To have even a remote chance of any significant and lasting impact—to help realize the aims of VISION 2020—an intervention must draw in many professional disciplines and resources. Surgeons, nurses, and administrators must be trained and have ongoing professional development. Equipment purchase, maintenance, and replacement must be organized. There must be ongoing ordering and supply of consumables. Financial sustainability through cost recovery must be secured. Patient cross-subsidization mechanisms need to be implemented to allow the very poor equitable access to care. Management capability must be developed. Members of the recipient community must be involved in conceiving the idea and planning its development. Through implementation and delivery of high-quality health care services, members of the recipient community must acquire ownership of the project. Of necessity, all of this can only be the product of donor/recipient consultation, often prolonged and intense. Integration and coordination of all these aspects and more are required to develop a successful, sustainable cataract blindness intervention.

> Brian G. Bringing the benefits of cataract surgery to the Third World. In: Spaeth GL, ed. Ocular surgery for the new millennium. Part II. *Ophthalmology Clin North Am.* 2000;13: 141–150.

Surgical Management of Cataract

To date, in addressing the problem of developing world cataract blindness, the international ophthalmic community has largely concentrated on the technicalities of the required surgery. Even in the late 1980s, many believed the status quo of intracapsular cataract extraction with aphakic spectacles sufficient for the needs of the developing world. However, some argued for no less a surgical intervention than was available elsewhere: extracapsular cataract extraction (ECCE) with posterior chamber lens implantation.

> Brian G, Beaumont J, Hollows F, et al. Intraocular lens implantation: a model for the Third World. *Aust N Z J Ophthalmol.* 1988;16:321–324.
> Brian GR, Hollows F. Pharmaceutical production and intraocular lens implantation: technology appropriate to the Third World. *Ophthalmic Surg.* 1989;20:820–822.
> Ruit S, Brian G, Hollows F. On the practicalities of eye camp cataract extraction and intraocular lens implantation in Nepal. *Ophthalmic Surg.* 1990;21:862–865.

Much of the discussion concerned the perceived impediments to providing routine posterior chamber intraocular lens implantation. As an advocate for this surgery on the grounds of vision outcome and equity issues, an Australian not-for-profit, nongovernmental development aid organization, The Fred Hollows Foundation, sought to identify and remedy these impediments. The first was the availability of good-quality, low-cost posterior chamber intraocular lenses.

In the mid-1990s, the Foundation built lens-manufacturing facilities in Eritrea and Nepal to produce lenses certified to the quality standards required in industrialized markets. By producing lenses at less than US$10, the facilities have contributed to a general market price reduction for this product and improved implant availability. In addition to their role in cataract management, the factories are examples of good manufacturing practice for other industries in the developing world. They also generate export income for these two countries, with the profits supporting blindness prevention.

In collaboration with Australian business, the Foundation has also developed a coaxial surgical microscope and YAG laser. These high-quality, low-cost robust devices are suitable for extracapsular cataract surgery and its attendant posterior capsule opacification. They can be transported safely in sturdy cases.

> Combe R, Watkins R, Brian G. Evaluation of the quality of generic polymethylmethacrylate intraocular lenses marketed in India. *Clin Experiment Ophthalmol.* 2001;29:64–67.
>
> Moran D, Gillies M, Brian G, et al. Low-cost intraocular lenses for cataract patients. *Lancet.* 1997;349:885–886.

Publication of rigorous assessments of developing world cataract surgery outcomes is uncommon. Postoperative vision results are frequently not as good and the complication rates are often greater than published data from the developed world. For example, a study of urban Indian surgery showed 21% of patients had a very poor outcome (presenting visual acuity of <20/200), with another 35% having poor outcome (20/60 to 20/200). In neighboring Nepal, which did a national blindness survey in 1981 and has had sizeable training and service inputs since, 21% also present postoperatively with visual acuity of <20/200 in both eyes. This improves to 7% with best correction.

> Dandona L, Dandona R, Naduvilath TJ, et al. Population-based assessment of the outcome of cataract surgery in an urban population in southern India. *Am J Ophthalmol.* 1999;127:650–658.
>
> Pokharel GP, Selvaraj S, Ellwein LB. Visual functioning and quality of life outcomes among cataract operated and unoperated blind populations in Nepal. *Br J Ophthalmol.* 1998;82:606–610.

Recently, an international cataract surgical standard has evolved. This consists of a complete preoperative eye examination, highly magnified cataract surgery using an operating microscope, a posterior chamber intraocular lens, and postoperative care that includes refraction.

The Fred Hollows Foundation System of Cataract Management

The Fred Hollows Foundation strives to develop systems of cataract management that deliver large-volume cataract surgery with good vision rehabilitation outcomes, fulfilling the aims of VISION 2020. In each country where the Foundation works—including

Nepal, Vietnam, China, Pakistan, and Eritrea—it seeks agreement concerning the responsibilities and expectations of government departments, national blindness prevention committees, and other interested agencies. These "country agreements" are the basis on which long-term relationships are forged at all levels. After they are signed, work starts.

The program offered to each country varies according to local circumstances, but it may consist of surgical and management training, supply of start-up capital equipment, and help in setting up of surgical audit, consumables resupply, and cost-recovery mechanisms.

Surgical training is given in the standardized Foundation procedure for ECCE with in-the-bag placement of a posterior chamber intraocular lens. This technique, based on considerable experience in Asia, avoids the high costs of overinstrumentation and expensive consumables, produces good-quality results, and is presented in the Foundation's standard operating procedure manuals and a video. This surgical training is provided during an initial intensive course, at which trainees get considerable experience in a short period. Where possible, local surgeons, previously trained by the Foundation, are used as teachers.

The surgeons are also reminded of the need to assess results and maintain surgical quality. They are instructed in surgical audit through the proper use of data collection and evaluation, using the Foundation's surgical tracking cards.

> Brian G, Ruit S, ul Mulk MK, et al. An approach to cataract surgery in the Third World (with Appendix 1). *Operative Techniques in Cataract and Refractive Surgery.* 2000;3:184–198.

At the conclusion of the initial course, which also emphasizes preoperative assessment, postoperative care, patient flow, and operating room management, most participants are sufficiently confident with straightforward cases of senile cataract that they are able to practice what they have learned when they return to their home facilities. They use a Foundation microscope and standard sets of surgical instruments selected by the Foundation for quality, cost, and suitability for the surgical technique taught. These are donated by the Foundation, as is a cache of intraocular lenses to prime cost recovery with profit generation to meet ongoing expenses. Initially, standard power intraocular lenses are used, but later an A-scan may be purchased and lenses individualized to improve the uncorrected postoperative vision.

> Connell B, Brian G, Bond MJ. A case-control study of biometry in healthy and cataractous Eritrean eyes. *Ophthalmic Epidemiol.* 1997;4:151–155.

Operating room nurses attend the initial training courses with their surgeons. This is seen as an opportunity to build a team approach. Tuition is given for training in microscope maintenance and trouble shooting and instrument handling, cleaning, and maintenance. Hospital administrators receive training in management issues concerning inventory maintenance and service sustainability through cost recovery. Help is given to identify suppliers of low-priced consumables.

After the initial course, the teachers make follow-up visits at varying intervals to each of the hospitals to which the "cataract teams" (surgeon, nurse, administrator) have returned. They use this opportunity to monitor surgical performance, as well as data and cost-recovery management skills. Supplementary training is given as requested and required.

> Ruit S, Brian G, Moran D, et al. Cataract intervention in the developing world: knock-on development through mentoring hospitals. *Clin Experiment Ophthalmol.* 2000;28:71–72.

Does This Deliver?

Cost estimates for cataract surgery vary, depending largely on local practice. For example, patient food and bed costs may be included where ambulatory surgery is not used, and vehicle expenses may figure in calculations for eye camps. In 1994, the unit cost for cataract surgery in an Indian eye camp was reported as US$23 and as US$56 (US$60 with IOL) for an African institution.

> Guillemot de Liniers F, Resnikoff S, Huguet P, et al. The cost of the surgical treatment of cataracts at the African Institute of Tropical Ophthalmology (Bamako, Mali). [Article in French] *Santé.* 1994;4:275–279.
>
> Murthy GV, Sharma P. Cost analysis of eye camps and camp-based cataract surgery. *Nat Med J India.* 1994;7:111–114.

A comprehensive analysis of the costs at two cataract surgery facilities in Nepal was undertaken by the Foundation. One was a metropolitan teaching facility with a large surgical load and extensive instrumentation. The other was a smaller volume provincial institution with meager equipment, more typical of the developing world. This study revealed total unit surgery costs of US$45 and US$13, respectively, including a US$6.60 intraocular lens.

Through the efforts of The Fred Hollows Foundation and others, there has been a substantial reduction in surgery costs due to cheaper consumables and economies associated with increased efficiencies. In addition, at the Nepalese metropolitan cataract surgery facility, high-quality cataract surgical outcomes have increased the demand for surgery by the middle classes, which has resulted in institutional profit. This profit pays facility, equipment, and consumables costs, as well as cross-subsidizing surgery for the poor. Thus, in 1998, 51% of patients paid US$88 and 7% paid US$58 for an operation costing US$45. The profit from these groups allowed 7% of patients to be charged US$29, with 33% receiving free surgery.

> McDonald MA. A cost recovery exercise in Nepal. In: Pararajasegaram R, Rao GN, eds. *World Blindness and Its Prevention.* Vol 6. Hyderabad, India: International Agency for the Prevention of Blindness; 2001:237–251.

Extracapsular cataract extraction with intraocular lens surgical outcomes are good and improving. A prospective, nonrandomized trial compared results at 2 months postsurgery for a Foundation partner's urban facility and for one of its remote rural eye camps, both in Nepal. The study involved 62 patients (100% follow-up) and 189 patients (91% follow-up), respectively. The urban center achieved 87% corrected visual acuity of 20/60 or better, compared with 74% of the eye camp cases.

> Ruit S, Tabin GC, Nissman SA, et al. Low-cost high-volume extracapsular cataract extraction with posterior chamber intraocular lens implantation in Nepal. *Ophthalmology.* 1999;106: 1887–1892.

There has been a shift in surgical culture in some countries in Asia. For example, in Vietnam, where The Fred Hollows Foundation has provided training courses, work by local partners has increased the cataract surgical rate fivefold in a decade. Extracapsular extraction with posterior chamber intraocular lens insertion is now the standard cataract procedure in Vietnam and Nepal. The same is increasingly true for some countries in Africa.

Through the use of tracking cards, outcome data are being collected and scrutinized. The result has been better patient care and informed surgical innovation. An example in Nepal is Tilganga Eye Centre's manual, smaller incision, sutureless cataract extraction technique. It uses only standard extracapsular instrumentation, without anterior chamber maintainer or routine viscoelastic. In a review of 362 consecutive completed sutureless surgeries at Tilganga, uncorrected distance visual acuity during the third to eighth postoperative week was available on 266 patients (73%); 10, 145, 101, and 10 had acuities of better than 20/30, 20/30 to 20/60, 20/80 to 20/200, and worse than 20/200, respectively. Of the 276 patients (76%) with recorded corrected distance acuity, 97, 165, 12, and 2 were in the same groups. Comparing postoperative to preoperative corneal astigmatism for each patient with postoperative information available (208), without regard to axis, the amplitude of astigmatism worsened by a mean of 0.94 D (± 0.17; 95% confidence; ± 1.23 standard deviation; 7.5 D maximum worsening; 2.5 D maximum improvement). As is often the case with developing country studies, these results are weakened by the failure of patients to return for follow-up and by incompletely recorded data.

Following an eye camp in Sikkim, 102 cases of completed ECCE with posterior chamber intraocular lens insertion were reviewed 1 month after surgery. Of these, 38 (37%) were by the Tilganga sutureless technique. A statistically significant difference (χ^2, 7 df; $\alpha = 0.05$, but not 0.01) between the unaided visual acuities for the sutureless (76% at 20/60 or better, with 5% at 20/200 or worse) and sutured groups (44% at 20/60 or better, with 17% at 20/200 or worse) was observed, with the latter performed by surgeons relatively new to the technique.

> Brian G, Ruit S, ul Mulk MK, et al. An approach to cataract surgery in the Third World (with Appendix 2). *Operative Techniques in Cataract and Refractive Surgery.* 2000;3:184–202.
> Ruit S, Paudyal G, Gurung R, et al. An innovation in developing world cataract surgery: sutureless extracapsular cataract extraction with intraocular lens implantation. *Clin Experiment Ophthalmol.* 2000;28:274–279.

Conclusion

Working with local partners in Asia and Africa, The Fred Hollows Foundation has developed a comprehensive approach for cataract management. This has not been without problems and local failures. However, through technical innovation and skill transfer, the cost of cataract surgery has been reduced and both the surgical quantity and outcome quality have been increased. With this input and the continuing hard work of local partners, self-sustaining programs of cataract management exist.

As of October 2001, more than 500,000 Hollows intraocular lenses have been implanted in patients with vision impaired by cataract, allowing most of them to function as productive members of their communities.

CHAPTER 32

Global Eye Banking and Corneal Transplantation

Background

The new frontier for eye banking and corneal transplantation in the developing world is to increase the availability of a safe tissue supply for corneal transplantation for all levels of society.

The World Health Organization (WHO) states that approximately 45 million people are bilaterally blind, with vision less than 3/60. An additional 135 million visually impaired individuals have vision in the range of 6/60 to 3/60. A total, therefore, of 180 million individuals are visually disabled, 60% of them located in sub-Saharan Africa, China, and India.

Corneal blindness in the developing world has a tremendous impact both on the quality of people's lives and on related economic issues. Corneal blindness affects more than 10 million people in the developing world (approximately 25%). Its epidemiology is diverse and dependent on endemic disease and the local environment. Classic causes of corneal blindness are related to trachoma, onchocerciasis, leprosy, ophthalmia neonatorum, and xerophthalmia. Emergent causes are related to ulceration, trauma, and complications involving the use of traditional medicines by nonmedically trained individuals.

>   Whitcher JP, Srinivasan M, Upadhyay MP. Corneal blindness: a global perspective. *Bull World Health Organ.* 2001;79:214–221.

Trachoma is the leading infectious cause of corneal blindness and morbidity. Currently, 146 million individuals in the developing world have trachoma; of these, 10 million have significant trichiasis and 5 million are completely blind. This disease can largely be prevented through public health projects. Large national programs are now under way, including WHO's S.A.F.E. (*s*urgery, *a*ntibiotics, *f*ace cleanliness, *e*nvironmental improvements) program, which will lessen the impact of trachoma for years to come. Unfortunately, this does not have an effect on the patient with corneal blindness.

Corneal ulceration has been labeled the "silent epidemic" cause of corneal blindness in the developing world. It occurs 30 to 70 times more often in the developing than in the developed world. Every year in the developing world, there are 1.5 to 2 million new cases. These cases have a high degree of morbidity due both to the high frequency of fungal disease and to the fact that large numbers of corneal ulcers have no treatment or treatment that is markedly delayed. In Nepal, an interesting nationwide corneal ulcer prevention program using prophylactic topical chloramphenicol for minor corneal trauma has been instituted in an effort to decrease the impact of corneal ulceration.

> Whitcher JP, Srinivasan M. Corneal ulceration in the developing world—a silent epidemic. *Br J Ophthalmol.* 1997;81:622–623.

Ocular trauma has been identified as the most important cause of unilateral loss of visual acuity in the developing world. Currently, 19 million people are unilaterally blind or have low visual acuity related to ocular trauma. In addition, 2.3 million have decreased visual acuity and 1.6 million are bilaterally blind due to ocular trauma. The etiology of the trauma varies from community to community. A vast majority of affected individuals are agricultural workers, followed by foundry workers and people who are injured by exploding land mines (eg, in Cambodia).

> Thylefors B. Epidemiological patterns of ocular trauma. *Aust N Z J Ophthalmol.* 1992;20: 95–98.

Every year in the developing world, there are 1 to 2 million new cases of blindness. This has profound human and socioeconomic consequences, with decreased life expectancy and decreased productivity. A unit of measure adopted by the World Health Organization is the disability-adjusted life-year (DALY), which reflects the time with disability in addition to premature mortality as the impact of blindness in the developing world. With the increase of noncommunicable disease as a cause of blindness, the impact of DALYs due to blindness will increase dramatically over the next 20 years.

Corneal blindness is the most common etiology of blindness among children. According to the WHO, approximately 73% of children who are blind live in the developing world, a total of approximately 1.4 million children. The causes include xerophthalmia, measles, ophthalmia neonatorum, herpes simplex keratitis, and the use of traditional eye medicines. Various forms of trauma, in particular exploding land mines, have an unfortunate impact on childhood blindness. Approximately 500,000 children per year become blind and half of these die within 1 to 2 years. The incidence of childhood blindness in the developing world is approximately 75 per 100,000, whereas in the developed world it is between 6 and 11 per 100,000. A significant percentage of the causes of childhood blindness is preventable or curable.

> Gilbert C, Foster A. Childhood blindness in the context of VISION 2020—The Right to Sight. *Bull World Health Organ.* 2001;79:227–232.

Corneal Transplantation in the Developing World

Millions of individuals in the developing world could benefit from corneal transplantation. The numbers will increase in the decades to come as cataract surgery becomes more frequent as a result of increasing levels of comprehensive eye-care delivery. Corneal transplantation and eye banking will play an important role. The delivery of successful corneal transplantation is much more complex than the delivery of cataract surgery in the developing world. Yorston, Wood, and Foster published a paper in 1996, regarding penetrating keratoplasty in Africa. The study was a retrospective analysis of more than 216 corneal transplants over 5 years using imported tissue. It demonstrated that penetrating keratoplasty could be successful when properly utilized in a developing world context. Another study, published in 1997 by Dandona and colleagues, followed more than 1200 transplants over an 8-year period in Hyderabad, India, using locally retrieved tissue. This paper demonstrated that corneal transplantation, when properly applied, can have a significant effect on decreasing blindness in the developing world.

> Dandona L, Naduvilath TJ, Janarthanan M, et al. Survival analysis and visual outcome in a large series of corneal transplants in India. *Br J Ophthalmol.* 1997;81:726–731.
>
> Yorston D, Wood M, Foster A. Penetrating keratoplasty in Africa: graft survival and visual outcome. *Br J Ophthalmol.* 1996;80:890–894.

The impact of corneal transplantation on patients was found to be at least 4 times more effective than cataract surgery in the reduction of DALYs. Eye banking and corneal transplantation have a role in visual rehabilitation in the developing world.

> Yorston D. Penetrating keratoplasty in East Africa: indicators and outcome. In: International Agency for the Prevention of Blindness, ed, *World Blindness and Its Prevention.* Vol. 5: 139–144. Hyderabad, India: International Agency for the Prevention of Blindness; 2001.

The purpose of this chapter is to review briefly the basic strategies that have been employed to establish successful corneal transplantation outcomes in conjunction with self-sustaining eye banking programs around the world. Unfortunately, in the past, the success of corneal transplantation in the developing world has been hampered by poor outcomes due to inadequate screening of donors, substandard tissue processing and tissue collection procedures, as well as a lack of sufficient medical and health care professional training programs. Fortunately, good models do exist now, and the future holds out a much stronger promise of success for those who would benefit from corneal transplantation.

National Eye Banking Programs

The Eye Bank Association of America (EBAA) is the gold standard organization for eye banking in the world. In 2000, more than 46,000 corneas were processed for corneal transplantation by its 100-plus US member eye banks. The EBAA is the prime example for medical standards, accreditation and certification programs, and training programs.

Several other national and international organizations have established innovative programs to increase the success of corneal transplantation and eye banking. The Australian Corneal Graft Registry was established in May 1985. This registry follows all donated tissue from the donor through surgery to the recipient to report long-term outcomes. Approximately 12,000 transplants are listed on this registry. An extensive analysis has been applied to the many issues that impact overall corneal transplant outcome. This program is unique in the world.

Brazil, which performs approximately 7000 corneal transplants per year, has statewide waiting lists that are state regulated. Patients are listed chronologically and are eligible for just one list. Tissue distribution is controlled by the executive secretary of health of the state where the patient is listed. The patient is able to access this list on the Internet and check his or her position.

Canada has established a unique program setting safety standards for cells, tissue, and organs for transplantation. The program is a collaborative effort among Health Canada, health care professionals from all areas of transplantation, and public advocates with the Canadian Standards Association. They have established a national Canadian General Standard for transplantation, which includes appropriate subsets of medical standards for areas such as stem cells, tissues, ocular tissues, solid organs, and tissues for assisted reproduction. Associated with this will be a comprehensive program of regulation, inspection, and accreditation. Approximately 2500 corneal transplants a year are performed.

The European Eye Bank Association stores approximately two thirds of all its tissue in organ culture at 36° Celsius, as opposed to cold storage at 4° Celsius, which is the accepted procedure in North America. This form of tissue storage has a tremendous positive impact on corneal transplantation, as the length of storage time can possibly be increased from 7 to 14 days to up to 1 month in cold storage.

The Japan Eye Bank Association is developing a national donor action plan in conjunction with the Japan Organ Transplantation Network and the Japan Transplantation Association. Over the last few years, the Japan Eye Bank Association, in conjunction with other organizations and the Japanese government, has been able to change the attitudes of Japanese citizens toward organ and tissue transplantation. In 1996, a national survey found that 10%–15% of individuals, if approached, would donate organs and tissues. The same study, undertaken in 2000, found that approximately 86% of the population would donate. This is an extremely positive outcome and demonstrates that, by approaching the issue in a culturally sensitive fashion, attitudes can be changed regarding organ and tissue transplantation.

The Eye Bank Association of India (EBAI) was established in 1989 and now represents an ongoing success story of corneal transplantation and eye banking in the developing world. In 1990, approximately 700 successful corneal transplants were performed in India. The frequency of primary graft failure was approximately 50%. In 2000, approximately 9000 corneal transplants were undertaken, with a much higher success rate and a dramatic decrease in incidence of primary graft failure. Currently, the EBAI has more than 150 eye banks, with performances varying greatly among these facilities. Eight eye banks collect 50% of all the tissue and another 20 eye banks collect an additional 25% of the tissue. The EBAI has a comprehensive set of medical standards, with an accreditation program under development, as well as ongoing training programs. The EBAI has set a goal of 25,000 corneal transplants per year by the year 2005.

Eye Banking

Establishing a successful corneal transplantation and eye banking program in the developing world depends first on establishing successful eye banking programs that are self-sustainable. The primary purpose of an eye bank is to acquire, evaluate, process, and distribute tissues for corneal transplantation and scleral grafts. The primary goal is to provide a clinical service to the public. The secondary role of eye banks is to undertake research. The eye bank acts as an important liaison among the donor families, the medical community, and the recipients.

Creating and adopting a comprehensive medical standard document is the most critical element in setting up a successful eye banking program. Standards establish baseline practices that improve the responsiveness of the system to new developments with a transparent scientific process covering all aspects of eye banking. The document must be comprehensive and dynamic in order to respond to current scientific knowledge. Furthermore, the medical standards must be realistic to the community they serve and take into account local financial considerations and the laws of the land. The medical standards document must be responsive to community issues, including regional legislation and cultural and religious sensitivities. An appropriate medical standards document facilitates uniform evaluation, standardized data collection, quality assurance, outcome analysis, and accountability. An example of an excellent medical standards document is that maintained by the Eye Bank Association of America.

> Medical Standards. Eye Bank Association of America, 1015 Eighteenth St. NW, Suite 1010, Washington, DC 20036.

Special procedures must be clearly defined for handling hazardous tissue infected with active viral hepatitis, acquired immune deficiency syndrome (AIDS), and prion disease (eg, Creutzfeldt-Jakob disease), not only to protect the recipient but also the health care professional involved in processing the tissue. A quality assurance program is critical as it ensures the routine application of medical standards (eg, establishing a baseline of serologic testing) to all donors. Ongoing outcome analysis must be established, looking particularly at the incidence of primary graft failure and any evidence of infectious disease transmission. These are indicators of the overall quality of tissue being supplied by an eye bank.

An accreditation program is required to demonstrate compliance with medical standards and federal and local laws, as well as to demonstrate proficiency in the performance of assigned duties via on-site inspections.

The "Best" Eye Bank Model

The elements of a "best" eye bank model are a professional organization with professional leadership and management, provision of education for health care professionals, and provision of public education through a coordinator-based system (a coordinator is a health care professional specifically trained in eye banking). The professional organization consists of a medical director, administrative director, and transplant coordinators. The professional organization, leadership, and management of an eye banking system determine the overall quality of tissue that is delivered. An organization maintains and improves the quality of tissue. When systems fail, it is generally due more to poor leadership than to technical deficiencies.

The medical director is responsible for ensuring that medical standards, which are usually developed by a national organization, are properly applied in that particular eye bank. The director is also responsible for developing medical policies and procedures that comply with these medical standards and that are consistent with the particular group. In addition, the medical director is responsible for technical staff training and supervision in the development of quality assurance programs.

Another characteristic of a comprehensive eye banking system is education of the health care workers both in the hospital and the community. Participation by local hospitals is critical to successful donation programs.

Public awareness is the third element of the best eye banking systems. This is important in clarifying general misconceptions and responding to the religious and cultural sensitivities of the area. The overall goal of these programs is to make donation a community expectation, not only for tissue but also for organs. Public education leads to long-term support and must be established after the professional organization is set up and appropriate professional health care education programs are begun. Public education is often undertaken too early in the development of an eye banking system to make a significant contribution to the success of that particular program. Donor cards are not an indicator of success of any program but may be used as a public relations tool.

Establishment of a coordinator-based system is the final element of the best eye banking systems. Coordinators are appropriately trained health care professionals who undertake many of the critical aspects of eye banking, including donor screening, recovery, processing, distribution, and tracking. The long-term self-sustainability of a program depends on these health care professionals, as they allow ophthalmologists to focus on patient care. Medical director oversight is required on a long-term basis. Opportunities for continuing education are important to the overall success of these programs.

Recipients, donor families, corneal surgeons, donor hospitals, and, ultimately, the public all benefit from well-established eye banking systems. Such systems maximize the impact of each eye donor, both for the community served by the eye bank and the recipient. This model is the most effective, both for short- and long-term delivery of suitable eye tissue for corneal transplantation and for the long-term development of successful eye banking systems.

Tissue Retrieval and Distribution Models

Four basic eye banking structures are used in the development model of tissue recovery and distribution. The first model has limited recovery of tissue and exclusive distribution to a particular surgeon; this is described as a "ma and pa" eye bank. Typically, these are small organizations with high costs per cornea. They are not self-sustaining and have poor long-term potential.

The second model has recovery from a large portion of the community but exclusive distribution to selected surgeons. This program is unethical for patients, as access is thereby restricted. It is also unethical for other qualified surgeons in the community. It encourages negative competition because others in the community will set up competing eye banks, which discourages community support.

The third model has limited recovery and community distribution. Limited recovery of tissue locally may be supplemented by tissue imported from areas with an excess tissue supply. This can be very effective for starting up eye banks, but it is a short-term solution.

Importing tissue may slow development of the community's own self-sustaining eye banking system. When tissue is imported, it is important to attempt to link it to local performance and local generation of tissue for corneal transplantation.

The fourth—and ideal—model for the development of a successful eye banking system is that of community recovery of tissue with community distribution. This system requires the cooperation of the ophthalmic community and hospitals in the region. It generates widespread community support and is by far the most cost-efficient model for long-term self-sustainability.

Government Participation

Local and national government participation is necessary for successful eye banking programs. Legislation, including required request laws, coroners' and medical examiners' laws, and routine notification laws, can help organ and tissue transplantation programs become successful. Negative participation or neglect can render any organ or tissue program unsuccessful. Governments may play an important role in the development of regulations, inspection, and accreditation programs. They are critical in the development of appropriate resources and the infrastructure necessary for successful eye banking systems. Regional laws and regulations, as well as cultural and religious sensitivities, must be taken into consideration. Governments may support the training of appropriate medical and paramedical health care professionals.

Strategy

The overall strategy for developing successful eye banking programs in the developing world will revolve around development of appropriate tertiary care centers with centralized eye banking systems. These centers will have appropriate medical standards and trained health care professionals. In selecting patients for transplantation, priority must be given to younger patients and to individuals with corneal blindness for whose disease—for example, keratoconus and dystrophies—transplants have shown a higher success rate. The maximum benefit is derived from performing transplantation on patients who are bilaterally blind. Patients must have access to appropriate follow-up and to appropriate topical medications on a long-term basis.

Fellowship training programs for ophthalmologists must be developed locally and then expanded if corneal transplant programs are to be successful. To obtain the appropriate and necessary skills to function as the medical director of an eye bank and/or perform corneal transplantation, individuals must be trained appropriately in a facility with an established eye bank. Training is absolutely necessary in dealing with postoperative complications of corneal transplantation. It is also critical that the fellowship-trained corneal surgeons have the skills to train their fellow ophthalmologists—especially those physicians living in geographic areas where patients have poor access to appropriate subspecialists—in patient follow-up. Fellowship training should also include opportunities for continuing education and training.

Eye Sight International (ESI) is a nongovernmental organization (NGO) involved in eye-care delivery in the developing world. In the area of eye banking and corneal transplantation, the organization serves as an example of how expertise can be developed by ongoing skills transfer. ESI personnel have been participating in ongoing eye bank and corneal transplantation programs since 1990. They have worked closely with the Eye Bank Association of India (EBAI) since its founding in 1989, establishing a proactive comprehensive medical standards document in coordination with an accreditation program. These education programs have included an annual eye bank coordinator training program and meetings with fellowship-trained corneal surgeons to discuss issues concerning corneal transplantation and eye banking. ESI personnel have functioned as advisors to the executive committee of the EBAI since 1997. In addition, ESI has sponsored fellowship programs in cornea and external disease. Similar programs have been undertaken with the Japan Eye Bank Association since 1993.

Conclusion

Corneal blindness has a very significant impact on morbidity and mortality in the developing world, where millions of people are presently denied access to corneal transplantation and therefore denied more productive lives. The development of comprehensive eye banking systems with fellowship-trained professionals can help change this situation (Table 32-1 provides a list of resources). Governments must play a positive role as well, with legislative assistance and appropriate infrastructure development. Almost all cultural and religious groups will donate organs and tissues if approached in a culturally sensitive manner. Usually, members of the local community define this approach. The challenge remains for global eye banking and transplantation to increase the availability of a safe tissue supply for corneal transplantation to all levels of society.

Table 32-1 Resources

World Health Organization: www.who.int
VISION 2020—The Right to Sight: www.v2020.org
Eye Bank Association of America (EBAA): www.restoresight.org
ORBIS: www.orbis.org
Tissue Banks International (TBI): tbionline.org
Centers for Medicare and Medicaid Services (CMS): cms.hhs.gov
Eye Bank Association of India: www.ebai.org
Food and Drug Administration (FDA): www.fda.gov
Pan American Association of Eye Banks (APABO): apabo@uninet.com.br
American Academy of Ophthalmology (AAO) Volunteer Registry: www.aao.org
Eyesight International: www.eyesightinternational.com
Children—Surgical Aid International (CSAI): www.csaintl.org

Credit Reporting Form

Basic and Clinical Science Course, 2004–2005
Section 13

The American Academy of Ophthalmology is accredited by the Accreditation Council for Continuing Medical Education to provide continuing medical education for physicians.

The American Academy of Ophthalmology designates this educational activity for a maximum of 30 category 1 credits toward the AMA Physician's Recognition Award. Each physician should claim only those hours of credit that he/she actually spent in the activity.

The American Medical Association has determined that non-US licensed physicians who participate in this CME activity are eligible for AMA PRA category 1 credit.

If you wish to claim continuing medical education credit for your study of this section, you may claim your credit online or fill in the required forms and mail or fax them to the Academy.

To use the forms:

1. Complete the study questions and mark your answers on the Section Completion Form.
2. Complete the Section Evaluation.
3. Fill in and sign the statement below.
4. Return this page and the required forms by mail or fax to the CME Registrar (see below).

To claim credit online:

1. Log on to the Academy website (www.aao.org).
2. Go to Education Resource Center; click on CME Central.
3. Follow the instructions.

Important: These completed forms or the online claim must be received at the Academy within 3 years of purchase.

I hereby certify that I have spent _____ (up to 30) hours of study on the curriculum of this section and that I have completed the Study Questions.

Signature: _____

Date

Name: _____

Address: _____

City and State: _____ Zip: _____

Telephone: (_____) _____ Academy Member ID# _____
area code

Please return completed forms to: **Or you may fax them to:** 415-561-8557
American Academy of Ophthalmology
P.O. Box 7424
San Francisco, CA 94120-7424
Attn: CME Registrar, Clinical Education

2004–2005
Section Completion Form

Basic and Clinical Science Course

Answer Sheet for Section 13

Question	Answer	Question	Answer
1	a b c d	17	a b c d
2	a b c d	18	a b c d
3	a b c d	19	a b c d
4	a b c d	20	a b c d
5	a b c d	21	a b c d
6	a b c d	22	a b c d
7	a b c d	23	a b c d
8	a b c d	24	a b c d
9	a b c d	25	a b c d
10	a b c d	26	a b c d
11	a b c d	27	a b c d
12	a b c d	28	a b c d
13	a b c d	29	a b c d
14	a b c d	30	a b c d
15	a b c d	31	a b c d
16	a b c d		

Section Evaluation

Please complete this CME questionnaire.

1. To what degree will you use knowledge from BCSC Section 13 in your practice?
   - ☐ Regularly
   - ☐ Sometimes
   - ☐ Rarely

2. Please review the stated objectives for BCSC Section 13. How effective was the material at meeting those objectives?
   - ☐ All objectives were met.
   - ☐ Most objectives were met.
   - ☐ Some objectives were met.
   - ☐ Few or no objectives were met.

3. To what degree is BCSC Section 13 likely to have a positive impact on health outcomes of your patients?
   - ☐ Extremely likely
   - ☐ Highly likely
   - ☐ Somewhat likely
   - ☐ Not at all likely

4. After you review the stated objectives for BCSC Section 13, please let us know of any additional knowledge, skills, or information useful to your practice that were acquired but were not included in the objectives. [Optional]

5. Was BCSC Section 13 free of commercial bias?
   - ☐ Yes
   - ☐ No

6. If you selected "No" in the previous question, please comment. [Optional]

7. Please tell us what might improve the applicability of BCSC to your practice. [Optional]

Study Questions

1. Which of the following statements about the program VISION 2020 is *not* correct?
   a. VISION 2020 is a global initiative to eliminate avoidable blindness by the year 2020.
   b. The program has targeted five disorders: cataract, refractive errors and low vision services, geographically focal diseases such as trachoma and onchocerciasis, glaucoma, and diabetic retinopathy.
   c. VISION 2020 emphasizes treatment strategies only and not disease prevention.
   d. Among the initial steps of VISION 2020 is a global campaign to raise awareness among peoples and governments about societal implications of vision loss.

2. Which of the following statements regarding evidence-based medicine is *not* correct?
   a. Evidence-based medicine is the application of clinical expertise and the best available clinical evidence.
   b. Evidence-based medicine is evidence obtained only by prospective, randomized clinical trials.
   c. Evidence-based medicine does not provide a blueprint for decision making for all patients.
   d. Quality scales for evaluating evidence have been developed and are useful as a systematic approach to include or exclude evidence.

3. Which of the following statements regarding cataract is *not* correct?
   a. Cataract is estimated to cause blindness in approximately 20 million people worldwide.
   b. The worldwide estimated annual cataract surgical rate is about 9–10 million surgeries.
   c. Cataract is estimated to cause blindness in approximately 6 million people worldwide.
   d. There is increasing evidence that for many patients visual outcomes are unsatisfactory.

4. Which of the following statements regarding worldwide vision impairment is *not* correct?
   a. The World Health Organization (WHO) estimates that 180 million people worldwide are visually impaired.
   b. The WHO estimates that 80% of global vision loss is avoidable.
   c. Cataract causes nearly one half of all visual loss.
   d. All of the above are correct.

5. All of the following are indicators that aid in measuring the burden of disease *except*
   a. Disability-adjusted life-years (DALY)
   b. Cost–utility analyses using cost per gains in quality-adjusted life-years ($/QALY)
   c. Utility values
   d. Outcome studies

6. Which of the following statements is *not* correct regarding meta-analysis?
   a. Two or more comparable randomized clinical trials are combined to enhance the estimate of the direction and the strength of an intervention effect.
   b. The most valid method of meta-analysis is to combine individual patient data from the original studies for a complete data reanalysis.
   c. There are four general methods for meta-analysis.
   d. One of the methods of meta-analysis is pooling, where the results are summarized to form one large study.

7. Which of the following about outcome studies is *not* correct?
   a. They don't need to include all relevant cases and be representative, both temporally and geographically, of actual clinical practice.
   b. They are dependent on clear endpoints.
   c. They are less costly than randomized clinical trials.
   d. They can measure the impact of disease, treatment cost-effectiveness, and the patient's functional status.

8. Which of the following statements regarding nonrandomized studies is *not* correct?
   a. They are observational studies that are designed to generate or test hypotheses.
   b. They have a clearly defined group or cohort that is studied prospectively or retrospectively.
   c. In a prospective cohort study, the investigator assembles the study groups based on clinical diagnosis or risk factors, records baseline data, and collects data over time.
   d. So that outcome events may be confirmed, the investigator should have no control over the data collection.

9. Which of the following statements about case-control studies is *not* correct?
   a. Risk or incidence of disease must be measured directly.
   b. This technique allows the relationship between risk factors and disease to be evaluated statistically.
   c. The population must have a comparison group that is disease-free to serve as controls.
   d. Selection bias is minimized when both cases and controls are selected from an unbiased sample of the same population.

10. Which of the following statements about observational studies is *not* correct?
    a. Their fundamental weakness is being unable to control for unknown confounding and sources of bias.
    b. Observational studies cannot provide evidence of effectiveness.
    c. They may be employed in the study of risk factors.
    d. The quality of the study improves by predetermined definitions.

11. Which of the following regarding efficacy versus effectiveness is *true*?
    a. The effectiveness of an intervention is the maximum reduction in a disease due to an intervention in the treatment arm of a randomized clinical trial (RCT).
    b. Efficacy is the benefit a larger population receives from application of an RCT's intervention to real health care situations in the community.
    c. Efficacy is frequently minimized in a randomized clinical trial.
    d. Major differences between efficacy and effectiveness of an intervention may be observed.

12. Which of the following is *not* a reason to stop a randomized controlled trial?
    a. When the study's interim data indicate a treatment benefit beyond a reasonable doubt ($P < .001$)
    b. When the new treatment is actually ineffective or insufficiently convincing to change clinical practice
    c. Unexpected high frequency of side effects from treatment
    d. Unexpected added benefits of treatment

13. Which of the following statements regarding the power of study (p_β) is *not* correct?
    a. Power is analogous to the sensitivity of a diagnostic test.
    b. The probability that an RCT will find a statistically significant difference when a difference exists is called its statistical power.
    c. A p_β of .20 means that a study has a 20% chance of missing a true difference in an RCT.
    d. It is a measure of the probability of a false positive result (type I, or α, error).

14. Which of the following statements about vision, as defined by the World Health Organization (WHO) in the 1970s, is *not* correct?
    a. Low vision is considered <20/60, <0.3, <6/18.
    b. Blindness is considered <20/400, <0.05, <3/60.
    c. The WHO classification has not been widely accepted.
    d. Vision is defined by a trichotomous scale (normal/low vision/blindness).

15. All of the following statements regarding surveys are true *except*
    a. A survey is an observational epidemiologic study based on examination of all persons in a given population and not in a specifically defined subgroup of the population.
    b. Surveys are most commonly used to estimate prevalence and incidence.
    c. Prevalence is estimated by cross-sectional studies that assess the presence of disease in a specific population at a point in time.
    d. Nonresponse biases occur if participants are not representative of the proposed study population due to selective nonparticipation.

16. Which of the following about case series epidemiology is *not* correct?
    a. Case series methodology is typically used to study diseases that have a low frequency of occurrence in the population and cannot be studied using large clinical trials.
    b. In most cases, the clinician must have the initiative to pursue these data without research funding.
    c. Diseases such as diffuse unilateral subacute neuroretinitis (DUSN), acute posterior multifocal placoid pigment epitheliopathy, multiple evanescent white dot syndrome, and acute retinal necrosis have been characterized using this approach.
    d. They tend to be more expensive than randomized clinical trials.

350 • Study Questions

17. Which of following statements regarding ophthalmia neonatorum is *not* correct?
    a. Ophthalmia neonatorum is an infection acquired postnatally that presents within 15 days of birth.
    b. In underdeveloped countries, such as in East Africa, the incidence increases to more than 10% of all births.
    c. *Chlamydia trachomatis* is the most frequent etiologic agent in most countries.
    d. In a clinical trial of more than 3000 babies in Kenya, povidone-iodine ophthalmic solution proved to be more effective than either silver nitrate ophthalmic solution or erythromycin ophthalmic ointment while being less toxic.

18. Which of the following statements regarding retinopathy of prematurity (ROP) is *not* correct?
    a. In a recent study, 49% of infants weighing ≤1251 grams developed ROP in some form and, of these, approximately 7% reached threshold, requiring treatment. Despite this intervention, one child developed bilateral stage 5 ROP with bilateral blindness.
    b. The process of normal retinal vascularization is complete by 16 weeks nasally and 20 weeks temporally.
    c. Regression, spontaneous healing of the lesion, occurs in over 90% of eyes afflicted with ROP by 48 weeks' gestational age.
    d. Plus disease, in combination with a significant extent of advanced ROP in the periphery, carries an ominous prognosis.

19. Which of the following statements regarding vitamin A deficiency disorders and xerophthalmia is *correct*?
    a. Night blindness is a late stage in xerophthalmia.
    b. Blindness is most likely due to retinal disease.
    c. Vitamin A supplementation is one of the most cost-effective preventive strategies that can be used to reduce mortality in young children in developing areas of the world.
    d. There is no evidence that immune function is impaired in vitamin A deficiency among young children.

20. Which of the following statements regarding amblyopia is *not* correct?
    a. Amblyopia is among the top three causes of monocular visual loss in the adult age group from 18 to 85 years.
    b. Estimates of the incidence and prevalence of amblyopia vary in the range of 1%–2.5% in children.
    c. Successful management is directly related to length of treatment.
    d. It is usually secondary to refractive error, strabismus, or both.

21. Which of the following statements regarding ocular trauma is *not* correct?
    a. The size of the wound is the most important variable influencing the prognosis of any eye injury.
    b. Penetrating injury is a single full-thickness laceration of the eye wall, usually caused by a sharp object, where no exit wound has occurred.
    c. The World Health Organization (WHO) Program for the Prevention of Blindness estimates that 55 million eye injuries occur globally each year.
    d. An important complication of corneal trauma is corneal infection caused by organisms from vegetative material.

22. Which of the following statements regarding epidemic optic neuropathy in Cuba is *not* correct?
    a. There was an initial bias toward a virus etiology by local experts studying the epidemic.
    b. Alcohol could not have played a role because consumption of rum was limited by the Cuban government to one bottle per family per month.
    c. There were almost 50,000 cases by the middle of 1993.
    d. The likely pathogenesis of this epidemic was a diet deficient in calories, protein, and vitamins and possibly including at least one form of toxin.

23. Which of the following statements regarding primary open-angle glaucoma (POAG) is *not* correct?
    a. The Barbados cohort has provided a measurement of incidence that supports the high risk of developing POAG in this population, with a 4-year incidence rate of 2.2%.
    b. The blindness rate could be up to 6 times higher among blacks than among whites with POAG.
    c. In Barbados, POAG accounted for 28% ($n = 42$) of bilateral blindness and was the leading cause of visual loss.
    d. The prevalence of POAG in Barbados is similar to that in black patients in Baltimore, MD.

24. Which of the following statements regarding sampling in observational, population-based studies is *true*?
    a. Use of a pilot study is not helpful in accurately projecting a reasonable sample size and assessing the feasibility of the survey.
    b. A sampling frame is required to identify eligible persons in the population.
    c. Examiners are not required to be standardized in all measurements prior to the beginning of a study.
    d. All detailed information should be obtained only by direct questioning and not by using standardized questionnaires given to participants.

25. Which of the following statements regarding assessment of childhood blindness in a population is *correct*?
    a. When only school-age children are considered, surveying schools may be a source of error.
    b. One of the most accurate methods for obtaining data is to survey the local schools for blind children.
    c. Reliable data collection can be obtained at a very low cost.
    d. School surveys have seldom been the source of information available in the literature.

26. Which of the following statements regarding the economics of retinopathy of prematurity (ROP) is *correct*?
    a. One percent of ROP cases are premature by definition: <2500 grams birth weight and 36 weeks' gestational age.
    b. In a recent study, 98% of infants with birth weight ≤1251 grams developed ROP in some form.
    c. Stage 5 ROP intervention always prevents bilateral blindness.
    d. The economic impact of ROP includes the lifetime costs of blindness to an individual and immediate family.

27. Which of the following statements about the cost of treatment and prevention of vitamin A deficiency disorders is *true*?
    a. Typical costs for high-dose vitamin A capsules are in the range of US$0.03/dose—less than US$0.10 for a treatment regimen of three doses.
    b. The costs of diagnosis and delivery of care are lower than the cost of vitamin A.
    c. Vitamin A supplementation is not a cost-effective preventive strategy.
    d. Vitamin A supplementation does not reduce mortality in young children in developing areas of the world.

28. Which of the following statements about blindness due to cataract is *true*?
    a. In the developed world, such as the United States and the United Kingdom, cataract is no longer a common cause of visual loss.
    b. Cataract surgery is ranked as one of the least cost-effective public health interventions for the developing world.
    c. An estimated 17 million persons are blind from cataract worldwide, making it the leading cause of visual loss.
    d. By the year 2020, it is estimated that 6 million people worldwide will have blinding cataract.

29. Which of the following statements about the economic impact of trachoma is *true*?
    a. Treatment is inexpensive because reinfections are very rare.
    b. Blindness from trichiasis is rare in those above 30 years old and even rarer in the elderly.
    c. Corrective surgery for trichiasis can be performed in about 15 minutes for approximately US$100–$200.
    d. Treatment efforts have to be directed toward a community and include the costs of identifying high-risk communities, educating these communities concerning the importance of hygiene, purchasing and distributing antibiotics, identifying trichiasis cases, and performing corrective surgery.

30. Which of the following statements regarding the economic impact of HIV is *true*?
    a. Modern treatment of HIV/AIDS includes long-term use of three or more antiretroviral agents, an approach termed combination therapy, or highly active antiretroviral therapy (HAART). The cost of such therapy currently exceeds $10,000 per year in the United States.
    b. Despite the cost, the vast majority of patients in the developing world with HIV/AIDS are fully treated.
    c. In countries of sub-Saharan Africa, HIV infection is rare and has produced little change in the overall life expectancy.
    d. Recent estimates suggest that there are over 10 million HIV-positive children and nearly 120 million HIV/AIDS orphans worldwide.

31. Which of the following statements about onchocerciasis is *correct*?
    a. *Onchocerca volvulus* is a gram-negative bacteria.
    b. It is transmitted by the vector *Simulium* spp, or blackfly, which breeds in fast-flowing rivers and streams.
    c. Two drugs have been available and are widely used for treating onchocerciasis: diethylcarbamazine (DEC), a microfilaricide, and suramin, a macrofilaricide.
    d. Because ivermectin is microfilaricidal, a short course is effective in curing the disease.

Answers

1. Answer—c. In February 1999, the International Agency for the Prevention of Blindness launched VISION 2020—The Right to Sight, a global initiative to eliminate preventable blindness by the year 2020. The program has targeted five disorders in its avoidable blindness campaign: cataract, refractive error and low vision services, geographically focal blinding diseases such as trachoma and onchocerciasis, glaucoma, and diabetic retinopathy. Prevention of blindness from these conditions was deemed feasible and affordable. The answer C is not correct because VISION 2020 does emphasize disease prevention and control. The initial step of VISION 2020 has been a global campaign to raise awareness among peoples and governments about the societal implications of vision loss and to mobilize a long-term commitment to eliminate avoidable blindness.

2. Answer—b. Evidence-based medicine is the application of clinical expertise and the best available clinical evidence to provide sound advice for health decisions. Evidence-based medicine does not provide a blueprint for clinical decision making, as decisions must be tailored to a patient's specific situation and needs. Quality scales have been established for evaluating the evidence. The highest quality evidence may come from prospective, randomized clinical trials, though they are not the only source of useful evidence for determining the effectiveness of care.

3. Answer—c. Cataract is estimated to cause blindness in approximately 20 million people worldwide. The worldwide estimated annual cataract surgical rate is about 9–10 million surgeries. Visual outcomes are less than satisfactory in some areas. It is important not only to increase the rate of surgeries but also to increase the quality of the surgical outcomes by incorporating thorough preoperative examinations and proper case selection, quality surgical techniques, postoperative follow-up, and refraction.

4. Answer—d. The WHO estimates that 180 million people worldwide are visually impaired, including approximately 45 million persons who have profound vision loss (visual acuity <20/400). The organization estimates that 80% of global vision loss is avoidable. The number of persons with vision loss is increasing and is expected to double by 2020 as world population and life expectancy increase. Vision loss impacts the affected individuals and their families and presents public health, social, and economic problems. Cataract causes nearly half the vision loss worldwide. Unfortunately, good intentions have created significant problems, such as blindness from complications of cataract surgery. In one study, almost half the patients operated on were dissatisfied with the outcome and more than one third were blind in the operated eye.

5. Answer—d. Among the indicators that aid in measuring the burden of disease are disability-adjusted life-years (DALY), cost–utility analyses using cost per gains in quality-adjusted life-years ($/QALY), utility values, and risk assessment. Outcome studies can be used to assess the benefits and complications of treatments but do not aid in measuring the burden of disease.

6. Answer—c. A meta-analysis is a method whereby two or more comparable randomized controlled trials (RCTs) are combined to enhance the estimate of the direction and the strength of an intervention effect. The most valid method of meta-analysis is to combine individual patient data from the original studies for a complete data reanalysis, although problems obtaining original data from trials have made this kind of meta-analysis rare. Option C is not correct because there are only two general methods for meta-analysis: pooling, where the

results are summarized to form one large study, and weighing individual studies against predetermined methodologic criteria, with the results reflecting the weighted value.

7. Answer—a. To be valid, outcome studies must include all relevant cases and be representative, both temporally and geographically, of actual clinical practice. Studies describing the outcome of treatment as actually delivered are of parallel value in establishing standards for clinical practice. Outcome studies with clear-cut endpoints, such as being alive or dead, reduce bias and misclassification. Outcome studies may be designed to measure the impact of disease, treatment cost-effectiveness, and the patient's functional status and quality of life. However, it is difficult to quantify the measurements of subjective aspects of outcome assessment.

8. Answer—d. Nonrandomized studies are observational and designed to generate or test hypotheses. A clearly defined group or cohort is studied prospectively or retrospectively. In a prospective cohort study, the investigator assembles the study groups based on clinical diagnosis or risk factors, records baseline data, and collects data over time. The investigator controls data collection so those outcome events may be confirmed. Only risk factors that have been defined and measured at the beginning of the study can be assessed. These studies are subject to many potential biases, a major weakness in this methodology.

9. Answer—a. The efficiency of a population-based study, randomized clinical trial, or observational study may be improved by designing case-control studies within the framework of the overall study. This technique allows the relationship between risk factors and disease to be evaluated statistically. The population must have a comparison group that is disease-free to serve as controls and a sample size sufficiently large to reduce the effect that chance may play in the observed results. Risk factors are the attributes associated with target conditions. They can help predict outcomes but may not cause the target condition. Most diseases require special methods of study to establish a relationship between exposure and disease. Risk or incidence of disease cannot be measured directly. Relative risk of exposure can be estimated by the odds ratio.

10. Answer—b. Well-designed observational studies may provide evidence of effectiveness. However, they may be more appropriately employed in the study of risk factors as determinants of disease. There are occasions when they may be useful in indicating the effect of health interventions, particularly in the prevention of disease. However, as in all such studies, the fundamental weakness of being unable to control for unknown confounding and sources of bias remains. A well-designed study with predetermined criteria and definitions is very important.

11. Answer—d. The efficacy of an intervention is the maximum reduction in a disease due to an intervention in the treatment arm of an RCT. Efficacy is frequently maximized in an RCT because patients are usually free of other confounding diseases and have excellent compliance with the protocol. Effectiveness is the benefit a larger population receives from application of an RCT intervention to real health care situations in the community. Major differences between efficacy and effectiveness may be observed, which makes getting realistic measures of effectiveness a challenge at times.

12. Answer—d. An interim analysis plan is always designed prior to the start of recruitment. An important function of the data-monitoring and ethics committee is to stop an RCT when the study's interim data indicate a treatment benefit beyond a reasonable doubt ($P < .001$) in order to avoid recruiting patients who will receive an inferior standard of treatment. The committee may stop the trial when the new treatment is actually ineffective or insufficiently convincing to change clinical practice or resolve important therapeutic issues. The committee must also carefully investigate the data for side effects of treatment to avoid putting patients

at risk. Unexpected added benefits of treatment would be a bonus but would not require cessation of the RCT.

13. Answer—d. Evaluation of an RCT with a negative outcome requires consideration of the role of chance and the probability of a false negative, also called a type II, or β, error. The risk of a false negative study is particularly large in small RCTs. The probability that an RCT will find a statistically significant difference when a difference exists is called its statistical power. Statistical power = $1 - p_\beta$. Power is analogous to the sensitivity of a diagnostic test. In other words, a study with high power has a high probability of detecting a difference of effect if a difference exists. In order to detect small differences in treatment outcome it is necessary to have a large sample size. A p_β of .20 is often chosen. This means that a study has a 20% chance of missing a true difference in an RCT. A type I, or α, error is a measure of the possibility of a false positive result, and not the power of the study.

14. Answer—c. A recent review of 50 surveys of vision loss showed that, a quarter of a century later, the WHO definitions have taken hold, with 95% reporting on the WHO definitions of low vision (<20/60, <0.3, <6/18) and blindness (<20/400, <0.05, <3/60). The WHO defines vision according to a trichotomous scale (normal/low vision/blindness).

15. Answer—a. A survey is an observational epidemiologic study based on examination of all persons in a given population or a specifically defined subgroup of the population. It is most commonly used to estimate the prevalence and incidence (if there is follow-up) of a disease. Prevalence is estimated by cross-sectional studies that assess the presence of disease in a specific population at a point in time. As such, prevalence studies provide information on the magnitude or impact of the condition in the population but do not determine incidence or risk of developing the disease. The study design must attempt to minimize the influence of biases that may result from the methods used to measure endpoints and risk factors, as they will affect the interpretation of the data collected. Nonresponse biases occur if participants are not representative of the proposed study population due to selective nonparticipation.

16. Answer—d. Diseases that have a low frequency of occurrence in the population cannot be studied using large clinical trials. In such cases of rare disease, case series methodology is useful in collecting data. Small numbers of patients, who are seen by only one or a few clinicians, are carefully identified and followed in order to develop an information database about the disease. In most such cases, the clinician must have the initiative to pursue these data without research funding. Case series epidemiology has made significant contributions to the discipline. Numerous diseases such as diffuse unilateral subacute neuroretinitis (DUSN), acute posterior multifocal placoid pigment epitheliopathy, multiple evanescent white dot syndrome, and acute retinal necrosis have been characterized using this approach.

17. Answer—a. Among the causes of pediatric blindness, ophthalmia neonatorum, or congenital conjunctivitis, is particularly dangerous because it can blind babies within 28–30 days of birth. Although found worldwide, the disease is more prevalent in geographic areas with a higher incidence of sexually transmitted diseases. Prominent among these areas are East Africa and Southeast Asia. In developing countries, such as in East Africa, the incidence of ophthalmia neonatorum increases to more than 10% of all births. *Chlamydia trachomatis* is the most frequent etiologic agent. In a clinical trial of more than 3000 babies in Kenya, povidone-iodine ophthalmic solution was compared with two control groups that received either silver nitrate ophthalmic solution or erythromycin ophthalmic ointment. Povidone-iodine proved to be more effective than the other two agents while being less toxic.

18. Answer—b. Normal retinal vascularization begins at 16 weeks' gestation and is complete nasally by 36 weeks' gestation and temporally by 40 weeks' gestation. Each year, 4 million infant births occur in the United States. Eight percent of these are premature by definition: <2500 grams birth weight and 36 weeks' gestational age. Of these, upward of 30,000 have extremely low birth weight (ELBW = <1000 grams) and less than 32 weeks' gestational age. It is this pool of infants that is at highest risk for developing the most severe, sight-threatening forms of the disease. In a recent study, 49% of infants ≤1251 grams developed ROP in some form and, of these, approximately 7% reached threshold, requiring treatment. Despite this intervention, one child developed bilateral stage 5 ROP with bilateral blindness. Regression, spontaneous healing of the lesion, occurs in over 90% of eyes afflicted with ROP by 48 weeks' gestational age. Plus disease, in combination with a significant extent of advanced ROP in the periphery, carries an ominous prognosis. Once the disease has reached this stage, little can be done except to treat it, as the likelihood of spontaneous regression is slim.

19. Answer—c. A longitudinal analysis by Sommer on risk factors for the appearance and disappearance of ocular signs of xerophthalmia found that "mild" xerophthalmia, previously thought to be important only as a predictor of populations at high risk for the blinding form of the disease, was associated with an increased risk of mortality. Vitamin A supplementation is one of the most cost-effective preventive strategies for reducing mortality in young children in developing areas of the world. Since the 1920s, there has been a recognized association of vitamin A deficiency and alterations in immune system function. Night blindness is the earliest and most prevalent form of vitamin A deficiency. The most severe stages of xerophthalmia involve loss of corneal stromal structure through corneal ulceration, most often without associated inflammation, or by necrosis of the stroma.

20. Answer—c. Estimates of the incidence and prevalence of amblyopia vary in the range of 1%–2.5 % in children. Amblyopia is among the top three causes of monocular visual loss in the adult age group from 18 to 85 years. This is a disconcerting finding, as these are the ages where the bilateral diseases of the older ages—cataract, macular degeneration, diabetic retinopathy, glaucoma—take their toll. It suggests that the condition persists well beyond the childhood years, resistant to therapy, leaving its victims vulnerable to the above-mentioned diseases in later life. It is almost always associated with the presence of strabismus, refractive error/anisometropia, a combination of both, or from deprivation early in life. The loss may be monocular or binocular. Success is inversely related to length of treatment—the shorter the duration, the more likely it is to be successful.

21. Answer—a. The World Health Organization (WHO) Program for the Prevention of Blindness estimates that 55 million eye injuries occur globally each year. Penetrating injury is a single full-thickness laceration of the eye wall, usually caused by a sharp object, where no exit wound has occurred. Variables that influence the prognosis of final vision outcome after ocular trauma include type of injury, grade of injury based on visual acuity at initial examination, the presence or absence of a relative afferent pupillary defect in the involved eye, and the zone of injury. Other important variables include the presence of vitreous hemorrhage, involvement of the lens, and the presence of endophthalmitis. An important complication of corneal trauma is corneal infection caused by organisms from vegetative material. The size of the wound may not be as important as the location.

22. Answer—b. An epidemic of blindness affecting as many as 50,000 patients in Cuba reached international attention in May 1993, when the Cuban government made a plea to the United Nations. The Cuban National Operative Group (NOG), a group consisting of about 1000 Cuban scientists and clinicians who had been investigating the epidemic for almost 1 year, had an initial theory for a viral etiology, suggested by the exponential increase in cases, a west to east geographic movement, and coxsackie growth in cerebrospinal fluid cultures. In the face of new evidence presented in May 1993, this theory was finally abandoned. The most striking risk factors may have been from diets deficient in calories, protein, and vitamins. Through detailed histories, it was found that patients made their own home-brewed rum, which was analyzed and found to contain almost 1.0% methanol. Because 15 to 30 mL of methanol constitutes a morbid or lethal dose, these concentrations were too low to produce acute methanol toxicity. The findings of the study, as well as those of subsequent investigations, suggested a complex interplay of nutritional and toxic issues that compromised, in particular, mitochondrial function.

23. Answer—d. Clinical impressions, as well as data from blindness registries, have long suggested that POAG and POAG-related blindness are more frequent in black than white individuals. The presence of racial differences in POAG is supported by prevalence studies in populations of African origin, where rates are generally much higher, especially in African Caribbeans. In Baltimore, POAG was responsible for 19% ($n = 14$) of all blindness among African Americans and 6% ($n = 3$) among whites. After age adjustment, the blindness rate was 6 times higher among black than among white participants, and POAG prevalence was 4 times higher. In Barbados, POAG accounted for 28% ($n = 42$) of bilateral blindness and was the leading cause of visual loss. Additional follow-up of the Barbados cohort provided a measurement of incidence that supports the high risk of developing POAG in this population, with a 4-year incidence rate of 2.2%. The prevalence of POAG in black Barbados Eye Study participants was higher (7.0%) than that reported for African Americans in Baltimore (4.2%).

24. Answer—b. Use of a pilot study may be helpful in projecting a reasonable sample size and assessing survey feasibility. Identification of the population sample with a sampling frame is required to identify eligible persons in the population. Some studies have used a household census conducted by trained interviewers to identify eligible residents, whereas others have successfully used large population databases to identify the population. Examiners should be standardized in all measurements before the study begins. Detailed information may be obtained by both direct questioning and use of standardized questionnaires.

25. Answer—a. Evaluating a large population to enumerate the rate of blindness in children would be expensive. Most investigations obtain data by surveying the local schools for blind children. However, there are two problems with this approach: only school-age children are considered, and, in some cultures, not all children attend school (especially if it is perceived that they have no future). Despite these reservations, school surveys have provided most of the information available in the literature. More reliable data collection is often too costly.

26. Answer—d. Each year, 4 million infant births occur in the United States. Eight percent of these are premature by definition: <2500 grams birth weight and 36 weeks' gestational age. Of these, upward of 30,000 have extremely low birth weight (ELBW = <1000 grams) and less than 32 weeks' gestational age. It is this pool of infants that is at the highest risk for developing the most severe, sight-threatening forms of ROP. In a recent study, 49% of infants ≤1251 grams developed ROP in some form and, of these, approximately 7% reached threshold, requiring treatment. Despite this intervention, one child developed bilateral stage 5 ROP with bilateral blindness. Without intervention, and sometimes despite it, ROP leading to blindness has staggering costs: the lifetime costs of blindness to an individual and immediate family; lost economic opportunities to the individual and to society; the dollars that are needed to provide the mobility, skills training, and education to fit the individual into a useful societal role; and the costs to provide the infrastructure to meet the needs of the visually handicapped for special educational benefits, social security, transportation, and other living needs.

27. Answer—a. Treatment for children with clinical xerophthalmia is very inexpensive. Typical costs for high-dose vitamin A capsules are in the range of US$0.03/dose—less than US$0.10 for a treatment regimen of three doses. Clearly, costs of diagnosis and delivery of care are much higher than the cost of vitamin A, but this varies greatly depending on the system of care delivery and on the strategy used to distribute the vitamin A supplements. For example, a number of countries have dramatically increased their coverage of the at-risk population in a cost-efficient fashion by linking vitamin A capsule distribution to national immunization days used in the polio eradication program. The most important message is that, regardless of the system of care delivery or distribution, vitamin A supplementation is an extremely cost-effective preventive strategy and can be used to reduce mortality in young children in developing areas of the world.

28. Answer—c. An estimated 17 million persons are blind from cataract worldwide, making it the leading cause of visual loss. In the developed world, such as the United States and the United Kingdom, cataract is still a common cause of visual loss, especially among African Americans and the elderly. By the year 2020, it is estimated that 40 million people worldwide will have blinding cataract. The economic impact in developing countries of vision loss from cataract is huge, including loss of jobs and increase in custodial care. It is estimated that 1500% of the cost of cataract surgery could be generated in 1 year through increased economic productivity. As such, cataract surgery is ranked as one of the most cost-effective public health interventions for the developing world.

29. Answer—d. Because reinfection is so common, it is not productive simply to treat individual cases of active trachoma. Rather, treatment efforts have to be directed toward a community and include the costs of identifying high-risk communities, educating these communities concerning the importance of hygiene, purchasing and distributing antibiotics, identifying trichiasis cases, and performing corrective surgery. Corrective surgery for trichiasis can be performed in about 15 minutes for approximately US$10–$20. Although blindness from trichiasis is rare in those under 30 years of age and much more common in the elderly, it can still be particularly costly to families and communities, as younger, productive members of the community have to care for the blind.

30. Answer—a. Modern treatment of HIV/AIDS includes long-term use of three or more antiretroviral agents, an approach termed combination therapy, or highly active antiretroviral therapy (HAART). The cost of such therapy currently exceeds $10,000 per year in the United States. High costs have limited the availability of both HAART and other HIV-related therapies to countries and regions where private or governmental health coverage is available to help meet the costs of therapy, most notably the United States, Western Europe, and selected countries in South America, such as Brazil and Argentina. The vast majority of patients with HIV/AIDS, who live in the developing world, go untreated. In some countries in sub-Saharan Africa, HIV infection is so common that overall life expectancy has dropped by more than 20 years over the past 2 decades, essentially reversing 50 years of social progress. Infection of large numbers of relatively young adults with HIV also affects children and future generations, both because a significant number of children born to HIV-positive women will themselves be infected by the virus and because many children, whether infected or not, will ultimately lose their parents to HIV disease. Recent estimates suggest that there are over 1 million HIV-positive children and nearly 12 million HIV/AIDS orphans worldwide.

31. Answer—b. Onchocerciasis is a parasitic infection caused by the filarial nematode *Onchocerca volvulus*. It is transmitted by the vector *Simulium* spp, or blackfly, which breeds in fast-flowing rivers and streams. Often called *river blindness,* it is a devastating, blinding disease that occurs in communities living along rivers, usually in remote, rural areas of tropical Africa, the Arabian Peninsula, and in foci in Latin America. Two drugs have been available for treating onchocerciasis: diethylcarbamazine (DEC), a microfilaricide, and suramin, a macrofilaricide. However, both cause very serious adverse reactions and are, thus, unsuitable for mass treatment. Ivermectin (Mectizan), a safe microfilaricide suitable for use in large-scale treatment, has proven an effective alternative. However, ivermectin is only microfilaricidal, so population treatment needs to continue during the entire lifespan of the adult worm, which can be up to 14 years.

Index

(i = image; t = table)

Absolute risk reduction (ARR), 23
Activities of daily living (ADL), 37
Acute retinal necrosis, 71
ADL. *See* Activities of daily living (ADL)
Affluence risk factor
   blindness and, 79
   ocular trauma and, 130
   prevention of blindness and, 150–151
African eye disease studies, 148–149t
African Programme for Onchocerciasis Control (APOC), 236i, 238, 250
Age
   cataracts related to, 161–162, 168t
   onchocercal eye lesions and, 243i
   PAC incidence and, 180i
   as vision impairment risk factor, 145–146, 146i, 147i
   visual acuity changes with, 45i
Age-related macular degeneration (AMD), 32–33, 147
Amblyopia
   clinical presentation and findings, 115–116
   context of, 111–112
   current treatment programs, 116–119
   economic impact of, 114
   epidemiology of, 112–114
   history of, 111
   pathogenesis, 114–115
   prevention, 116
   probability of therapy success, 117t
   weeks after first patching stopped, 119i
AMD. *See* Age-related macular degeneration (AMD)
American Society for Testing and Materials, 131
Ancylostoma caninum (dog hookworm), 69
Andhra Pradesh Eye Disease Study
   comparison to other studies, 144t, 145t
   gonioscopy used during, 61
   ocular examination data in, 59
   on prevention, 151
   rate of severe visual impairment reported in, 143–145
   references listed for, 62
Anterior uveitis, 246
Aravind Eye Care System (India)
   background of, 291–292
   challenges in scaling-up process for, 302
   demand generation clinical service model of, 294, 295i
   division of labor in, 299–300
   economies of scale and, 298
   as equitable development model, 292–293
   financial viability of, 300
   in-house technology used in, 301
   LAICO expansion of, 300–301
   local ownership/financial self-sufficiency of, 295–296
   number of surgeries under, 293
   output per hour under different scenarios, 299t
   quality assurance of, 300
   social marketing of, 296–298
   standardization of, 299
Aravind Eye Hospital (India)
   blindness prevention model of, 8
   in-house technology used by, 301
   studies on ocular trauma and occupation by, 129
Archives of Ophthalmology (journal), 25
Arlt's line, 209–210i
ARR (absolute risk reduction), 23
Asian eye disease studies, 148
The Asian Foundation for the Prevention of Blindness, 9
Astigmatism, 157
Auditing outcomes, 36
Australian Corneal Graft Registry, 337
Auto accident injuries, 133–134

Baltimore Eye Survey
   comparison to other studies, 143–145, 144t, 145t, 146i, 147
   ocular examination data in, 59
   references listed for, 63
   sampling issues in, 57–58
Barbados Eye Study (BES)
   comparison to other studies, 143–145, 144t
   on primary open-angle glaucoma (POAG), 174–176
   references listed for, 63
   sampling issues in, 58
Baylisascaris procyonis (raccoon ascarid), 68
Beaver Dam Eye Study
   comparison to other studies, 144t, 145, 145t, 147i
   ocular examination data in, 59
   references listed for, 63
   sampling issues in, 57–58
Bias
   detection, 56
   in meta-analysis, 28–29
   nonresponse, 55–56
   recall, 56
   sampling, 56
Bilateral ocular injuries, 128–129
Birth trauma, 81
Blindness. *See also* Pediatric blindness; Vision impairment; Vision loss
   comparing causes of adult, 140t
   contribution of HIV/AIDS to global, 232
   definitions of, 40, 42–43t, 143
   individual contributions to reducing avoidable, 9–14
   international efforts to reduce avoidable, 5–9
   ocular trauma and, 121–134
   prevalence of avoidable, 5
   WHO definition of, 43t, 77
   WHO estimates on bilateral, 335
Bloch, CE, 99
Blue Mountains Eye Study
   ocular examination data in, 59
   references listed for, 63
   sampling issues in, 57–58
Brazil. *See also* CFZ (cataract-free zone) projects (Brazil)
   CFZ projects, supporting organizations/agencies in, 327
   national campaign for prevention of blindness (1998) in, 327

national eye banking program in, 337–338
recommendations for future programs in, 327–328
Brazilian Council of Ophthalmology, 327
British Diabetic Association, 194
British ophthalmologist distribution, 7
Buffon, Comet de, 111
Burden of disease
cost-benefit analysis of, 34
cost-effectiveness analysis of, 34–36t
cost-utility analysis of, 34–35
using DALYs to measure, 33–34

CAHA. *See* Canadian Amateur Hockey Association (CAHA)
Canadian Amateur Hockey Association (CAHA), 132
The Canadian National Institute for the Blind, 9
Canadian Ophthalmological Society, 134
Canadian Standards Association, 338
The Carter Center, 9
Case-control studies, 31–32
Case series epidemiology
description of, 65–66
in diagnosis, 66–68
in treatment, 69–71
Case series studies, 32–33
Casteldaccia Eye Study, 144t, 145, 146i
Cataract. *See also* CFZ (cataract-free zone) projects
background of, 161–162
clinical research currently under way on, 170
economic impact of, 162–163
epidemiology of, 166–169
extracapsular cataract extraction (ECCE) technique used for, 327, 333, 334
magnitude of problem, 162
mortality and, 169
pediatric blindness from, 80
quality of life and, 165–166
risk factors, 166–169, 167t, 168t
Cataract management (developing countries)
background of, 329–330
Fred Hollows Foundation system of, 331–334
surgical, 330–331
Cataract surgery
outcome studies on, 30, 165
prevalence rates of, 164t
quality of, 165
VISION 2020 goal for accessible, 166
Ceftriaxone, 89
Central America eye disease studies, 148
CENTRAL database, 25
Centre for Eye Research Australia (CERA), 283
Centre for Rehabilitation of Blind and Visually Impaired (LV Prasad Eye Institute), 308t
Centre for Sight Enhancement (LV Prasad Eye Institute), 308t
CEON. *See* Cuban epidemic optic neuropathy (CEON)
CFZ (cataract-free zone) projects (Brazil). *See also* Brazil
accomplishments of, 325–326
backlog of unoperated cataract and, 322
development of, 323
magnitude of problem facing, 321
personnel training for, 323
public health system/available eye care and, 322

surgical techniques used in, 326–327
waiting line for, 324i
CFZ (cataract-free zone) projects (Peru)
community support of, 324–325
workers and patients of, 325i, 326i
Chemotherapy, for onchocerciasis, 248–250
Children. *See also* Pediatric blindness
assessing refractive errors in, 157
corneal blindness among, 336
ETDRS standard chart for, 50
ocular trauma risk factors for, 128
preschool screening for amblyopia, 113, 116–117
screening for refractive error in, 158
Snellen's original chart (1862), symbols for, 47–49
trachoma risk factors for, 207–208
trachoma treatment for, 211
Chlamydia trachomatis, 87, 205, 209, 212
Chlamydial conjunctivitis, 87, 89t
Chorioretinitis, 246–247i
Choroidal neovascular membranes (CNVM), 32–33
Christoffel-Blindenmission (Christian Blind Mission International [CBM]), 10, 317–318, 319i
Closed-globe injury classification, 125t
CME. *See* Cystoid macular edema (CME)
CNVM. *See* Choroidal neovascular membranes (CNVM)
Cochrane, Archie, 19
Cochrane Database of Systematic Reviews, 26, 27
Cochrane Library, 19, 29
Cogan, DG, 92
Cohort studies, 30–31
Collaborative research
on Cuban epidemic optic neuropathy (CEON), 261–270
Glaucoma Inheritance Study in Tasmania (GIST), 271–275
Hong Kong Vision Study (HKVS), 283–286
ophthalmia neonatorum research paradigm for, 257–259
on sickle cell retinopathy in Jamaica, 277–282
Consanguinity, 80
CONSORT (Consolidated Standards of Reporting Trials) statement, 25
Contact lenses, 158–159
Corneal blindness
background on, 335–336
resources on, 342t
Corneal opacity (CO), 212i
Corneal transplantation. *See also* Eye banks
in the developing countries, 336–337
establishing eye banking programs for, 338–339
national eye banking programs for, 337–338
Corneal ulceration "silent epidemic," 335
Cost-benefit analysis, 34
Cost-effectiveness analysis, 34–36t
Cost-utility analysis, 34–35
Cryotherapy for ROP Trial, 96
Cuban epidemic optic neuropathy (CEON)
clinical presentation and findings, 263–264i
concentration of cases, 265i
context of, 262
current treatment of, 268
economic impact of, 262–263
epidemiology, 263–266

Index • 363

government policies and scientific bias impact on, 262
history of, 261
lessons learned from, 269–270
optic nerve pathology in, 268*i*
pathogenesis of, 266–267
prevention of, 268
research currently under way on, 269
risk factors for, 263, 266
Cystoid macular edema (CME), 28
Cytomegalovirus (CMV), 223, 225
Cytomegalovirus retinitis, 232–233

Dadaab Refugee Camp surgery (East Africa), 311*i*
DALYs. *See* Disability-adjusted life-years (DALYs)
Dark & Light, 10
Data collection
 interview, 58–59
 ocular examination, 59
 ophthalmic survey methodology and, 58–59
Data-monitoring and ethics committee, 24
DCCT. *See* Diabetes Control and Complications Trial (DCCT)
Detection bias, 56
Developed countries
 contact lens use in, 158–159
 economic impact of uncorrected refraction error in, 154
 factors influencing vision impairment in, 140–141
 prevention of eye injuries in auto accidents in, 133
 quality of cataract surgery in, 165
 retinopathy of prematurity (ROP) in, 80, 94*t*
Developing countries
 cataract management in, 329–334
 central corneal ulcers in, 217*t*
 corneal transplantation in, 336–337
 difficulties using ETDRS standard charts in, 50
 economic impact of uncorrected refraction error in, 154
 epidemiology applicable to, 5
 factors affecting pediatric blindness in, 79–81
 factors influencing vision impairment in, 140–141
 ophthalmia neonatorum research paradigm for studies in, 257–259
 prevalence of pediatric blindness in, 77–78*i*
 providone-iodine prophylaxis considered for, 89–90*i*
 quality of cataract surgery in, 165
Diabetes Control and Complications Trial (DCCT), 23–24, 29*i*, 190, 194
Diabetes mellitus
 measuring DALYs for, 34
 measuring risk and benefits in treatment of, 23–24
 prevalence of blindness in Iceland due to, 196*i*
 prevalence of diabetic retinopathy and duration of, 192*i*, 193*i*
 risk factors, 194
 screening for, 193–194
Diabetic retinopathy
 DCCT report on treatment of, 194
 DRS findings on epidemiology of, 191–193*i*
 Iceland programs for, 195–199
 masked photographic grading for measuring, 61
Diabetic Retinopathy Study (DRS)
 background of, 189–190

epidemiology, 191–193*i*
pathogenesis, 190
Diethylcarbamazine (DEC), 248
Diffuse unilateral subacute neuroretinitis (DUSN)
 description of, 66–67
 diagnosis of, 67–69
 treatment of, 69–71
Disability-adjusted life-years (DALYs)
 as global disease measurement, 33–34
 vitamin A deficiency and, 100
Division of Maternal and Child Health (U.S. Public Health Service), 113
DM. *See* Diabetes mellitus
DMEC. *See* Data-monitoring and ethics committee
DRS. *See* Diabetic Retinopathy Study (DRS)
DUSN. *See* Diffuse unilateral subacute neuroretinitis (DUSN)

Early Treatment Diabetic Retinopathy Study (ETDRS), 189–190
Early Treatment for ROP Trial, 96
EBAA (Eye Bank Association of America), 337, 339
EBAI (Eye Bank Association of India), 338, 342
EMB. *See* Evidence-based medicine
Endogenous infections, 80
Epidemiology
 amblyopia, 112–114
 applicable to developed and developing nations, 5
 case series, 65–71
 cataract, 166–169
 Diabetic Retinopathy Study (DRS) findings on, 191–193*i*
 of HIV/AIDS affecting vision, 228–232*i*
 of Kikuyu Eye Unit, 311–312
 ocular trauma, 126–128
 onchocerciasis, 240–244*i*
 ophthalmia neonatorum, 86
 primary angle-closure glaucoma (PACG), 179–181
 primary open-angle glaucoma (POAG), 171, 174
 retinopathy of prematurity (ROP), 79–80, 93–95, 94*t*
 sickle cell retinopathy (Jamaica), 278
 trachoma, 206–209*i*
 uncorrected refraction error, 155–157
 vitamin A deficiency disorders, 101–102
Erythromycin ophthalmic ointment, 88, 89
ESI (Eye Sight International), 341–342
ETDRS. *See* Early Treatment Diabetic Retinopathy Study (ETDRS)
ETDRS standard charts
 choice of test distance for, 50, 51*i*
 data collection using, 59
 developing countries and difficulties with, 50
 measuring visual acuity loss with, 40, 41
 scoring on non-ETDRS charts vs., 50
Ethical methodology standards, 57
Ethnic differences. *See also* Populations; Risk factors
 cataract and, 161, 167*t*, 168*t*
 eye disease studies on, 141–142, 148–150
 ophthalmia neonatorum and, 86
 prevalence of myopia in, 155–156
 in primary open-angle glaucoma (POAG), 171–176
 trachoma and, 209
 vision impairment studies on age and, 146*i*, 147*i*
 vitamin A deficiency, 103

European Eye Bank Association, 338
Evidence-based medicine, 19–36
  auditing outcomes and, 36
  described, 19–20
  grading scales of evidence for, 20–21
  hierarchy of preprocessed evidence for, 20t
  levels of evidence used in, 21t
  measuring burden of disease, 33–36t
  observational studies in, 30–33
  randomized controlled trials and, 21–25
  systematic reviews and meta-analysis of, 25–29
  US Preventive Services Task Force rating evidence, 20t
External validity, 56
Extracapsular cataract extraction (ECCE), 326, 327, 333, 334
Eye Bank Association of America (EBAA), 337, 339
Eye Bank Association of India (EBAI), 338, 342
Eye banks. See also Corneal transplantation
  elements of "best" models for, 339–340
  establishing successful, 338–339
  existing national programs, 337–338
  government participation in, 341
  strategies for developing successful, 341–342
  tissue retrieval and distribution models for, 340–341
Eye care. See also Ophthalmologic examination
  evidence domains relevant to delivery of, 21
  levels of evidence used in evidence-based, 21t
Eye Sight International (ESI), 341–342

Finland ocular trauma studies, 129
Flynn, J, 75
Foster, A, 137, 336
Foundation of the American Academy of Ophthalmology, 83
The Fred Hollows Foundation, 10–11
  estimates of cataract surgery costs, 333
  overview of cataract management by, 331–334
  training programs conducted by, 333–334
Functional vision, 37

Gass, JDM, 67, 70
Gaza, 80
Gentamicin, 89
Geographic/environmental/social factors. See also Risk factors
  Cuban epidemic optic neuropathy (CEON) and, 263–266
  HIV/AIDS and, 229–232
  microbial keratitis and, 217
  onchocerciasis and, 242–244
  ophthalmia neonatorum and, 86
  prevalence of myopia and, 155–156t
  study findings on vision impairment and, 148–150
  trachoma and, 207–209
  vitamin A deficiency and, 102–103i
Glaucoma. See also Primary angle-closure glaucoma; Primary open-angle glaucoma
  assessed using gonioscopy, 61
  ethnic differences in primary open-angle, 171–176
Glaucoma Inheritance Study in Tasmania (GIST)
  agreement between family history/actual diagnosis in, 273t
  background on, 271

comparative size of pedigrees/diagnostic status of family members, 272i
design of, 271–272
findings of, 274–275
future treatment recommendations of, 275
social concerns and, 275
study methodology used in, 273–274
Gonioscopy, 61, 183
Gonococcus, 87, 87i, 89t
Group purchasing organizations (GPOs), 301

HAART. See Highly active antiretroviral therapy.
Haemophilus, 87
Handicap aspect, 37
Health care delivery systems
  Aravind Eye Care System (India), 291–302
  for cataract management in developing countries, 329–334
  CFZ (cataract-free zone) projects, 321–328
  for global eye banking/corneal transplanation, 335–342
  Kikuyu Eye Unit (Kenya), 311–319
  LV Prasad Eye Institute (LVPEI) [India], 303–310
Helen Keller Worldwide, 11
Herpes simplex virus, 87
Herpes zoster ophthalmicus (HZO), 223
Highly active antiretroviral therapy (HAART), 223–225, 227, 229i, 233–234
HIV/AIDS
  clinical presentation/findings on ocular complications of, 232–233
  common forms of retinitis observed in patients with, 230i
  contribution to global blindness by, 232
  economic impact of, 223–226
  epidemiology of, 228–232i
  HAART treatment for, 223–225, 227, 229i, 233–234
  history and context of, 223
  natural history of HIV infection, 227i
  pathogenesis of, 226–228i, 228t, 229i
  population living with (2001), 224i
  prevention of, 233
  risk factors, 229–232
  screening for, 233
Hockey injuries, 132–133t
Hong Kong Vision Study (HKVS)
  background of, 283
  clinical presentation of, 284
  findings from, 284–285
  pathogenesis, 284
  prevalence/degree of myopia in comparable studies, 285t
Hospital ocular trauma studies, 127t
HOTV test, 48
HZO (herpes zoster ophthalmicus), 223

IAPB. See International Agency for the Prevention of Blindness
ICD. See International Statistical Classification of Diseases, Injuries, and Causes of Death (ICD)
Iceland
  diabetes mellitus treatment programs in, 195
  incidence of diabetic retinopathy in, 193i
  prevalence of legal blindness due to diabetes in, 196i

program strengths and weaknesses in, 198
screening for diabetic retinopathy in, 195–199
utilization of eye-care services in, 198
ICF (International Classification of Functioning), 37
ICIDH. *See* International Classification of Impairments, Disabilities and Handicaps (ICIDH)
ICO (International Council of Ophthalmology), 8, 11–12
IFOS (International Federation of Ophthalmological Societies), 5, 12
India. *See also* Aravind Eye Care System (India); LV Prasad Eye Institute (LVPEI) [India]
Andhra Pradesh Eye Disease Study in, 59, 61, 62, 143–145, 151
distribution of ophthalmologists in, 7
models of blindness prevention/treatment in, 8–9
Indirect ophthalmoscopy, 61
Individual patient data (IPD) meta-analysis, 27
Infectious keratitis, 159
Informed consent, 57
Institutional Review Board, 24
Internal validity, 56
International Agency for the Prevention of Blindness (IABP), 5–6, 12
International Centre for Eyecare Education, 12
International Classification of Functioning (ICF), 37
International Classification of Impairments, Disabilities and Handicaps (ICIDH), 37
International Cochrane Collaboration, 26
International Council of Ophthalmology (ICO), 8, 12
International Federation of Ophthalmological Societies (IFOS), 5, 11–12
International Statistical Classification of Diseases, Injuries, and Causes of Death (ICD), 60
Interview data collection, 58–59
IPD (Individual patient data meta-analysis), 27
Isenberg, Sherwin J, 256
Ivermectin
DUSN treatment using, 70
onchocerciasis treatment using, 249–250

Japan Eye Bank Association, 338, 342

Kaplan-Meier analysis, 118
Kenya, 258–259, 311–318
Kenyatta National Hospital, 313
Keratitis, 245, 246*i*
Kikuyu Eye Unit (KEU) [Kenya]
background of, 311
Christoffel-Blindenmission (CBM) work with, 10, 317–318, 319*i*
epidemiology of, 311–312
finances of, 317–318*t*
operations performed under direction of, 311*i*, 314*i*
ophthalmic infrastructure of, 312
outreach services of, 316–317*i*
personnel of, 313–314
physical structure of, 312–313
services by department, 314–315
teaching and research programs at, 315–316
Koch's postulates (1882), 67*t*
Kumamoto University Study, 194

Landolt Cs (or Landolt broken rings), 49
Laser in situ keratomileusis (LASIK), 159

LCR (ligase chain reaction), 211
Lea symbols, 47
Legally sighted/legally blind scale, 40–41
Lens Opacities Classification System (LOCS), 60, 161
Ligase chain reaction (LCR), 211
Lighthouse International, 12
Lions Aravind Institute of Community Ophthalmology (LAICO), 300–301
Lions Clubs International Foundation, 12
"Lizard skin," 244
LOCS III, 60
LOGIC syndrome, 81
LogMAR (logarithm of the minimum angle of resolution) scale, 41
Lumbini Eye Hospital (Nepal), 302
LV Prasad Eye Institute (LVPEI) [India]
background of, 303
basic research projects at, 307*t*
challenges faced by, 304–310
eye bank maintained by, 307
financial expenditures and resources of, 304–307
origins and development of, 303–304
outpatients and surgeries served by, 305*i*, 306*i*, 309*t*
personnel training at, 307–308
quality assurance at, 309–310
rehabilitation services offered by, 308*t*
services in underserved areas by, 308–309
Lymphatic system, onchocerciasis and, 244

McCollum, EV, 99
Macula evaluation, 60
Masked photographic grading, 61
Mazzotti reaction, 248
Measles/vitamin A deficiency comorbidity, 106
Mectizan Donation Program, 249
Mectizan Expert Committee, 249
Medical therapy cost-effectiveness comparison, 36*t*
MEDLINE, 25
Melbourne Visual Impairment Project. *See also* Visual Impairment Project
ocular examination data in, 59
references listed for, 63
sampling issues in, 58
Meta-analysis
bias in, 28–29
described, 25, 27–28
individual patient data, 27
Microbial keratitis
clinical presentation and findings, 218–219*i*
clinical research currently under way, 220–221
current treatment/screening programs for, 219–220
economic impact of, 215–216
epidemiology of, 216–217*t*
history and context of, 215
pathogenesis of, 216
prevention of, 219
risk factors, 217
Middle East eye disease studies, 150
Migration patterns, 81
Minimal/mild vision loss range, 44
Moderate vision loss range, 46
Myopia
clinical presentation and findings, 157
clinical research currently under way, 160

current treatment programs, 158–159
prevalence of, 155–156t
prevention of, 157
risk factors for, 155–156
study on Hong Kong population, 283–286
surveys to determine prevalence of, 156–157

National Eye Institute, 40
National Program for Control of Blindness (India), 7
National Study of Cataract Outcomes, 165
NDF (Neutral Density Filter Test), 109
Near vision tests, 50–52i
Near-blindness range, 46
Near-total vision loss range, 46
Neisseria gonorrhoeae, 89t
Neonatal intensive care units, 79–80
Neutral Density Filter Test (NDF), 115–116
NGOs (nongovernmental organizations), 8
NNT. *See* Number needed to treat
Nonresponse bias, 55–56
The Noor Al Hussein Foundation, 13
Normal vision range, 44
Normal vision/low vision/blindness classifications, 40
Nuclear cataract, 169
Number needed to treat, 23

Observational studies
  case-control, 31–32
  case series, 32–33
  cohort, 30–31
  defining, 30
  outcomes, 30
Occupation/ocular injuries link, 129
Ocular examination
  automated perimetry data using, 59
  data collection using, 59
  refraction data using, 59
Ocular trauma
  auto accidents and, 133–134
  classification system for, 122, 123i, 125t
  context of, 121
  data collection on, 130
  economic impact of, 122
  epidemiology of, 126–128
  hospital studies on, 127t
  as important cause of visual acuity loss, 336
  pathogenesis, 131
  prevention standards, 131–134
  proposed terminology of, 124t
  risk factors, 128–130
  sports and, 130, 131, 132–133t
  terminology issues of, 122
Odds ratio, 23
Onchocercal nodules, 244
Onchocerciasis
  clinical presentation and findings on, 244–246
  clinical research currently under way on, 250–251
  current treatment/screening programs for, 247–250
  described, 235
  diagnosis of, 244
  economic impact of, 238–239
  epidemiology of, 240–244i
  global control programs for, 235, 236i, 239, 240–242, 248, 249–250

history and context of, 236, 238
Onchocerca volvulus and, 69, 237i, 239–240, 244
pathogenesis and immune response, 239–240
prevention of, 247
risk factors, 242–244
Onchocerciasis Control Programme (OCP), 235, 236i, 239, 240–242, 247–248, 250
Open-globe injuries
  classifications of, 125t
  zones of, 126i
Operation Eyesight Universal, 13
Ophthalmia neonatorum
  background of, 85
  clinical presentation and findings, 81i, 82, 86–87i
  economic impact of, 85
  epidemiology of, 86
  pediatric blindness due to, 81, 81i, 82
  prevention of, 88
  prophylaxis administered to prevent, 82, 82i
  treatment of, 89–90, 89t, 90i
  work-up of, 88–89, 88t
Ophthalmia neonatorum research
  algorithm for planning, 258t
  background of, 257
  findings of, 259
  mechanisms for preparing foreign study, 258–259
  pilot data of, 257–258
Ophthalmic survey methodology
  data collection in, 58–59
  design issues of, 55–56
  ethical standards and informed consent, 57
  interpretation of, 56
  sampling issues, 57–58
  using standardized exam/international classification/ grading system, 60–62
Ophthalmologic examination. *See also* Eye care
  data management/analysis of, 62
  document summarizing results of, 62
  gonioscopy used during, 61
  importance of complete, 140
  indirect ophthalmoscopy during, 61
  using international classifications/grading system during, 60–62
  LOCS III for lens, 60
  macula assessment during, 61
  masked photographic grading methods during, 61
  stereophotography used during, 61
  VCDR for optic nerve assessment, 60
Ophthalmologists
  British distribution of, 7
  South African distribution of, 7
  utilization of volunteer, 8
  VISION 2020 goal for distribution of, 312
Ophthalmology (journal), 25
Optic nerve VCDR assessment, 60
OR. *See* Odds ratio
Oral antihelminthic drugs, 69–71
ORBIS International (Headquarters), 13
Organisation pour la Prévention de la Cécité, 13
Oulu Study, 144t, 145, 146i
Outcome studies, 30
Ovid Evidence-based Medicine Reviews database, 25
Oxford Clinical Cataract Classification and Grading System, 161–162

PACG. *See* Primary angle-closure glaucoma
Participation methodology issues, 58
Pashby, TJ, 133
Paulus Sextineus, 111
PCR (polymerase chain reaction), 211
Pediatric blindness. *See also* Blindness; Children
   amblyopia and, 111–119
   causes of, 79
   estimates by world region, 77–78*i*
   factors in particular regions affecting, 79–81
   global prevention and treatment efforts for, 75–76
   methods for assessing population, 79
   ophthalmia neonatorum and, 81*i*, 85–90*i*
   ordered approach to dealing with world, 77
   retinopathy of prematurity (ROP) and, 80, 91–97
   suggestions for reducing, 82–83
   WHO statistics on global, 3
Pediatric blindness risk factors
   affluence, 79
   availability of neonatal intensive care units, 79–80
   cataracts, 80
   consanguinity, 80
   endogenous infections, 80
   migration patterns, 81
   perinatal factors, 81
   rural vs. city setting, 80
Perinatal risk factors, 81
Perkins School for the Blind, 13
Peruvian Society of Ophthalmology, 325
Peto odds ratio, 23–24
Phacoemulsification, 326–327
Photorefractive keratectomy, 159
Pictures (as optotypes), 49
Pilot study, 57
POAG. *See* Primary open-angle glaucoma (POAG)
Polymerase chain reaction (PCR), 211
Populations. *See also* Ethnic differences
   identification of sample in, 57–58
   living with HIV/AIDS (2001), 224*i*
   methods for assessing childhood blindness in, 79
   ocular trauma studies based on, 128*t*
   participation issues for sample, 58
   prevalence of myopia in various, 156*t*
   sample selection issues, 57–58
   study on myopia in Hong Kong, 283–286
   summary of POAG studies on ethnic, 172*t*–173*t*
Posterior subcapsular cataract (PSC), 162
Povidone-iodine prophylaxis, 89–90*i*
Preventable infectious causes of vision impairment. *See also* Vision impairment
   HIV/AIDS, 223–234
   microbial keratitis, 215–221
   onchocerciasis, 235–251
   trachoma, 205–213, 335
Prevention of blindness programs, 9–13
Primary angle-closure glaucoma (PACG)
   age- and sex-specific incidence of, 180*i*
   assessed using gonicoscopy, 61, 183
   asymptomatic patients and, 186–187
   clinical presentation and findings, 182–183
   context of, 177–179
   epidemiology of, 179–181
   ethnicity and, 179–180
   history of, 177

pathogenesis, 179
   prevention, 183–186
   pupillary block and non-pupillary block in, 179
   recommendations for research into, 178–179
   research currently under way on, 187
   risk factors, 181–182
   screening for, 183–184, 185*i*, 186*i*
   sequence of events triggering, 182
   treatment, 185–186
Primary open-angle glaucoma (POAG)
   Barbados Eye Study on, 174–176
   comparisons among studies on, 174
   epidemiology, 171, 174
   ethnic differences in, 171–176, 172*t*, 173*t*
   risk factors for, 181–182
   summary of population-based studies on, 172*t*–173*t*
PRK surgery, 159
Profound vision loss range, 46
Prospective cohort study, 30–31
Protective eyewear
   shotgun injuries and, 131
   sports and, 130, 131–133

Quality-adjusted life-year (QALY), 34, 35

Radial keratotomy (RK), 159
Randomized controlled trials (RCTs)
   auditing outcomes, 36
   clinically useful measures of effects of treatment, 24*t*
   CONSORT statement on, 25
   efficacy vs. effectiveness outcomes of, 22–23
   evidence gathering standards established by, 21–22
   measuring burden of disease, 33–35
   measuring risks and benefits, 23–24
   meta-analysis of, 25, 27–29
   methodology of, 21–22
   observational studies used in, 30–33
   reporting adverse events in, 23
   registries, 25
   role of data-monitoring and ethics committee in, 24
   systematic reviews of, 25–26
Recall bias, 56
Refractive surgery, 159
Relative risk, or risk ratio (RR), 23–24
Relative risk reduction (RRR), 23
Research Ethics Committee, 24
Retinopathy of prematurity (ROP)
   clinical presentation of, 95
   clinical research on, 96–97
   current treatment of, 96
   economic impact of, 92
   epidemiology of, 79–80, 93–95, 94*t*
   history of, 91
   neonatal intensive care units availability and, 79–80
   pathogenesis of, 92–93
   prevention of, 95
   rural vs. city setting and, 80
Retrolental fibroplasia. *See* Retinopathy of prematurity
Retrospective cohort study, 31
Ridley's fundus, 246, 247*i*
Risk factors. *See also* Ethnic differences; Geographic/environmental/social factors
   age, 145–146*i*, 147*i*
   for cataract, 166–169, 167*t*, 168*t*

for Cuban epidemic optic neuropathy (CEON), 263–266
for diabetes mellitus, 194
for HIV/AIDS, 229–232
influencing vision impairment, 140–141
for microbial keratitis, 217
for ocular trauma, 128–130
for onchocerciasis, 242–244
for ophthalmia neonatorum, 86
for pediatric blindness, 79–81
for primary angle-closure glaucoma (PACG), 181–182
for primary open-angle glaucoma (POAG), 176
for trachoma, 207–209
for uncorrected refraction error, 155–156
for vitamin A deficiency disorders, 102–103i
River blindness. *See* Onchocerciasis
RK (Radial keratotomy), 159
ROP. *See* Retinopathy of prematurity (ROP)
Rotterdam Eye Study
compared to Hong Kong Vision Study (HKVS), 283, 285
comparison to other studies, 144t, 145, 145t, 146i, 147i
RR (relative risk, or risk ratio), 23–24
RRR (relative risk reduction), 23
Rural Outreach Program (LV Prasad Eye Institute), 308–309, 309t
Rural vs. city setting, 80

Sackett, David L, 21
S.A.F.E. strategy, 212
Salisbury Eye Evaluation Project
comparison to other studies, 144t, 145t, 147i
references listed for, 63
sampling issues in, 58
Sampling issues
bias as, 56
for ophthalmic survey methodology, 57–58
Screening
for amblyopia, 113, 116–117
for diabetes mellitus, 193–194
for diabetic retinopathy (Iceland), 195–197
for HIV/AIDS, 233
for microbial keratitis, 219–220
for onchocerciasis, 247–248
for primary angle-closure glaucoma (PACG) and PAC, 183–184, 185i, 186i
for refractive error, 158
for trachoma, 211–212
Seva Foundation, 13
Severe vision loss range, 46
Sex-specific incidence of PAC, 180i
Shotgun injuries, 131
Sickle cell (SS) disease
anemia due to, 277
global distribution of, 277i
Sickle cell retinopathy (Jamaica)
background of, 277–278
clinical findings in, 279–281, 279i, 280i
epidemiology of, 278
natural history of, 278–279i, 280i
treatment and prevention of visual loss due to, 281
Sight Savers International, 14

Smoking/cataract relationship, 166–167, 168t
Snellen eye chart (1862), 46–48, 48t, 50
Sofia Study, 144t
Sommer, A, 75, 99, 150
South Africa ophthalmologist distribution, 7
South America eye disease studies, 148
South Pacific eye disease studies, 150
Sport injuries
American Society for Testing and Materials on, 131
hockey and ocular, 132–133t
ocular trauma and, 130
Sri Lanka, 80
Staphylococcus aureus, 87
Stereophotography, 61
Stockholm Diabetes Intervention Study, 27
Studies of Ocular Complications of AIDS (SOCA), 232
Systematic review, 25–26

Thailand prevention of blindness programs, 7
Thiabendazole, 70
Tielsch, J, 75
Tilganga Eye Centre (Nepal), 334
Total blindness range, 46
Toxocara canis infection, 68, 69
Toxoplasmosis macular scarring, 80
Trachoma
clinical presentation and findings, 209–210
clinical research currently under way on, 213
economic impact of, 205–206
epidemiology of, 206–209i
history and context of, 205
as leading cause of corneal blindness/morbidity, 335
pathogenesis of, 206i, 207i
prevention, 210–211
risk factors, 207–209
screening for, 211–212
treatment programs for, 212–213
WHO grading system for, 211t
Tumbling Es test, 48

UKPDS (United Kingdom Prospective Diabetes Study), 190, 194
Uncorrected refractive error
clinical presentation and findings, 157
clinical research currently under way, 160
context of, 153
current treatment programs, 158–159
economic impact of, 154
epidemiology of, 155–157
history of, 153
prevention, 157
Unilateral wipe-out syndrome, 66
United Kingdom Prospective Diabetes Study (UKPDS), 190, 194
United Nations Programme on HIV/AIDS (UNAIDS), 223, 225t
University of Campinas (UNICAMP) [Brazil], 323, 325–326
University of Nairobi Kenyatta National Hospital [Kenya], 313
Urban Slum Program (LV Prasad Eye Institute), 308
US Preventive Services Task Force, 20t
Users' Guide to the Medical Literature, 20
Utility theory, 35

Validity
    described, 56
    internal and external, 56
VanNewkirk, M, 76, 137
Vector control (OCP countries), 248
Vertical cup–disc ration (VCDR), 60
Vinger, P, 76
VISION 2020—The Right to Sight
    cataract surgery accessibility goal of, 166
    launching of, 6
    LVPEI successful embodiment of, 310
    ophthalmologist distribution goal, 312
    partners of, 6t
Vision field loss ranges, 41, 43t
Vision impairment. *See also* Blindness; Preventable infectious causes of vision impairment
    age-related macular degeneration (AMD) and, 32–33, 147
    cataract and, 162–170
    comparable studies on, 143, 144t, 145t, 146i, 147i
    comparing causes of, 140t, 146–147
    comparison of eye disease studies on, 141–142, 144–145t
    context of, 140
    diabetic retinopathy studies and application to, 189–199
    economic impact of, 142–143
    factors influencing causes of, 140–141
    history of, 139
    importance of eye examinations to prevent, 140
    prevalence of profound and severe, 143–145
    primary angle-closure glaucoma (PACG) and, 61, 177–187
    primary open-angle glaucoma (POAG) and, 171–176
    socioeconomics of, 8
    uncorrected refractive error and, 153–160
Vision loss. *See also* Blindness
    acuity measurement of, 40–41, 42t, 46–53
    aspects of, 37–38t
    causes and consequences of test choices, 38–39
    individual contributions to preventing, 9–14
    international efforts to reduce avoidable, 5–9
    prevalence of avoidable, 5
    ranges of, 40–41, 42t–43t, 44–45i, 46
    scales of, 40, 42t–43t
    various interventions in case of, 39t
    visual field loss, 41, 43t
Visual acuity
    age and changes in, 45i
    amblyopia and loss of, 111–119
    loss ranges of, 40–41, 42t
    measurement of, 46–53
    ocular trauma as cause of loss in, 336
Visual acuity measurement
    choice of test distance for, 50–51i
    formulas for calculating, 52–53
    presentation in chart form for, 49–50i
    scoring on non-ETDRS vs. ETDRS charts, 49–50
    Snellen's chart layout used for, 46–48, 48t

tests for near vision, 51–52i
Visual function measurements, 37
Visual Impairment Project, comparison to other studies, 143–145, 144t, 145t, 146i, 147, 147i
Vitamin A deficiency disorders. *See also* Xerophthalmia
    clinical presentation and findings, 103–106
    clinical research currently under way, 108–109
    cost of treatment/prevention, 100
    comorbidity of measles and, 106
    context of, 100
    current treatment recommendations, 108
    economic impact of, 100
    epidemiology of, 101–102
    history of, 99
    pathogenesis of, 101
    prevention of, 107
    risk factors, 102–103i
    in rural areas of Philippines, 80

Wang, PH, 28, 29
WBU (World Blind Union), 6
WESDR (Wisconsin Epidemiologic Study of Diabetic Retinopathy), 190, 197–198
West Bank, 80
WHO. *See* World Health Organization
Wilmer Grading System, 162, 163i
Wisconsin
    incidence of blindness in diabetic patients in, 197–198
    incidence of diabetic retinopathy in, 193i
Wisconsin Cataract Grading System, 161
Wisconsin Epidemiologic Study of Diabetic Retinopathy (WESDR), 190, 197–198
Wood, M, 336
World Bank study (1990), 34
World Blind Union, 14
World Health Organization (WHO)
    blindness as defined by, 77
    on childhood blindness, 3
    chorioretinal diseases data compiled by, 285
    contact information for, 14
    efforts to reduce avoidable vision loss, 6
    estimates of bilateral blindness by, 335
    estimates on prevalence of blindness in India by, 291
    estimates on trachoma prevalence/incidence, 206
    international diagnostic classification/grading systems recommended by, 60
    Program for the Prevention of Blindness, 6, 121
    trachoma grading system by, 211t
    vision loss classifications by, 37
    xerophthalmia treatment recommendations by, 108

Xerophthalmia. *See also* Vitamin A deficiency disorders
    clinical classification of, 104t
    clinical presentation of, 103, 106
    stages of, 105i

Yorston, D, 336

Zones of open-globe trauma, 126i